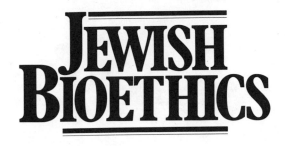

JEWISH BIOETHICS

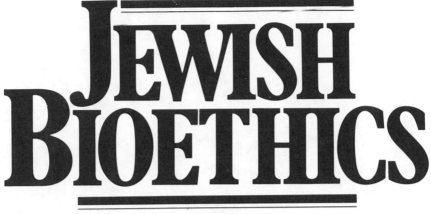

JEWISH BIOETHICS

Edited by

FRED ROSNER & J. DAVID BLEICH

with essays by

Menachem M. Brayer
Immanuel Jakobovits
Norman Lamm
Nachum L. Rabinovitch
Azriel Rosenfeld
David S. Shapiro
Aaron Soloveichik
Moshe Halevi Spero
Moses D. Tendler

Sanhedrin Press

New York · London

Sanhedrin Press

a division of Hebrew Publishing Company
80 Fifth Avenue
New York, N.Y. 10011

Library of Congress Cataloging in Publication Data

Main entry under title:

Jewish bioethics.

    Includes bibliographical references.
    1.   Medical ethics.   2.   Medicine and Judaism.
3.   Ethics, Jewish.   I.   Rosner, Fred.   II.   Bleich,
J. David.
R724.J48   174'.2   79-23330
ISBN 0-88482-934-0
ISBN 0-88482-935-9 pbk.

PRINTED IN THE UNITED STATES OF AMERICA

Contents

PREFACE   vii

INTRODUCTION
The *A Priori* Component of Bioethics   xi
    J. David Bleich

THE PRACTICE OF MEDICINE
  1. The Obligation to Heal in the Judaic Tradition:
     A Comparative Analysis   1
     J. David Bleich
  2. The Physician and the Patient in Jewish Law   45
     Fred Rosner

SEXUALITY AND PROCREATION
  3. Be Fruitful and Multiply   59
     David S. Shapiro
  4. Test-tube Babies   80
     J. David Bleich
  5. Contraception in Jewish Law   86
     Fred Rosner
  6. Population Control — The Jewish View   97
     Moses D. Tendler
  7. Artificial Insemination in Jewish Law   105
     Fred Rosner
  8. Jewish Views on Abortion   118
     Immanuel Jakobovits
  9. Abortion in Halakhic Literature   134
     J. David Bleich
10. Tay-Sachs Disease: To Screen or Not to Screen   178
     Fred Rosner
11. Transsexual Surgery   191
     J. David Bleich
12. Judaism and the Modern Attitude to Homosexuality   197
     Norman Lamm

MENTAL HEALTH AND DRUGS
13. Psychiatry, Psychotherapy and Halakhah   221
    Moshe HaLevi Spero
14. Drugs: A Jewish View   242
    Menachem M. Brayer

DEATH AND DYING
15. The Jewish Attitude Toward Euthanasia   253
    Fred Rosner
16. The Quinlan Case: A Jewish Perspective   266
    J. David Bleich
17. Establishing Criteria of Death   277
    J. David Bleich
18. The Halakhic Definition of Death   296
    Aaron Soloveichik
19. Neurological Death and Time of Death Statutes   303
    J. David Bleich
20. Suicide in Jewish Law   317
    Fred Rosner
21. Autopsy in Jewish Law and the Israeli Autopsy Controversy 331
    Fred Rosner

ORGAN TRANSPLANTATION
22. What is the Halakhah for Organ Transplants?   351
    Nachum L. Rabinovitch
23. Organ Transplantation in Jewish Law   358
    Fred Rosner

HUMAN EXPERIMENTATION
24. Medical Experimentation on Humans in Jewish Law   377
    Immanuel Jakobovits
25. Experimentation on Human Subjects   384
    J. David Bleich
26. Judaism and Human Experimentation   387
    Fred Rosner

GENETIC ENGINEERING
27. Judaism and Gene Design   401
    Azriel Rosenfeld
28. Genetic Engineering and Judaism   409
    Fred Rosner

BIOGRAPHICAL NOTES   423

Preface

Recent advances in biomedical technology and therapeutic procedures have generated a moral crisis in modern medicine. The vast strides made in medical science and technology have created options which only a few decades earlier would have been relegated to the realm of science fiction. Man, to a significant degree, now has the ability to exercise control not only over the ravages of disease but even over the very processes of life and death. With the unfolding of new discoveries and techniques, the scientific and intellectual communities have developed a keen awareness of the ethical issues which arise out of man's enhanced ability to control his destiny. In response to the concern for questions of this nature there has emerged the rapidly developing field of bioethics.

Jews, to whom all such questions are quests not simply for applicable humanitarian principles but for divine guidance, must, of necessity, seek answers in the teachings of the Torah. "The Torah of God is perfect" (Psalms 19:8) and in its teachings the discerning student will find eternally valid answers to even newly-formulated queries. As physicians and patients turn to rabbinic authorities for answers, Jewish scholars seek to elucidate and expound the teachings of the Torah in these vital areas of concern.

A significant body of literature reflecting Jewish scholarship in the field of bioethics has appeared. Nevertheless, many areas have not, as yet, been investigated adequately and the Jewish attitude to some pressing issues has not yet been fully formulated. This book is an attempt to present within the covers of a single volume a representative selection of materials of significance which have appeared thus far. Needless to say, since this book is designed to present the teachings of the rabbinic tradition, only material reflecting traditional Jewish scholarship has been selected. In some areas, notably mental health and gene design, the paucity of material which has been published to date renders these selections less complete than would have been desired. It is our fervent hope that publications such as this, precisely because of their inherent deficiencies, will spur scholars to redouble their efforts in investigating these issues from the perspective of Torah scholarship.

Much of the present work has previously been published in various scientific and religious journals or books. We are indebted to their editors and/or publishers, as well as to the individual authors, for permission to

vii

reprint their material. Many of the articles have been updated by their authors for this book and some contain new material. The opinions expressed by the various authors of articles in this book are their own and are not necessarily those of the editors; in some areas even the editors have divergent views.

For the sake of consistency, the system of transliteration has been made uniform throughout. In addition, footnotes have been renumbered where necessary in order to avoid confusion, and obvious typographical errors have been corrected.

We are deeply grateful to Mr. David M. L. Olivestone, editor-in-chief of Hebrew Publishing Company, for his enormous contributions and assistance both in the preparation of the work and in the various stages of its publication. We are indebted, too, to Mrs. Sophie Falk and Mrs. Miriam Regenworm for secretarial assistance.

Fred Rosner, M.D.
Rabbi J. David Bleich, Ph.D.

New York, September 1978
Elul 5738

Introduction

Introduction: The *A Priori* Component of Bioethics

J. DAVID BLEICH

Every comprehensive ethical system must contain within itself, either implicitly or explicitly, a conceptual skeletal framework for the categorization of every human deed, barring none. Value quotients are then either assigned, or are readily assignable, to every action and to every character trait on the basis of a comparison of the deed or trait and its proper pigeonhole in the conceptual scheme. Examination of diverse ethical systems reveals that virtually every system of ethics implicitly recognizes five distinct ethical categories which may be listed and defined:

1. The morally imperative — actions which are morally incumbent upon an individual; actions which are obligatory and mandatory as distinct from those which are voluntary or discretionary. "Honor thy father and thy mother" is an example of a moral imperative recognized as such by most ethical traditions. Truth-telling is another.

2. The morally commendable — actions which are not obligatory or mandatory in the usual sense of those terms; actions which cannot be compelled on moral grounds but which are worthy of approbation. Such actions are recognized as laudatory and praiseworthy not simply on subjective personal grounds but because the ethical value inherent in the deed renders the act commendable. Arguments urging performance of such deeds are usually not compelling in nature; frequently they are horatorical in

Reprinted from *Jewish Life* (Summer/Fall, 1978). Copyright © 1978 by the Union of Orthodox Jewish Congregations of America.

thrust. Acts of philanthropy fall into this category. The term "philanthropy" must be employed in this context rather than "charity" because although many systems of ethics recognize charity as being a moral imperative, all ethical systems posit limits to the extent of such obligations. It is at that limit that charity becomes philanthropy: highly laudable but hardly obligatory.

3. The morally neutral — actions which are devoid of moral significance, either positive or negative. Eating spinach is probably as good an example as any. Total abstinence from alcohol, unless one subscribes to a value system which posits teetotalism as a value, is a more significant example. Although overindulgence and drunkenness may indeed be odious in nature, imbibing alcohol in moderation is morally neutral.

4. The morally odious — actions which evoke moral disapprobrium. Schematically, the morally odious directly parallels the morally commendable. The morally commendable is greeted with approbation although it cannot be commanded; the morally odious is viewed with disapprobrium although it cannot be banned categorically. The conduct of litterbugs falls into this category. Actions which have deleterious ecological effects are usually viewed as being of this nature, although many ethicists now take an even more serious view of such actions.

5. The morally proscribed — actions which are condemned on ethical grounds; actions which are viewed as *malum in se,* i.e., evil by virtue of their very nature. "Thou shalt not kill" is perhaps the best example of an expression of such an ethical judgment.

This schematization is, of course, useful and applicable only if applied to a specific action evaluated in isolation from the *realia* of human life. Life would be so much easier for ethicists as well as for ordinary mortals if all issues were black and white. The ethicist may resort to the expedient of creating his own universe of discourse by positing a *ceteris paribus* clause asserting that "all things being equal" the moral judgment is thus and so. Real life is, however, quite different. "Honor thy father and thy mother" is a moral maxim which obligates one to provide for the physical comfort of one's parents. But what if one's father suffers from chronic emphysema and wishes to be supplied with cigarettes? How does a moral individual react when confronted by a situation which imposes two conflicting moral imperatives? On the one hand, he is obliged to honor his father's wishes; on the other, he is constrained by the commandment "Thou shalt not kill" not to aid and abet the wanton destruction of human life. How does a person escape from between the horns of a moral dilemma of such a nature while preserving intact ethical commitments?

Physicists are well aware of the phenomenon of antagonistic vector forces which, when totally equal, cancel each other out. When one force is stronger than the other, the prevailing force is equal to that of the greater minus that of the lesser. When the velocity of an object hurled into space is greater than the force of gravity, it escapes the earth's gravitational pull; when weaker, it falls back to earth; when velocity and the force of gravitational attraction are exactly equal, the object remains suspended in orbit.

Ethical systems operate in much the same manner. Every ethical system must, of necessity, posit not only a set of ethical values but must also either arrange those values in a hierarchical order or develop a system of rules to be applied in resolving conflicts between values. Moral vectors operate in a manner which parallels the behavior of vector forces. The weaker moral value must give way to the stronger. The ethicist is charged not only with the identification and labelling of moral values but also with assessing and determining the relative weight to be assigned to each moral value *vis-à-vis* all others. Ethical conduct often requires adjudicating between competing moral claims.

An excellent, although perhaps seldom recognized, example of this process is contained in the Robin Hood narrative. Preservation of human life is certainly a moral goal and so is preservation of property rights. Robin Hood finds himself confronted with a moral dilemma arising from two different and conflicting moral claims which cannot be reconciled. His obligation to preserve human life compels him to do whatever is necessary in order to assuage the hunger of starving widows and orphans; his obligation to respect the property rights of others restrains him from expropriating for this purpose any object of material value under the jurisdiction of the Sheriff of Nottingham. What is required is a ranking of values so that the moral agent may be guided in his conduct and enabled to preserve or promote the higher moral value. Robin Hood's conduct is predicated upon a determination that the sanctity of human life represents a higher moral value than preservation of property. Perhaps the most significant aspect of the Robin Hood tale is the role of Friar Tuck who, as "professor of moral theology", as it were, gives ecclesiastic sanction to Robin Hood's value judgment and subsequent course of action.

How can one arbitrate between conflicting moral claims? How is one to determine which value takes priority over another and under what circumstances? In actuality, such questions are simply the recasting of a more fundamental question concerning the nature and basis of all moral claims. Throughout the history of philosophy the formulation of moral imperatives has virtually always been predicated upon some form of one or another of the following theories:

1. Ethical relativists maintain that moral values are little more than conventions accepted by society at large. Hence, society remains

the sole arbiter of good and evil. Different societies may adopt different and even conflicting moral systems without doing violence to the logic of morality. According to this view, there can be no appeal to ultimate moral truth; there is no absolute good toward which one must aspire. Since objective right or wrong does not exist one may attempt to alter ethical mores only by attempting to convince a society or culture that there are good (in the non-moral sense of the term) and sufficient reasons for modifying or rejecting a heretofore accepted moral code.

2. The religionist perceives moral values as being determined by the Deity as a manifestation of divine wisdom or divine will. Frequently, the doctrine of *imitatio Dei* is invoked in urging men to engage in certain activities and to eschew others in emulation of God. The postulates of a religio-moral system are most frequently presented as the subject of divine revelation as incorporated in sacred writ. Ethical discourse is thus rooted primarily in scriptural exegesis and theology.

3. Intuitionist systems are far more prevalent in classical ethics. Common to all such systems is their derivation from notions of moral consciousness. Moral values are perceived as having an *a priori* basis in the human intellect, and, accordingly, can be established without reference to empirical data. The intuitionist can no more be dissuaded from the cogency of his value system than he can be dissuaded from his affirmation of the proposition "Seven plus five equals twelve". For the intuitionist, moral principles have the same cognitive status as the postulates of mathematics and logic.

The notion of a moral intuition in one guise or another, while formally denied by many, is ubiquitous. Indeed, relativists, who in the philosophy classroom deny this category of moral cognition, nevertheless, in day to day life and conversation, frequently talk and behave as if prompted in their actions by a moral conscience. Certainly, Western democratic societies profess the belief that the basic moral principles upon which they are founded are *a priori* in nature and that moral intuition serves as a viable basis for distinguishing between right and wrong. Indeed, under Anglo-Saxon common law, insanity is defined as the inability to distinguish between right and wrong. A person may be "normal" and rational in every respect other than with regard to the ability to distinguish between right and wrong and yet be judged legally insane. Although individuals may differ with regard to the content of these dichotomous categories and be quite sane, the absence of an ability to fathom the significance of these antithetical categories is indicative of the absence of a component crucial to the definition of moral responsibility. Total absence of the moral faculty renders a person legally insane.

Of course, non-intuitionists deny that there exist *a priori* concepts of good and bad, right and wrong. The intuitionist can no more convey the content of his moral consciousness to such a person than he can convey the concept of color to the sightless person who has been blind from birth. In a somewhat different context Prof. W. K. Frankana, in an incisive essay entitled "The Naturalistic Fallacy" (*Mind,* 48, 1939), has remarked that the intuitionists can but view the non-intuitionist as being afflicted with moral blindness. Conversely, the non-intuitionist diagnoses the malady of the intuitionist and pronounces him to be suffering from moral hallucinations.

The crucial problem in bioethics is not identification of values. Regardless of our ethical orientation we are all fairly well agreed on the nature and definition of those values. A problem arises only when one value comes into conflict with another. The crucial questions arise in attempting to order those values in a hierarchical series or in attempting to devise rules for purposes of establishing conditions under which one value supersedes another.

In order to elucidate the nature of such conflicting value claims it may be instructive to cite the preamble of the Declaration of Independence: "We believe these truths to be self-evident: that all men are created equal, that they are endowed by their Creator with certain inalienable rights, that these are life, liberty and the pursuit of happiness". The sentiments expressed in this historic document were prompted by the moral theory of John Locke who believed that moral laws are discoverable by "the light of nature", i.e., reason alone. Another incident in the annals of American history demonstrates dramatically that the claims of different "inalienable rights" may, at times, be in conflict with one another, and that some means must be found to adjudicate between them. Life and liberty are enumerated as specific rights which are discernable by reason. It is not always possible to possess both. The inability to possess both prompted Patrick Henry to declaim, "Give me liberty or give me death". In a subsequent age a different and conflicting adage gained currency: "Better Red than dead".

The question to which we must address ourselves is not that of self-preservation versus martyrdom in the name of liberty. Rather, it is the conflict between preservation of life and other human values which is the fulcrum of much of current bioethical debate. In the bioethical context the question is which of the two values is to be promoted over the other. In its most extreme formulation the question to be answered is, "Does commitment to the preservation of life preclude the liberty to commit suicide or does a person enjoy absolute autonomy to the extent that preservation of life is subservient to the principle of liberty?" In the context of the ongoing euthanasia debate, the libertarian motto has now become "Give me liberty *and* give me death".

The question of legalization or non-legalization, prevention or non-prevention, of suicide is hardly the burning issue of the day, but withdrawal of treatment and euthanasia in a variety of different guises are currently the subjects of heated debate. In other instances, particularly in the case of a patient who is unconscious and incapable of exercising self-determination or of a defective newborn who has not attained the age of reason, the question is not that of adjudicating a conflict between contradictory claims of liberty and preservation of life, but rather between preservation of life and the third value of the triad of values recognized by the founding fathers of this country, namely, happiness. The most compelling argument in support of allowing such a patient to die is that a life of pain should not be prolonged; life itself in such circumstances is antithetical to the pursuit of happiness. Sometimes the pain is that of the patient, not infrequently it is that of the family whose members experience considerable anguish. There is also an additional value involved, albeit the promotion of this value sometimes constitutes a hidden rather than an open agenda, viz., the allocation of the resources of society. It might be well to point out that in the original catalogue of rights discoverable by the "the light of nature" which appears in the writings of John Locke, the cardinal values are expressed as life, liberty and the right to enjoy property. The latter was transformed by the authors of the Declaration of Independence into the notion of the pursuit of happiness. The conflict between these two Lockean values is an omnipresent one. When confronted with a question involving preservation of life versus preservation of material wealth which of the two must take precedence over the other? Does promotion of either value place limitations upon the other?

It should be clearly recognized that this dilemma is not limited to treatment of terminal patients or of defective newborns. Precisely the same issue and the same moral claims must be confronted, for example, in the case of custodial care of the incurably insane. Shall life be preserved even at the expense of pain, pain of the mentally deranged himself, of his keepers and of society? Is preservation of the lunatic's life worth a not inconsiderable expenditure of the taxpayers' funds? Which shall we conserve, the life of the mentally deranged, a life useless to himself or to others, or the financial resources of society which can be put to use so well in other ways in order to promote social welfare and happiness?

When couched in crass terms of life versus money virtually all men of good will profess what is tantamount not only to an *a priori* awareness of preservation of life as a cardinal moral value but also to an *a priori* ordering of values which places preservation of life above Locke's notion of the enjoyment of property. Moreover, our *a priori* ordering of moral values places preservation of life above the pursuit of happiness so that when the two conflict we intuitively believe — at least in the abstract — that the unhappy life is better than no life at all.

To be sure ethical theorists who deny *a priori* moral perceptions will categorize these comments as a projection of what Frankana termed moral hallucinations. One can but answer that if perception of preservation of life as a cardinal value be a hallucinatory experience rather than a veridical moral perception it seems to be endemic to most of Western society. There have indeed existed legal and moral systems in which preservation of life was not regarded as the highest of all moral values. In some systems preservation of life is subordinate to loyalty to the State or to obedience to law. Thus, for example, Socrates, who believed himself unjustly condemned to execution as a result of a miscarriage of justice, is afforded the opportunity to avoid this fate. The door to his prison cell is open; a chariot awaits outside. But to the astonishment and chagrin of his disciples Socrates refuses to avail himself of the opportunity for escape. His explanation is devastatingly simple. As a citizen of Athens he must obey the law, even when the law is unjust. It remained for Hobbes to declare that no law can bind a person to surrender his life. Resolution of the dilemma posed by the conflict between the opposing duties of obedience to law and preservation of life hinges upon proper ranking of these values.

Of course, it may be argued that even for Plato obedience to law takes precedence over self-preservation, not because it is intrinsically a higher value, but because Plato deemed obedience to law to be the only means of preventing anarchy and with it the cheapening of all human life. Nevertheless, this position was carried to an obscene extreme in Nazi Germany which subscribed to a hierarchical ordering of human values which to our minds appears grossly immoral, to say the least. In Nazi Germany the edict of the Fuehrer had the effect of law and obedience to law was viewed as the supreme moral value. Obedience to law was a moral desideratum sufficiently weighty to serve as sanction for genocide. This defense of German atrocities as being firmly rooted in the accepted moral code of the German social order is the central thesis of Hannah Arendt's thought-provoking book, *Eichmann in Jerusalem*.

But is this defense morally cogent? Some may remember a motion picture called "Judgment at Nuremberg". It is doubtful that the producers thought of themselves as conducting a moral debate of the highest significance. But that is precisely what is embodied in this motion picture film and, for that matter, in the arguments at the Nuremberg trials themselves. The defense offered an apologia firmly rooted in ethical relativism. The prosecution rebutted this argument by claiming that the argument was a sham. The prosecution contended that obedience to law is not sufficient justification for wantonly snuffing out innocent human life. In effect, runs the argument, there is a moral obligation to disobey an unjust law. But, much more significantly, the prosecution was forced to argue that this is a matter regarding which there cannot be honest disagreement. Otherwise, how can a person be called to task and condemned by a court of law for following the dictates of his moral conscience, particularly when those moral principles are enshrined in the law of the land? The Nuremberg trials were predicated upon acceptance of the sanctity of life as a compelling and overriding human value. But more than this — the charges against the defendants were predicated upon the acceptance of the sanctity of life as a self-evident, undeniable, irrefutable, *a priori* cardinal value. As such, it takes precedence not only over obedience to law but over virtually all other human values as well.

Since mankind recognizes the notion of the sanctity of life as an overriding and *a priori* moral value, the crucial question is whether the quality of life to be preserved plays any role whatsoever in the formulation of this *a priori* concept. No one, to my knowledge, has argued that there exist *a priori* grounds for such a distinction. Certainly, man instinctively feels called upon to preserve a life which is endangered and does not find himself pausing to ponder whether the life to be saved will be a happy one or not. Life as such, from the moment it comes into existence and as long as it continues to exist, demands preservation. Any limitations which may be intuitively applied to the obligation to preserve life are not predicated upon the quality of the life which requires therapeutic intervention for preservation but are born of the nature of the action required to preserve that life. Thus, as it is reflected in Jewish law, it is the intrinsic sanctity of every moment of human life which prompts the conclusion that hazardous procedures need not be employed in treating the terminally ill or the defective neonate. The certainty of a short span of life must be weighed against the possibility of cure or long-term remission, if successful, but imminent death if unsuccessful. The decision against aggressive intervention in such circumstances is not a decision that the quality of life to be preserved is not of sufficient value to warrant the therapy in question, but a decision that even fleeting periods of life are too precious to be lightly gambled away.

The *a priori* nature of the obligation to preserve human life has found expression in a judicial decision handed down in *J.F.K. Memorial Hospital vs. Heston*. In that landmark case the court ruled that there exists a compelling State interest in the preservation of the life of each of its citizens. It is quite apparent that the court was not affirming a State interest in the sheer numbers of its citizenry. There is no inherent incompatibility between that decision and demographic concern with regard to population explosion or even advocacy of zero population growth. All that the court intended was an affirmation of an *a priori* obligation which is based upon concepts of natural law and — again to use Locke's delightful phrase — the "light of reason".

For Jews committed to guiding their conduct on the basis of a divinely revealed corpus of law, the question of the validity of an *a priori* moral cognition is largely irrelevant. An ethical system predicated upon divine revelation need not be overly concerned with the *a priori* since divine fiat supersedes all such considerations. An examination of whether intuitive cognitions are sufficient to establish binding obligations in the absence of revelation is beyond the scope of this endeavor. However, since divine law and man's human conscience are in full agreement with regard to such salient matters ought one not to conclude that man was endowed by God with a moral consciousness precisely in order that God's will be immediately known to man?

The Sages clearly recognized that the ethical moment of Halakhah consists of commandments which, "Had they not been written, it would have been proper that they be written." Thus R. Yonatan states that in the absence of a revealed Torah "we would have learned modesty from the cat, aversion to robbery from the ant, marital faithfulness from the dove, and conjugal deportment from the rooster" (*Eruvin* 100b). Basic moral values are universal and not contingent upon sectarian claims. This is so, despite the fact that following revelation at Sinai such matters are, for Jews, encompassed within the parameters of Halakhah.

To be sure, not all bioethical problems are questions of black and white. There are many gradations of gray, questions to which answers are not immediately and intuitively available. A person who seeks to find answers within the Jewish tradition can deal with such questions in only one way. He must examine them through the prism of Halakhah for it is in the corpus of Jewish law as elucidated and transmitted from generation to generation that God has made His will known to man.

The Practice of Medicine

1
The Obligation to Heal in the Judaic Tradition: A Comparative Analysis

J. DAVID BLEICH

Introduction

Until relatively recently, medical science offered all or nothing in its treatment of virtually all illnesses and defects. Either the patient responded to treatment, when treatment was available, and was cured, or else he succumbed as a result of his malady. Such dichotomous situations generated few moral dilemmas for the medical practitioner. Patients, by and large, sought treatment and physicians strained to do all that was in their power in order to effect a cure. To be sure, theologians and ethicists agonized over questions such as the moral legitimacy of euthanasia for patients who found continued existence too painful to bear and the extent to which the patient was obliged to seek extraordinary measures in effecting a cure; but the number of people with regard to whom such perplexities were germane was rather small.

In recent years medical science and technology have made tremendous strides. Some diseases have been virtually eradicated; for others effective remedies have been found. Concomitantly, ways and means have been

Reprinted from Chester A. Swinyard (ed.), *Decision Making and the Defective Newborn*. Copyright © 1978 by Charles C. Thomas, Publisher, Springfield, Illinois.

developed which enable physicians to sustain life even when known cures do not exist. Maladies and deformities often appear in associated syndromes. While heretofore untreatable conditions now respond to medical ministration such response is often less than total. Particularly in the case of defective newborns, methods now exist which make it possible to correct certain problems only to leave the patient in a deformed or debilitated state. In such cases questions with regard to the value of the life which is preserved become very real.

The physician's practical dilemma can be stated in simple terms: to treat or not to treat. In deciding whether or not to initiate or maintain such treatment the physician is called upon to make not only medical, but also moral, determinations. There are at least two distinguishable components which present themselves in all such quandaries. The first is a value judgment. Is it desirable that the patient be treated? Should value judgments be made with regard to the quality of life to be preserved? The second question pertains to the physician's personal responsibilities. Under what circumstances and to what extent is the physician morally obligated to persist in rendering aggressive professional care? It is instructive to analyze some of the legal aspects of these questions and to examine the physician's legal responsibilities and his moral duties as enunciated within the Catholic tradition before proceeding to an analysis of Jewish moral teaching with regard to these issues.

Anglo-American Law

Under the Anglo-Saxon system of law a physician has no greater obligation to treat or advise a person in need of medical attention than has any other individual. The physician-patient relationship is viewed in common law as a contractual relationship based upon consensual agreement. While it is true that such contracts need not be expressly verbalized and exist even when the physician's services are rendered gratuitously, no obligation exists with regard to the provision of medical care unless the patient wishes medical assistance and the physician offers such treatment. The Code of Ethics of the American Medical Association states quite clearly, "A physician may choose whom he will serve." Although the same Code states that "In an emergency, however, he should render service to the best of his ability" it is recognized that this constitutes a moral, as distinct from a legal, duty. It is only after a patient is accepted for treatment that certain obligations devolve upon the physician. By appearing in a physician's office or at the emergency room of a hospital and submitting himself to examination and treatment, the patient impliedly grants permission for medical treatment and impliedly agrees to pay such professional fees as are customary and usual. By treating the patient the physician impliedly promises to continue such treatment until his professional services are no longer needed or desired by the patient. Also, since the patient seeks the physician because the latter possesses skills and knowledge which the patient lacks, the law places an obligation upon the physician which goes beyond the obligation assumed in the usual contract for services. The physician is obligated not only to exercise reasonable care but also reasonable skill in the treatment of his patient. Thus, the physician-patient relationship is based upon a contract implied-in-fact. The physician-patient contract implies that the physician will not abandon the patient. As stated in the Code, "Having undertaken the care of the patient, he may not neglect him; and unless he has been discharged, he may discontinue his services only after giving adequate notice."

In terms of law, a physician, despite his skill and licensure, is under no obligation to practice medicine, nor is he under a legal duty to render aid to another in distress. It has been conclusively established that a physician is not legally obligated to accept a patient for treatment.

Moreover, except in emergency situations, the physician is under legal constraint not to minister to the needs of the sick unless there is a clear indication on the part of the patient that treatment is desired by him. Under the common law the freedom from intentional unauthorized touching of the body is one of the basic freedoms enjoyed by every person. While unavoidable trespasses such as unintentional touching in a crowded bus or elevator or the intentional grasping of a friend's arm in order to attract his attention are accepted as part of casual social intercourse and do not constitute a personal indignity, medical procedures such as a hypodermic injection, a proctological examination or the lancing of an abscess constitute an invasion of the integrity of the person and, when unauthorized, any such action becomes an act of assault and battery. A patient who voluntarily consults a physician and voluntarily submits to treatment relying entirely upon the physician's skill and care gives general consent by implication to at least such operation or treatment as may be reasonably necessary. The patient may at any time withdraw or limit such permission. Furthermore, the courts have ruled that if consent is given for one procedure the physician may not perform another procedure without specific consent. A leading case in this area of law, *Mohr v. Williams*,[1] involved a patient who had an earache and consulted a physician who examined both ears and recommended an operation upon the right ear. Under anesthesia the doctor discovered that the condition of the left ear was even more serious than that of the right ear. Consequently, he operated on the left ear for which he had no consent. The court held that the operation on the left ear was not authorized and, therefore, constituted an act of assault and battery upon the patient. Even though the operation was skillfully performed and benefitted the patient, the court ruled that going beyond the consent or authorization of the patient constitutes a trespass to the person and that the physician may be subjected to exemplary or punitive damages.

It has been established that prior consent of the patient is not required in life-threatening situations. In emergencies, when the patient requires immediate care to preserve life and health, the physician is reasonably privileged to treat the patient.[2] Such action is usually justified on the basis of a hypothetical assumption that were the patient competent and were it possible to seek consent without jeopardizing the patient such consent would be willingly forthcoming.

The law with regard to a physician's right to proceed *against* the expressed wishes of a fully competent patient in life-threatening situations is somewhat unsettled. Patients afflicted with terminal illnesses may, at times, express a desire for palliative treatment but indicate that they have no desire for life-prolonging therapy. In practice physicians are often reluctant to be guided by a patient's desire under such circumstances because of fear not only of potential civil liability but also because of possible criminal charges. Even though the physician acts in a purely passive manner, the omission of treatment under certain circumstances constitutes manslaughter. As stated in one judicial decision:

> The law recognizes that under some circumstances the omission of the duty owed one individual to another, where such omission results in the death of one to whom the duty is owing, will make the other chargeable with manslaughter.[3]

The physician's culpability for such omission proceeds directly from the contractual obligation owed the patient who has been accepted for treatment.

Criminal culpability in the omission of treatment for defective newborns is a question which, to my knowledge, has never been adjudicated. The crucial legal issue is whether or not the newborn has been accepted by the physician as a patient. The matter can be argued both ways. It may be argued that the physician-patient contract exists only between the doctor and the mother; the obstetrician has contracted only to attend the mother during pregnancy and to deliver her child. In fact, care of the infant falls within the province of another practitioner, the pediatrician. On the other hand it may be argued that certain aspects of pre-natal care are designed primarily for the benefit of the fetus,[4] that in delivery itself the child is treated as a patient and that ministration to the infant following parturition confirms his status as a patient. Indeed the infant may well be regarded as an intended third-party beneficiary of the contract between the mother and her physician.[5] Certainly, once therapeutic procedures, however minimal those may be, have been instituted, it would appear that a physician-patient contractual relationship has been established and hence the physician is bound by the terms of his contract not to abandon the patient. The physician who, subsequently, suspends treatment of a defective newborn may well be guilty of manslaughter. Several jurisdictions have adopted legislation which provides that live born fetuses are to be treated as persons and that failure to take reasonable steps to preserve the life of the fetus shall result in civil and criminal liability.[6] These stipulations are clearly grounded upon the assumption that a physician-patient relationship exists *vis-à-vis* the fetus and *a fortiori* with regard to a child delivered in the course of natural childbirth.

At least one legal authority[7] has argued that even in the absence of a physician-patient relationship the physician is criminally liable for failing to treat an infant on the basis of the assumption-of-care doctrine as well as by virtue of the physician's role in creating the child's peril. The physician, in assuming responsibility for treatment of the newborn infant, has clearly created a situation in which other physicians will not come to the rescue of the endangered child. Creation of a situation in which others will not perceive the necessity of coming to the rescue of an endangered individual entails assumption-of-care liability. The same authority argues somewhat tenuously that the physician who delivered the baby is, in a legal sense, the "cause" of its subsequent peril. If not for his act the child would not face the prospect of mistreatment. Having placed the infant in danger, the physician is legally obligated to protect it.

It has long been assumed that a showing by the physician that the patient had relieved him of all further responsibility, thus terminating the contract, would constitute a complete defense:

> The rule of law is always based on the proposition that the duty neglected must be a legal duty and not a mere moral obligation. It must be a duty imposed by law or by contract. . . .[8]

Yet, more recently, in a note appended to the court's decision in *Application of the President and Directors of Georgetown College, Inc.,* the court declared: "Whether or not a waiver signed by a patient *in extremis* would protect the hospital from civil liability it could not be relied upon to prevent criminal prosecution. Death resulting from failure to extend proper medical care, where there is a duty of care is manslaughter in the District of Columbia."[9]

If this decision becomes a precedent to be followed in other jurisdictions, it may well have ramifications with regard to treatment of defective newborns as well. If a moribund but mentally competent patient cannot relieve a physician from criminal culpability by discharging him it is difficult to see how a physician may be relieved of his responsibility to continue treatment of a deformed or defective infant.[9a]

Assuming that there exists no criminal culpability for omission of treatment on the part of the physician who has been relieved of his obligation by the patient, does the physician have the right to proceed in instituting measures designed to save the life of the patient against the wishes of the latter?

Quite a number of such cases have come before the courts via the petition of a physician or of hospital officials seeking a court order to proceed with such treatment. The vast majority of such cases involve patients who have refused medical treatment, usually in the form of blood transfusions, on religious grounds. When presented with situations in which the patient is a mentally competent adult and the resultant death will not turn the patient's children into wards of the state, the courts, for the most part, have refused to intervene.[10] Such cases involve potential abridgment of constitutionally protected freedom of religious practice. The courts, in refusing to intervene, have ruled that, in the absence of a clear and present danger to society, the right to religious liberty must prevail. It is, however, firmly established that the courts are empowered to order compulsory medical treatment of minor children despite the opposition of parents based upon religious con-siderations.[11] The state acting *parens patriae* possesses authority to guard the general interest of a child's well-being. This authority is not nullified by virtue of a conflicting religious claim. In another case, the court indicated that the parents of a dependent child may not refuse treatment even for themselves on the basis of religious conviction.[12] Since the parent has a responsibility to the community to care for the infant, argued the court, the state has an interest in preserving the life of the parent. Accordingly, the state may legitimately intervene in order to prevent the abandonment of the child.

In recent years, a number of decisions have been issued in which the stance traditionally adopted by the judiciary has been reversed. As a result the legal situation with regard to court directed intervention contrary to the wishes of the patient solely for the purposes of preserving his life remains somewhat unsettled. The legal arguments for intervention have been made on four grounds: 1. Refusal of life-saving treatment is tantamount to suicide. This argument is of course germane only in jurisdictions in which suicide or attempted suicide are violations of the criminal code. 2. Consent on the part of the victim is no defense to a homicide prosecution. This is predicated upon society's interest in the life of an individual. An individual has no right to consent to his own death for the sake of euthanasia; a natural concomitant of this view is that he has no right to withhold consent for the administration of life-saving medical treatment. 3. Any exception to the general principle of the sanctity of any form of human life will necessarily result in the cheapening of all human life. 4. Society has an interest in preserving the lives of its members. The State recognizes the value of each individual life as being so great as to constitute a "compelling in-terest" taking precedence over any other right or liberty which might be claimed by the individual.

In *Erikson v. Dilgard,* a lower New York court while affirming ". . . that it is the individual who is the subject of medical decision who has the final say and that this must necessarily be so in a system of government which gives the greatest possible protection to the individual in the furtherance of his own desire,"[13] nevertheless recognized the paradox involved in sanctioning the withholding of treatment even while banning suicide. In that case, the court circumvented the issue of the suicidal nature of the patient's refusal of a transfusion by advancing the somewhat specious argument that there is always some question as to whether or not the medical decision is correct. In another case, a Washington, D.C. court noted that it is doubtful that suicide is a crime in the District of Columbia but indicated that the suicide argument might be a compelling one and that if suicide were indeed a crime even the principles of religious freedom would be insufficient to support non-intervention.[14] Thus, in *Application of the President and Directors of Georgetown College, Inc.,* the court noted, ". . . where attempted suicide is illegal by the common law or by statute, a person may not be allowed to refuse necessary medical assistance when death is likely to ensure without it."[15] The distinction between an active versus a passive act or between misfeasance or nonfeasance is dismissed as a "quibble." But, most significantly, the court in the same case argued that a patient may not relieve a physician from his obligation to preserve life. "The normal principle that an adult patient directs his doctor is based on notions of commercial contract which may have less relevance to life-or-death emergencies. It is not clear just where a patient would derive her authority to command her doctor to treat her under limitations which would produce death."[16] The court declined to accept as persuasive the argument that this authority is part of a constitutionally protected liberty.

In a later case, *U.S. v. Elishas George and Elizabeth George,*[17] the U.S. District Court in Connecticut cited with approval Judge Wright's memorandum in *Application of the President and Directors of Georgetown College, Inc.,* and introduced yet another weighty consideration. Whereas Judge Wright argued that a patient cannot, under the guise of personal liberty and self-determination, demand a protocol of treatment or nontreatment which would lead to death, the District Court in *U.S. v. George* for the first time recognized the existence of a compelling moral, as distinct from legal, obligation which compels a specific course of action on the part of the physician. The court asserted that "the doctor's conscience and professional oath" must be viewed with a gravity equal to the seriousness of religious conscience:

> In the difficult realm of religious liberty it is often assumed only the religious conscience is imperiled. Here, however, the doctor's conscience and professional oath must also be respected . . . to require these doctors to ignore the mandates of their own conscience, even in the name of free religious exercise, cannot be justified under these circumstances.[18]

Judge Zamano, in this opinion, carefully distinguishes between a situation in which a patient knowingly declines treatment and one in which he demands mistreatment, *viz.*, the omission of blood transfusions, and stresses that in the case under consideration "the patient voluntarily submitted himself to and insisted upon medical care." This distinction, which is not made on considerations of tort liability or violation of criminal statutes, but upon moral grounds, is presumably drawn from the Code of Ethics of the American Medical Association.

This line of reasoning is strikingly similar to that employed by the U.S. Supreme Court in ruling that deeply held moral convictions, even when not grounded upon professed religious beliefs, satisfy the criteria for exclusion from conscription on the grounds of conscientious objection. This argument would apply with even greater force in a situation in which the doctor's desire to proceed with treatment is grounded in religious belief regarding the sanctity of human life, rather than upon a code of professional ethics, and in which the patient bases his refusal upon a subjective preference for death over life, rather than upon religious exceptions to the mode of treatment. If this decision is accepted as a judicial precedent it may be inferred that a patient suffering from a debilitating illness may not demand of a physician as a matter of right, "Just give me something for the pain." Having submitted himself to the care of the physician, the physician may treat the patient in accordance with his professional oath without fear of legal sanctions.

The judicial decisions and lines of reasoning adopted in both *Application of the President and Directors of Georgetown College, Inc.,* and *U.S. v. George* are predicated upon the fact that the patient in question *did* seek medical treatment. Neither establishes an obligation or right which would enable a physician to institute treatment even in emergency situations contrary to the express desire of a competent patient.

A recent case in this area and a case which speaks most directly to the issue of initiation of treatment under such circumstances is *John F. Kennedy Memorial Hospital v. Heston.* Writing for a unanimous court Chief Justice Weintraub declared, "It seems correct to say there is no constitutional right to choose to die."[19] The State, argues Chief Justice Weintraub, has a legitimate interest in the preservation of the lives of its citizens. It is from this interest that not only suicide statutes but also statutes such as those mandating the use of protective devices by motorcyclists (or the use of seat belts in automobiles) derive their legitimacy. As in *Application of Georgetown* the court rejected an argument seeking to differentiate between "passively submitting to death and actively seeking it"[20] stating that "If the State may interrupt any mode of self-destruction it may with equal authority interfere with another."[21] In extremely broad language the court apparently sanctions intervention in any and all situations[22] save those in which "the medical option itself is laden with the risk of death or of serious infirmity" . . . . Otherwise, "the State's interest in sustaining life in such circumstances is hardly distinguishable from its interest in the case of suicide.''[23] The State's interest in preservation of life is viewed as sufficiently compelling to warrant intervention even when such intervention prevents the full exercise of religious practices as established in *Reynolds v. U.S.*[24] In reaching those conclusions, the New Jersey court took note of earlier judicial decisions to the contrary. Specific reference is made to the decision handed down in *In re Estate of Brooks,*[25] in which the Supreme Court of Illinois ruled that a transfusion could not be administered against the religious objections of the patient. The Illinois court held that only the presence of ''a clear and present danger'' warrants interference with a patient's religious scruples. The New Jersey court, in its opinion, stated that apart from the question of the counterposed moral scruples of the physician the correct criterion to be applied is that of ''compelling State interest.''[26] Although it does not define the issue as sharply as in *U.S. v. George,* this decision also takes cognizance of the moral obligation devolving upon members of the medical profession and notes that in light of the profession's consecration to preserving life, failure to administer treatment constitutes malpractice in the moral sense even if there exists no legal culpability.

The State's interest as enunciated by the courts is in the preservation of life *per se* and is not qualified in any way by virtue of the quality of the life which is preserved. The court, in this decision, did indeed explicitly recognize that a patient need not submit to treatment which would produce a serious infirmity and in *Georgetown* the court noted that the proposed treatment did not involve ''a dangerous or crippling operation.'' Presumably, under such circumstances, the Court would not have mandated treatment contrary to the wishes of the patient.[27] However, the context in which these distinctions are made does not indicate that the considerations which are operational are value judgments with reference to the quality of the life which is preserved. In each of these cases the court has simply presented a reaffirmation of the classic distinction between ordinary and extraordinary therapeutic measures. Indeed, consideration of the quality of life to be preserved was expressly rejected in a later decision handed down by the Massachusetts Supreme Judicial Court. In *Superintendent of Belchertown State School et al. v. Joseph Saikewicz* the court found it necessary to qualify one of the considerations cited in favor of withholding treatment from a mentally defective terminal patient with the forceful statement, ''To the extent that this formulation equates the value of life with any measure of the quality of life, we reject it.''[28]

The position, expressed in a decision of the Supreme Court of the State of New Jersey in *John F. Kennedy Memorial Hospital v. Heston,* has been significantly modified by a later decision of the same judicial body. In its widely known decision in the case of Karen Quinlan[29] permitting the removal of the respirator upon which the patient was believed to be dependant, the New Jersey Supreme Court affirmed the principles enunciated in *Heston* but found that the situations were not analogous. The court reasoned that the State has no compelling interest in prolongation of the life of an individual if the patient is "only to vegetate a few measurable months with no realistic possibility of returning to any semblance of cognitive or sapient life." In *In re Quinlan,* the court explicitly recognized both a constitutional right to privacy and an extension of that right to encompass refusal of medical treatment and the withdrawal of life support therapy but also recognized that the individual's right to privacy is ordinarily subservient to the State's compelling interest in preservation of life. Accordingly, the court reaffirmed its position in *Heston,* but with a significant limitation: The legal requirement for medical intervention is recognized as absolute in cases where the medical procedure indicated constitutes a minimal bodily invasion and the chances of recovery and return to functioning life are very good. However, the court held that "the State's interest *contra* weakens and the individual's right to privacy grows as the degree of bodily invasion increases and the prognosis dims. Ultimately, there comes a point at which the individual's rights overcome the State's interest."[30]

The extent of the bodily invasion required to overcome the State's interest is not defined in *Quinlan.*[31] Moreover, the combined factors of significant bodily invasion and dim prognosis must be present before the individual's right of privacy overcomes the State's interest in preservation of life. In *Quinlan,* a determination of dim prognosis was made on the basis of a description of the patient as being in a chronic and persistent vegetative state with no reasonable prospect of returning to a cognitive or sapient state. At the same time the court expressly indicated that its finding with regard to the individual's right to privacy was not necessarily limited to the circumstances of the case and its considerations but failed to give detailed examples of other medical situations in which the individual's rights would overcome the State's interest.[32] The principle enunciated in *Quinlan* was amplified and extended by a lower court in New Jersey in a recent ruling. The Morristown Memorial Hospital petitioned the Morris County Court for the appointment of a guardian for the purpose of obtaining consent for the amputation of the gangrenous legs of an elderly patient who refused to authorize the procedure without which the patient faced imminent death. There was every medical reason to anticipate that amputation, if performed, would be successful in averting death. In *In re Quackenbush,*[33] the court found the patient mentally competent and ruled that "the extensive bodily invasion involved here — the amputation of both legs above the knee and possibly amputation of both legs entirely — is sufficient to make the State's interest in the preservation of life give way to Robert Quackenbush's right of privacy to decide his own future regardless of the absence of a dim prognosis."[34] In *Quackenbush* the patient's right to privacy was found to be paramount on the basis of extensive bodily invasion alone, despite the absence of a dim prognosis.[35]

An even more significant limitation of the State interest in preservation of life is embodied in the *Saikewicz* decision. The question before the court was the appointment of a guardian on behalf of a mentally retarded individual suffering from terminal leukemia with authority to agree to the withholding of chemotherapy. In the *Saikewicz* case, the court ruled that the State's interest in effecting "a brief and uncertain delay in the natural process of death" was not sufficiently strong to warrant that the patient be compelled to assume the traumatic cost of that prolongation. The individual's right to bodily integrity and privacy were viewed, under such circumstances, as empowering him to reject the physical and emotional burdens of a rigorous regimen of drug therapy. In effect, the court ruled that the State has no compelling interest in minimal prolongation of the life of a patient afflicted with a terminal malady.

John F. Kennedy v. Heston establishes a significant procedural matter as well. In issuing its decision, the court stated that a court order need not necessarily be sought in order to institute treatment. The questions of law and of compelling State interest are regarded by the court as settled. Significantly, no determination need be made regarding the quality of life which is preserved in this manner. The sole remaining question is whether or not it is probable that death will ensue if life-sustaining medical procedures are not initiated. An application to the court is viewed as appropriate for determination of this fact but such application need be made only if the nature of the emergency is such that the unavoidable delay entailed by such a procedure is medically acceptable.

The Catholic Tradition

Although Scripture depicts life as a gift of God, Catholic tradition does not teach that there exists an overriding and all encompassing obligation to preserve human life. Certainly the fifth commandment forbids the taking of life and, by implication, acts which are seriously injurious to life and perhaps even risks which involve an unreasonable likelihood of such injury. However, affirmative actions obliging one to protect and preserve bodily life or to effect a cure for debilitating illnesses and procedures designed merely to prolong life are a different matter entirely. Some such obligations may be implied in Paul's admonition to husbands to love their wives as their own bodies predicated upon the assertion that "no man ever hates his own flesh, but nourishes and cherishes it" (Eph. 5:29). Thomas Aquinas teaches that an obligation to exercise proper care over the body is contained in the law of charity and hence a man should love his own body with the love of charity.[36] However, Matthew 6:25–34 and Luke 12:22–34 have apparently been understood as cautioning man against losing sight of higher values as a result of a pervasive concern with the preservation of life. Pius XII explicitly counselled that "Life, health, all temporal activities are in fact subordinated to spiritual ones."[37] Since preservation of life is seen as a value, but not as a paramount or overriding value, Catholic moralists teach that the obligation embraces only the use of ordinary means for the preservation of life. Life is a relative good and the duty to preserve it is a limited one. However, employment of ordinary means is an absolute moral requirement. Failure to supply ordinary means of preserving life, albeit an act of nonfeasance, is equated with euthanasia.[38] Ordinary means are defined in the papal pronouncement as those "that do not involve any grave burden for oneself or another." In addition to being "too burdensome for most men" a more strict obligation, in the Catholic view, "would render the attainment of the higher, more important good too difficult." Extraordinary means in the preservation of life and health, i.e., measures which involve excessive difficulty by reason of physical pain, repugnance, danger or expense, etc., while not mandated by Catholic teaching, are not forbidden as long as the person employing such means "does not fail in some more serious duty." Even when not strictly obligatory, they are described as often being of great value for gaining merit, atoning for sins and giving good example for others. Hence they are not only permissible but frequently laudable.[39] Some moralists caution against withholding of extraordinary means in certain circumstances because such conduct may be construed in the minds of some as a form of euthanasia.[40] In other circumstances, it may impede the perfection of medical skill and techniques.[41]

The categories of ordinary and extraordinary are relative ones and are recognized in the papal pronouncement as varying "according to circumstances of persons, places, times and culture." In the absence of definitive concrete examples it is quite difficult to determine precisely where the point of demarcation between the two is to be drawn. Earlier authors have listed criteria which, presumably, are still applicable, e.g., leaving one's home for a more healthful climate, the amputation of a limb, all very costly treatments[42] and procedures which involve great pain.[43] Any procedure entailing grave danger of death must be considered extraordinary.[44] Other measures, once considered extraordinary, would under contemporary conditions be considered ordinary, e.g., a maiden's repugnance at being treated by a male physician or surgeon. There is no doubt that reclassification of treatment of a woman by a male as ordinary rather than extraordinary is warranted in light of changed cultural mores. Such examination is simply no longer offensive or repugnant. It is, however, highly significant that the repugnance attached to the innocent, nay therapeutic, violation of feminine modesty, when present, renders medical attention an extraordinary matter. In pre-anesthetic days the excruciating pain attendant upon surgery was sufficient reason for all such procedures to be classified as extraordinary. One authority suggests that submission to general anesthesia is itself an extraordinary measure because it deprives the patient of the use of reason at least temporarily.[45]

The notion of ordinary means is a relative concept, determined by societal or situational considerations. The concept is nevertheless a norm established by society as a whole rather than by the individual as a subjective value. Thus one theologian speaks of extraordinary means as those which "exceed the moral strength of men in general."[46] The judgment of ordinary versus extraordinary is to be made on the basis of how the majority of individuals would react in a given situation, allowing for the objectification of situational and subjective variables.

There does, however, appear to be some disagreement with regard to whether or not, in a practical sense, there is, in addition to a relative norm, an absolute norm by means of which medical procedure may be measured as ordinary or extraordinary. Joseph V. Sullivan writes quite clearly, "There is an absolute norm beyond which means are *per se* extraordinary."[47] Edwin F. Healy, S.J., not only states that means may become extraordinary either in the relative or absolute sense of the term but actually, in terms of financial burden, sets a dollar amount upon expenses which must be considered ordinary in terms of an absolute norm. Writing in 1956, Healy states that if, "in normal times," the treatment required for the cure of a fatal disease would cost $2,000 or more, such treatment must be considered to be extraordinary and even a wealthy person would not be obligated to afford so large a sum in order to effect a cure.[48] In the case of a poor person the relative norm would be applicable and the dollar figure would be much lower. Another moralist, Charles J. McFadden, O.S.A., disagrees:

> It would be most difficult for me to understand how a man who owns a palatial permanent residence, another home at the seashore, two or three cars, possibly a little cabin cruiser, enjoys periodic vacations abroad and sponsors lavish parties at home, would not be morally obligated to spend more than $2,000 to save his life. . . . Surely, it would be hard to believe that a man would not be morally bound to spend as much to save his life as he habitually and unconcernedly throws away on trivialities.[49]

Although McFadden concedes that in theory there "may be some absolute amount beyond which a man would not have to go" he professes disbelief at the possibility that "any kind of needed and otherwise ordinary medical care could possibly come anywhere near what such an amount would have to be."[50] Hence, McFadden reasons that speculation with regard to the amount which might constitute an absolute norm is of little practical value.

Healy makes a very curious point in the course of a discussion of one of the cases which he presents for purposes of illustration. Mr. A. is told by his physician that in order to save his life he must undergo a costly operation. Mr. A, however, is a veteran and entitled to hospitalization in the veteran's hospital in the city where he resides. In his analysis of the case Healy comments, ". . . a patient is not free to appeal to the principle of the absolute norm if the state, county, city, or Federal Government is ready to provide without cost to him all the medical services that may be necessary."[51] Healy offers no further explanation. In the absence of such elucidation it may be assumed that governmental provision of health care changes the moral consideration simply by virtue of the changed reality of the situation. Since financial aid is freely forthcoming the patient need assume no financial burden whatsoever; he may not spurn treatment which places no ordinary, much less extraordinary, imposition upon him.

If, however, we examine governmental or societal responsibility in this matter a different perspective presents itself. Society has no obligation in charity to make extraordinary means available. Hence governments are not *obligated* to assume the expenditure of sums for medical care of its citizens which are in excess of the objective norm as it is determined. According to Catholic teaching, expenditure of extraordinary sums is discretionary both for the individual and for society.

The implication in terms of the treatment of both defective newborns and the chronically ill is obvious. It would appear that if one accepts the moral reasoning upon which these distinctions are made, it would follow that medical practitioners may be granted discretionary authority to withhold costly procedures when such care is provided through the use of public funds.

Significantly, mere prolongation of life is not a Catholic value. Two specific cases are discussed by the 17th century Spanish Cardinal, Juan de Lugo.[52] A man is unjustly condemned to death by starvation but somehow his friends manage to get some nourishment to him. Is he obligated to eat and thereby ward off death temporarily? A man is about to be burned to death, but has a sufficient quantity of water to quench the flames which are now raging. Is he obliged to quench the fire, knowing full well that it will be rekindled by the executioner? The Cardinal answers that a person is obligated to save his life if he is capable of doing so, but he is under no obligation to put off death. Thus the condemned man is obligated to eat only if he has prospects of obtaining food on a regular basis; he must put out the flames only if there is hope that the fire will not subsequently be rekindled. De Lugo applies the principle *parum pro nihilo reputatur* and declares, "The duty of preserving one's life through ordinary means does not include the duty of using means that will prolong life so briefly that they may be morally considered as nothing."

The crucial question which De Lugo does not explore is the determination of the minimum threshold of life potential which is endowed with moral meaningfulness. McFadden, in a somewhat different context, indicates that an operation which would add "only a few weeks" of life is extraordinary and thus optional.[53] This, however, does not warrant the conclusion that natural means such as food and drink are not obligatory in order to prolong life for an equivalent period of time.

In a somewhat fuller discussion, Healy advances the position that in determining what constitutes ordinary means of preserving life in any given case there must be a just proportion between the good effects to be anticipated and the negative effects, including cost, pain, and inconvenience, attendant upon use of the processes in question. He then argues that means utilized by men in general even when no danger is present such as food and drink are always (or nearly always) to be considered ordinary means. De Lugo obviously considered the prolongation of life for a short period of time by even such ordinary and usual measures as not being a matter of moral consequence. Healy asserts that a person in the terminal stages of illness whose life can be prolonged for only a short time, defined by Healy as "a week or two," must utilize only natural means, i.e., food, drink, and the like, for the conservation of life but need not use artificial means such as intravenous feeding, oxygen, blood transfusions or chemical stimulants to prolong life.[54] Elsewhere Healy states that respirators, oxygen tents (and presumably I.V. bottles as well) need not be employed as "permanent adjuncts" in keeping a patient alive and hence supportive therapy involving utilization of these adjuncts need not be instituted if their use is deemed to be permanent. Healy defines permanence as being a period of six months or more.[55]

Some Catholic theologians assert that only natural means are to be classified as ordinary and that all artificial means must be deemed extraordinary.[56] Others ignore the distinction between artificial and natural in favor of the criterion of that which is commonly used.[57] Healy, as we have seen, and Thomas J. O'Donnell, S.J.,[58] adopt an intermediate position in maintaining that developed techniques of artificial life support are to be distinguished from commonplace natural means such as eating, drinking and sleeping. According to the latter, use of such modern means shall be weighed against the quality of life which may be preserved by employing such means. One theologian sharply disagrees with the view that would regard intravenous feeding in particular as other than an ordinary means. Joseph P. Donovan, C.M., insists that recourse to intravenous feeding entails neither a physical nor moral impossibility; it is therefore an ordinary means of acquiring nourishment.[59]

With regard to the inconvenience or difficulty of surgery when weighed against prolongation of life, Healy is both cryptic and imprecise. He remarks that "unless the life expectancy is at least three or four months, the operation is not obligatory."[60] Since there is no obligation with regard to use of means whose effectiveness is only probable rather than certain the operation is mandatory only if the patient will *certainly* survive for three or four months after the operation, even though he will probably live for a much longer time. However, in the very next sentence, Healy concludes, "If the surgery would ensure the patient six or more months of life, it must be considered as ordinary means and one that is obligatory."[61] There is quite apparently some equivocation in Healy's mind with regard to whether it is a three, four, or six-months survival period which establishes a reasonable proportion between the bad effects relating to surgery, which in the case discussed was an appendectomy, and the good effect, i.e., the prolongation of life.

Not only are therapeutic measures which themselves produce pain deemed to be extraordinary, but even otherwise ordinary measures may become extraordinary when prolongation of the life of a severely ill patient is accompanied by excessive pain. An interesting problem arises in the treatment of a patient suffering from two illnesses, one painful, the other not, e.g., cancer and diabetes. If insulin is withheld the patient will quickly lapse into a diabetic coma and die an easy death; continued use of insulin will prolong life but leave the patient racked with pain. One theologian, Fr. J. McCarthy, has argued that the duty of administering insulin must be considered independently of the moral considerations which must be weighed in treating the malignancy.[62] Since the use of insulin is a normal means of treating diabetes its use is obligatory despite the fact that cancer makes the patient's life painful. Thus, McCarthy states that insulin may be withdrawn only if it becomes an extraordinary means by virtue of expense or if its administration in itself becomes too painful. Significantly, McCarthy points out that, according to Catholic teaching, even when extraordinary means are withdrawn it is not permissible to "intend the shortening of life as the immediate object of the act." Pope Pius' statement implies much the same limitation. In speaking of the permissibility of attempts at resuscitation, the principle of double effect and of *voluntorium in causa* is invoked.

One basic difficulty presents itself with regard to McCarthy's reasoning. Although nonfeasance is tantamount to euthanasia, nontreatment of cancer or interruption of attempts at resuscitation is justified as a licit application of the double effect theory: the primary purpose is not to kill but to refrain from inflicting or prolonging pain. Precisely the same rationale is involved in withdrawal of insulin. The physician treats the patient, not the disease. This is true from the theological vantage point no less than from the medical perspective. Hence it would seem that all factors, including the presence of other physiological conditions, must be weighed in reaching a determination with regard to whether any proposed therapy is extraordinary relative to the condition of the patient. Nevertheless, it is clearly McCarthy's position that a proposed mode of therapy is to be judged ordinary or extraordinary relative solely to the condition it is designed to treat.[63]

This point would appear to be extremely important in terms of decision-making with regard to the treatment of defective newborns. The crucial question is whether ordinary versus extraordinary is to be determined relative to each procedure and the condition it is designed to remedy or whether this decision is to be made relative to the situation in its totality. Insofar as considerations pertaining to the quality of life to be preserved are concerned, McFadden states quite clearly that ordinary means of sustaining life are obligatory even in cases of monstrosities.[64] Healy, in one of his case discussions, comments, "Whatever a physician would be obliged to do for a normal child, he must do for a hydrocephalic."[65] If, however, the situation is viewed in its totality there may well be room to argue that such methods are extraordinary when measured against the quality of life which is preserved. Richard McCormick, S.J., clearly follows this mode of reasoning in arguing that not only do the classical examples of situations involving pain and great hardship to the patient create conditions in which preservation of life is extraordinary but that the absence of potentiality for human relationship creates a situation in which all attempts to preserve life become extraordinary.[66] His position, however, appears to constitute a marked departure from that of earlier Catholic moralists.

The Judaic Tradition

1. The Supreme Value of Human Life   The value with which human life is regarded in the Jewish tradition is maximized far beyond the value placed upon human life in the Christian tradition or in Anglo-Saxon common law. In Jewish law and moral teaching the value of human life is supreme and takes precedence over virtually all other considerations. This attitude is most eloquently summed up in a Talmudic passage regarding the creation of Adam: "Therefore only a single human being was created in the world, to teach that if any person has caused a single soul of Israel to perish, Scripture regards him as if he had caused an entire world to perish; and if any human being saves a single soul of Israel, Scripture regards him as if he had saved an entire world."[67] Human life is not a good to be preserved as a condition of other values but as an absolute basic and precious good in its own stead. The obligation to preserve life is commensurately all-encompassing.

Life with suffering is regarded as being, in many cases, preferable to cessation of life and with it elimination of suffering. The Talmud, *Sotah* 22a, and Maimonides, *Hilkhot Sotah* 3:20, indicate that the adulterous woman who was made to drink "the bitter waters" (Numbers 6:11–31) did not always die immediately. If she possessed other merit, even though guilty of the offense with which she was charged, the waters, rather than causing her to perish immediately, produced a debilitating and degenerative state which led to a protracted termination of life. The added longevity, although accompanied by pain and suffering, is viewed as a privilege bestowed in recognition of meritorious actions.[68] Life accompanied by pain is thus viewed as preferable to death.[69] It is this sentiment which is reflected in the words of the Psalmist: "The Lord has indeed punished me, but He has not left me to die" (Psalms 118:88).

A most eloquent exposition of the nature of theological restraint against disposing of human life, even of one's own, is presented by Plato in the *Phaedo*. Socrates in a farewell conversation with his students prior to his execution speaks of the afterlife with eager anticipation. Thereupon, one of his disciples queries, if death is so much preferable to life, why did not Socrates long ago take his own life? In a very apt simile Socrates responds that an ox does not have the right to take its own life because it thereby deprives its master of enjoyment of his property. Man is the chattel of the gods, says Socrates. Just as "bovicide" on the part of the ox is a violation of the proprietor-property relationship, so suicide on the part of man constitutes a violation of the Creator-creature relationship.

The 16th century rabbinic scholar R. David ibn Zimra demonstrates that God's proprietary interest in the life and body of each of his creatures is a fundamental concept of Jewish law. The laws of jurisprudence provide that the statement of a defendant is given absolute credence when contrary to the defendant's self-interest. Accordingly, judgment is rendered against a defendant who accepts liability even if the defendant's confession is contradicted by the testimony of a hundred unimpeachable witnesses. In criminal law, however, a diametrically opposite principle is applied. According to the laws of evidence as postulated by Halakhah, not only cannot an accused be forced to testify against himself, but should he confess to a crime or implicate himself by his own mouth the defendant's testimony must be completely disregarded.

R. David ibn Zimra[70] raises the obvious question. If a person's testimony with regard to his own liability is given credence in matters of financial liability why should the same principle not be operative with regard to criminal culpability as well? His answer is incisive. In matters of financial responsibility and obligation, answers Ibn Zimra, the court is not at all concerned with the veracity of the defendant's self-incriminatory statement. His wealth and material resources are his to dispose of as he wishes. Should he desire to do so, he has full power to make a gift of his possessions to the plaintiff. If he chooses to do so via the medium of judicial proceedings the *Bet Din* will accommodate him in fulfilling his desire. Self-incrimination leading to corporal or capital punishment is, however, an entirely different matter. Criminal liability presages a punishment which the accused has no right to impose upon himself for "man's life is not his possession but the possession of the Holy One, blessed be He."[71] Since man lacks proprietary rights over his body, the confessed criminal cannot direct the court to inflict punishment upon him. Such punishment can be meted out only in accordance with the law of God. Man's body is not his to dispose of at will.

The selfsame concept was earlier formulated by Maimonides in a somewhat different context. Maimonides, *Hilkhot Roze'ah* 1:4, succinctly explains that ransom cannot be accepted from a murderer as a substitute for execution even with the consent of the victim's kin or blood avenger. The explanation offered by Maimonides is that the life of the victim "is not the property of the blood-avenger but the property of the Holy One, blessed be He."[72]

Man does not possess absolute title to his life or to his body; title to human life is vested in the Creator, and man is but the steward of the life which he has been privileged to receive. Man is charged with preserving, dignifying and hallowing that life. He is obliged to seek food and sustenance in order to safeguard the life he has been granted; when falling victim to illness or disease he is obliged to seek a cure in order to sustain life. Never is he called upon to determine whether life is worth living—this is a question over which God remains the sole arbiter.

The value placed upon human life is reflected in Halakhah, the corpus of Jewish law, which provides for the suspension of all religious precepts (with the exception of the prohibition against commission of the three cardinal sins: idolatry, murder and certain sexual offenses) when necessary in order to save life.[73] Even the mere possibility of saving human life mandates violation of such laws "however remote the likelihood of saving human life may be."[74] The quality of life which is thus preserved is never a factor to be taken into consideration. Neither is the length of the survivor's life expectancy a controlling factor. Judaism regards not only human life in general as being of infinite and inestimable value, but regards every moment of life as being of infinite value.[75] Obligations with regard to treatment and cure are one and the same whether the person's life is likely to be prolonged for a matter of years or merely for a few seconds. Thus, even on the Sabbath, efforts to free a victim buried under a collapsed building must be maintained even if the victim is found in circumstances such that he cannot survive longer than a brief period of time.[76] Sectarians such as the Sadducees who lived during the period of the Second Commonwealth and the Karaites of the Geonic period who challenged these provisions of Jewish law and, by implication, the value system upon which they are predicated, were branded heretics.[77]

Defective newborns are known and discussed in rabbinic literature. *Sefer Ḥasidim,* no. 186, a 13th century compendium authored by R. Judah the Pious, describes the case of a child born with the severest of physical deformities and mental deficiencies — a monster-like creature which obviously had no human potential whatsoever. A question was raised as to whether or not the monster-birth might be destroyed. The answer was an emphatic negative. The answer is not at all surprising. Noteworthy is the question. The desire to destroy this creature was predicated upon the fact that the monster-like child was born with ferocious looking teeth and an elongated tail. In light of these characteristics and in view of the general demeanor of the monster-birth it was felt by some that this creature constituted a life-threatening menace to the community. In circumstances of lesser gravity it would not have occurred to anyone to raise the question. An early nineteenth-century responsum authored by R. Eleazar Fleckeles, *Teshuvah me-Ahavah,* I, no. 53, makes much the same point in connection with a somewhat less dramatic situation. A child born of a human mother, despite the possession of animal-like organs and features, is a human being whose life must be protected and preserved.[78] Such a creature may not be killed, nor may it, despite its deformity, be permitted to die as a result of benign neglect.[79]

The obligation to save the life of an endangered person is derived by the Talmud from the verse, "Neither shalt thou stand idly by the blood of thy fellow" (Leviticus 19:16).[80] The Talmud and the various codes of Jewish law offer specific examples of situations in which a moral obligation exists with regard to rendering aid. These include the rescue of a person drowning in a river, assistance to one being mauled by wild beasts and aid to a person under attack by bandits.

2. Medical Intervention: The Theological Dilemma   Application of this principle to medical intervention for the purpose of preserving life is not without theological and philosophical difficulties. It is to be anticipated that a theology which ascribes providential concern to the Deity will view sickness as part of the divine scheme. A personal God does not allow His creatures, over whom He exercises providential guardianship, to become ill unless the affliction is divinely ordained as a means of punishment, for purposes of expiation of sin or for some other beneficial purpose entirely comprehensible to the Deity, if not to man. Thus, while the ancient Greeks regarded illness as a curse and the sick as inferior persons because, to them, malady represented the disruption of the harmony of the body which is synonymous with health, in Christianity suffering was deemed to be a manifestation of divine grace because it effected purification of the afflicted and served as an enobling process. Since illness resulted in a state of enhanced spiritual perfection, the sick man was viewed as marked by divine favor.

Human intervention in causing or speeding the therapeutic process is, then, in a sense, interference with the deliberate design of providence. The patient in seeking medical attention betrays a lack of faith in failing to put his trust in God. This attitude is reflected in the teaching of a number of early and medieval Christian theologians who counseled against seeking medical attention.[81] The Karaites rejected all forms of human healing and relied entirely upon prayer. Consistent with their fundamentalist orientation they based their position upon a quite literal reading of Exodus 15:26. A literal translation of the Hebrew text of the passage reads as follows: "I will put none of the diseases upon thee which I have put upon the Egyptians, for I am the Lord thy physician."[82] Hence, the Karaites taught that God alone should be sought as physician.[83]

This view was rejected in normative Jewish teaching, but not without due recognition of the cogency of the theological argument upon which it is based. Rabbinic teaching recognized that intervention for the purpose of thwarting the natural course of the disease could be sanctioned only on the basis of specific divine dispensation. Such license is found, on the basis of Talmudic exegesis, in the scriptural passage dealing with compensation for personal injury:

> And if men quarrel with one another and one smiteth the other with a stone or with the fist and he die not, but keep his bed . . . he must pay the loss entailed by absence from work and cause him to be thoroughly healed (Exodus 21:18–19).

Ostensibly, this passage refers simply to financial liability incurred as the result of an act of assault. However, since specific reference is made to liability for medical expenses it follows that liability for such expenses implies Biblical license to incur those expenses in the course of seeking the ministrations of a practitioner of the healing arts. Thus the Talmud, *Bava Kamma* 85a, comments, "From here [it is derived] that the physician is granted permission to cure." Specific authorization is required, comments Rashi, in order to teach us that ". . . we are not to say, 'How is it that God smites and man heals?' " In much the same vein, *Tosafot* and R. Solomon ben Adret state that without such sanction, "He who heals might appear as if he invalidated a divine decree."[84]

An eloquent midrashic narrative reflects both recognition of man's inherent lack of authority to tamper with physiological processes since, *prima facie,* such intervention would be construed as a violation of the natural order as well as awareness that permission to practice the medical arts is a matter of specific divine dispensation:

> It occurred that R. Ishmael and R. Akiva were strolling in the streets of Jerusalem accompanied by another person. They were met by a sick person. He said to them, "My masters, tell me by what means I may be cured." They told him, "Do thus and so until you are cured." He asked them, "And who afflicted me?" They replied, "The Holy One, blessed be He." [The sick person] responded, "You have entered into a matter which does not pertain to you. [God] has afflicted and you seek to cure! Are you not transgressing His will?"

[R. Akiva and R. Ishmael] asked him, "What is your occupation?" He answered, "I am a tiller of the soil and here is the sickle in my hand." They asked him, "Who created the vineyard?" He answered, "The Holy One, blessed be He." R. Akiva and R. Ishmael said to him, "And you enter into a matter which does not pertain to you! [God] created [the vineyard] and you cut His fruits from it." He said to them, "Do you not see the sickle in my hand? If I did not plow, sow, fertilize and weed nothing would sprout." They said to him, "Foolish man! Have you never in your life heard that it is written 'as for man, his days are as grass; as grass of the field, so he flourishes' (Psalms 103:15). Just as if one does not weed, fertilize and plow, the trees will not produce [fruit] and if fruit is produced but is not watered or fertilized it will not live but die, so with regard to the body. Drugs and medicaments are the fertilizer and the physician is the tiller of the soil."[85]

The analogy between the physician and the farmer is drawn with utmost precision. Prior to the flood man was forbidden to eat the flesh of animals. Only after Noah emerged from the Ark did God tell Noah "Every moving thing which lives shall be for food for you; as the green herb have I given you all" (Genesis 9:3). The Gemara, *Sanhedrin* 59b, points out that Adam was not permitted to eat meat but was restricted to the produce of the field. Permission to eat growing things is granted to Adam in the verse "And God said: 'Behold, I have given you every herb yielding seed which is upon the face of all the earth and every tree . . . to you it shall be for food' " (Genesis 1:29). In the absence of this dispensation Adam would have been forbidden to partake in any way of the bounty of the Garden of Eden. Any attempt on his part to do so would have been an act of theft.

Before Adam sinned it was not necessary for him to till the soil. "With the sweat of your face will you eat bread" (Genesis 3:19) is indeed a curse, but it is a dispensation as well. Without such dispensation Adam would have had no right to plow the field or to uproot thorns and thistles. One who enters his neighbor's field and engages in such acts is an intruder and usurper. Since the land was created by God, Adam had no right to till the soil unless given specific dispensation. In declaring "By the sweat of your brow shall you eat bread" God at one and the same time grants dispensation for tilling the soil and indicates that henceforth it is the divine will that Adam do so. Adam may no longer simply rely only upon the largesse of God; he *must* till the soil for sustenance.

The analogy drawn by the Midrash is an obvious one. The sick man viewed therapeutic intervention as a contravention of divine will and application of medicaments as illicit interference with the natural processes of the human body which is the chattel of God. Indeed this is so, but by the same token fields and vineyards are the property of God as well and man has no natural right to till the soil or to pluck the fruits which the land produces. Man may do so, not as a matter of right, but by virtue of specific divine dispensation. Man is similarly granted dispensation to practice the medical arts. Just as God grants dispensation to till the soil and to reap the harvest in order that man shall not perish, so also does He grant dispensation to seek medical assistance in order to restore the body to health.

3. The Halakhic Imperative   Non-therapeutic life-saving intervention is Talmudically mandated on independent grounds. The Talmud, *Sanhedrin* 73a, posits an obligation to rescue a neighbor from danger such as drowning or being mauled by an animal. This obligation is predicated upon the scriptural exhortation with regard to the restoration of lost property, "And thou shalt return it to him" (Deuteronomy 22:2). On the basis of a pleonasm in the Hebrew text, the Talmud declares that this verse includes an obligation to restore a fellow-man's body as well as his property. Hence, there is created an obligation to come to the aid of one's fellow man in a life-threatening situation. Noteworthy is the fact that Maimonides,[86] going beyond the examples supplied by the Talmud, posits this source as the basis of the obligation to render medical care. Maimonides declares that the Biblical commandment "And thou shalt return it to him" establishes an obligation requiring the physician to render professional services in life-threatening situations. Every individual, insofar as he is able, is obligated to restore the health of a fellow man no less than he is obligated to restore his property. Maimonides views this as a binding religious obligation.

Noteworthy is not only Maimonides' extension of this concept to cover medical matters but also his failure to allude at all to the verse "And he shall cause him to be thoroughly healed." It would appear that Maimonides is of the opinion that without the granting of specific *permission* one would not be permitted to tamper with physiological processes; obligations derived from Deuteronomy 22:2 would be limited to prevention of accident or assault by man or beast. Dispensation to intervene in the natural order is derived from Exodus 21:20; but once such license is given, medical therapy is not simply elective but acquires the status of a positive obligation.[87] As indicated by *Sanhedrin* 73a, this obligation mandates not only the rendering of personal assistance as is the case with regard to the restoration of lost property, but, by virtue of the negative commandment, "You shall not stand idly by the blood of your neighbor" (Leviticus 19:16), the obligation is expanded to encompass expenditure of financial resources for the sake of preserving the life of one's fellow man. This seems to have been the interpretation given to Maimonides' comments by Rabbi Joseph Caro who, in his code of Jewish law, combined both concepts in stating:

> The Torah gave permission to the physician to heal; moreover, this is a religious precept and it is included in the category of saving life; and if the physician withholds his services it is considered as shedding blood.[88]

Naḥmanides also finds that the obligation of the physician to heal is inherent in the commandment, "And thou shalt love thy neighbor as thyself" (Leviticus 19:18).[89] As an instantiation of the general obligation to manifest love and concern for one's neighbor, the obligation to heal encompasses not only situations posing a threat to life or limb or demanding restoration of impaired health but also situations of lesser gravity warranting medical attention for relief of pain and promotion of well-being.[90]

Despite the unequivocal and authoritative rulings of both Maimonides and Rabbi Joseph Caro, there do exist within the rabbinic tradition disonant views which look somewhat askance at the practice of the healing arts. Abraham ibn Ezra[91] finds a contradiction between the injunction "And he shall cause him to be thoroughly healed" and the account given in II Chronicles 16:12. Scripture reports that Asa, King of Judah, became severely ill and in his sickness "he sought not to the Lord, but to the physicians." Of course, this passage can readily be understood as implying that Asa was deserving of censure because he relied upon mortal physicians exclusively and failed to seek divine help through penitence and prayer. If the verse in question is interpreted in this light it contains no disparaging reference whatsoever with regard to either physicians or to the practice of medicine. Rabbinic scholars, including exegetes such as *Meẓudat David* and legal authorities such as R. Joel Sirkes, *Bayit Ḥadash, Yoreh De'ah* 336, do indeed interpret this passage in precisely this way. Alternatively, the passage may be understood as censuring Asa for not recognizing that the physician and his ministrations are merely vehicles for divine healing and that all healing ultimately comes from God.[92] However, Ibn Ezra, and later Naḥmanides as well, understand this verse as teaching that Asa was censured for seeking medical assistance. According to Ibn Ezra, Asa was taken to task for not placing his trust in God alone to the exclusion of endeavors to effect a cure through the vehicle of medical science.[93] Seen in this light, there is a clear contradiction between II Chronicles 16:12 and Exodus 21:19. Ibn Ezra resolves this difficulty by examining the contextual reference of each passage. Exodus refers to an act of physical assault. The healing to which specific reference is made is treatment of a presumably external wound which is humanly inflicted. II Chronicles speaks of sickness undoubtedly resulting from "natural" physiological processes. According to Ibn Ezra, Scripture grants license for therapeutic intervention only for treatment of external wounds. Wounds inflicted by man, either by design or by accident, may legitimately be treated by any means known to mankind. That which has been inflicted by man may be cured by man. However, internal wounds or physiological disorders, according to this view, are not encompassed in the injunction "and he shall cause to be thoroughly healed." Such afflictions are presumed to be manifestations of divine rebuke or punishment and only God, who afflicts, may heal.

Needless to say, Ibn Ezra's position was rejected by normative Judaism as is most eloquently demonstrated by the ruling recorded in *Shulḥan Arukh, Oraḥ Ḥayyim* 328:3. Jewish law not only sanctions but requires suspension of Sabbath restrictions for treatment of a person afflicted by a life-threatening malady. *Oraḥ Ḥayyim* 328:3 rules blanketly that all "internal wounds" are to be presumed to be life-threatening for purposes of Halakhah. Quite obviously, Jewish law as codified mandates treatment of even internal disorders by means of all available therapeutic techniques. R. Ẓemaḥ Duran, while acknowledging Ibn Ezra's outstanding competence as a Biblical exegete, had little regard for the latter's legal acumen and dismisses him as "not having been proficient in the laws."[94]

Of greater relevance in the formulation of Jewish thought are the comments of Naḥmanides in his commentary on the Bible, Leviticus 26:11:

> The principle is that when [the people of] Israel are perfect and numerous their affairs are not at all conducted in accordance with nature, neither with regard to their persons nor their land, neither collectively nor individually. For God will bless their bread and their water and remove illness from their midst to the point that they will have no need of a physician and [no need] to safeguard themselves by any medical means whatsoever as [Scripture] states, "for I am the Lord your healer."
>
> So did the righteous do in the days of prophecy; even when a transgression occurred to them so that they became ill they did not seek to physicians but only to prophets as was the case of Asa and Hezekiah when [Asa] became ill; Scripture says "Even in his sickness he sought not to the Lord but to the physicians." If the matter of physicians was customary among them for what reason does [Scripture] mention the physicians? The guilt would have been solely because he did not seek the Lord. . . . However, one who seeks God through a prophet does not seek physicians.
>
> What portion is there unto physicians in the house of those who do the will of God since He has vouchsafed "and He will bless your bread and your water and I will remove sickness from your midst?" The function of physicians is only with regard to food and drink, to admonish and to instruct with regard to them. So declared the Sages: "Throughout the twenty-two years during which Rabbah the son of Rabbi Joseph reigned, he did not even call a physician to his home (*Berakhot* 64a; *Horayot* 14a). . . . Such is their dictum (*Berakhot* 60a): "For it is not the nature of mankind [to make use of] medical cures, but they have accustomed themselves [to do so]."
>
> For if they were not wont [to seek] cures, a person would become ill, in accordance with the punishment for his sin which is upon him and would be healed at the will of God. But [men] have become accustomed to medical cures and God has left them to the chance occurrences of nature. This was the intent [of the Sages] in their declaration " 'And he shall surely heal'—from here it is derived that the Torah gave the physician dispensation to heal." They did not state, "The Torah gave permission to

the sick to become healed"; rather since the sick person has become ill and seeks to be cured since he has been accustomed to medical cures, for he is not of the community of God whose portion is life, the physician should not restrain himself in the cure [of the patient] either because of fear lest [the patient] die under his hand . . . or because [the physician] might say that God alone is the healer of all flesh, for they have already accustomed themselves [to medical treatment]. Therefore, [with regard to] individuals who strive and smite one another with a stone or fist there is a claim against the assailant for medical compensation, for the Torah does not predicate its laws upon miracles . . . but when the ways of man find favor unto God he has no traffic with medical cures.

It might be argued that, according to Naḥmanides, the patient may justifiably reject medical treatment and, when he is prompted to do so because he has placed his trust in God, renunciation of further therapy is even meritorious. In apparent striking contrast to the comments of Naḥmanides stand the diametrically opposed words of Maimonides in his commentary on the Mishnah, *Pesaḥim* 4:9. *Pesaḥim* 56a and *Berakhot* 10b record that King Hezekiah performed a number of exemplary and meritorious acts. It is with reference to these actions that Hezekiah prays "Remember . . . how I have walked before You in truth and with an able heart and that which is good in Your eyes I have done" (Isaiah 38:3). The first of the enumerated actions is the suppression of a certain *Book of Cures*. Rashi, *Pesaḥim* 56a, comments that Hezekiah was motivated to act in this manner because individuals falling ill might consult this book and find an immediate cure for their illnesses. The result of such speedy care was that "their hearts did not become subdued as a result of their illness." Maimonides, in his commentary on the Mishnah, cites a slightly different version of this explanation and states that the concern was that the afflicted failed to place their trust in God. He proceeds to denigrate this interpretation in the harshest of terms. If this reasoning is cogent, argues Maimonides, partaking of nourishment should also serve to undermine faith in God. Following this line of reasoning, were a person to become hungry and seek bread he would undoubtedly become cured of the severe malady of hunger and would no longer rely upon God. In actuality, declares Maimonides, just as one gives thanks to God upon eating for having created food with which one may assuage hunger, so will one give thanks to God for having created the cure for one's illness. Maimonides himself opines that the work in question was either idolatrous in nature or contained directions for the use of dangerous drugs and was suppressed because the drugs were misused with adverse results. It is clear that Maimonides himself sees no more disopprobrium in the use of drugs than in the consumption of food. Food and medicine were both created by God for the benefit of man.

Naḥmanides' statements, if taken literally, are contradicted by a number of Talmudic dicta. *Sanhedrin* 17b declares that a scholar dare not reside in a city which lacks a physician. In an aggadic statement, *Avodah Zarah* 55a declares, "Afflictions which befall a person are foresworn not to depart other than through a specific drug administered by a specific [physician] on a specific day and at a specific hour." *Gittin* 56b reports that Rabbi Yoḥanan ben Zakkai requested of Vespasian that a doctor be sent to attend Rabbi Zadok. *Bava Meẓia* 85b speaks of a certain Samuel who is referred to as the personal physician of R. Judah the Prince and describes the manner in which he treated an ophthalmological condition from which his patient suffered. The clear meaning of these references is not only that the physician is duty-bound to render treatment but also that the patient is obligated to seek medical remedies. Moreover, Naḥmanides himself apparently contradicts his own comments. In his authoritative halakhic work, *Torat ha-Adam,*[95] Naḥmanides states unequivocally that the "permission" or "dispensation" of which the Talmud speaks is in actuality a "commandment" or obligation (*hai reshut reshut de-mitzvah hi*).[96] In this work Naḥmanides clearly views the seeking of medical treatment as obligatory on the part of the patient. The sole latter-day scholar to permit a patient to follow the option of Naḥmanides in refusing medical attention is Rabbi Zev Nahum of Biala.[97]

These difficulties are, however, readily resolved if it is understood that Naḥmanides' remarks in his commentary on the Bible are intended only as a description of conditions prevailing in a spiritual utopia. In developing his theory of providence, Maimonides explains that the quality of providential guardianship extended to man is directly correlative with man's spiritual attainment. To the extent that man is lacking in perfection his condition is regulated by the laws of nature.[98] Thus a pious person privileged to be the recipient of a high degree of providential guardianship would not require medication, but might expect to be healed by God directly. Other individuals, not beneficiaries of this degree of providence, are perforce required to seek a cure by natural means. In doing so they incur no censure whatsoever. Indeed, Naḥmanides prefaces his comments with a reference to such times when the people of Israel "are perfect" and specifically states that failure to seek medical attention was normative only "for the righteous" and even for them solely "during the time of prophecy." Lesser individuals living in spiritually imperfect epochs are duty-bound to seek the cures made available by medical science. Understood in this manner, there is no contradiction between Naḥmanides and the Talmudic references cited, or, for that matter, between Naḥmanides and Maimonides.[99] In terms of normative Jewish law, there is no question that there exists a positive obligation to seek medical care.[100]

However, in the absence of specific scriptural license to practice and to seek the benefits of the healing arts, the Jewish faith-community would be a community of faith healers.[101] Thus, despite the serious nature of the halakhic imperative with regard to the preservation of human life, it is not surprising that this imperative is somewhat circumscribed insofar as therapeutic preservation of life is concerned. The limited situation in which treatment may be withheld must be carefully delineated.

4. Experimental Therapy and Hazardous Procedures   There is no basis in Jewish teaching for a distinction between ordinary versus extraordinary forms of therapy *per se,* and, in fact, no rabbinic authority draws such a distinction. There does, however, exist a different type of distinction which is of great relevance. A patient may be compelled to submit to medically indicated therapy. However, declares R. Jacob Emden, *Mor u-Kezi'ah, Orah Hayyim* 328, a distinction must be made between therapeutic procedures of proven efficacy and those of unproven therapeutic value. Acceptance of a therapeutic procedure of known efficacy, known as *refu'ah bedukah,* is a moral and halakhic imperative. The patient may not terminate or shorten his life either actively or passively. Since God grants dispensation to seek medical cure, use of medicaments or acceptance of surgical intervention in such situations is mandatory. Man may no more abstain from the use of drugs to cure illness than he may abstain from food and drink. However, if the proposed therapy is of unproven value the patient may legitimately refuse treatment. This is true not only when the treatment itself is potentially hazardous but even if there is no reason to suspect that the proposed treatment may be harmful in any way. In such instances treatment is discretionary; the patient may licitly decline treatment and rely exclusively upon divine providence. R. Emden declares that one who consistently abstains from such modes of therapy "and does not rely upon a human healer and his cure but leaves the matter in the hands of the trustworthy . . . Healer" is praiseworthy. R. Emden, an eighteenth-century authority, himself believed that all medical procedures designed to cure internal afflictions were of the latter category. While R. Emden's position must undoubtedly be modified in the light of present-day medical knowledge the underlying principle is entirely applicable. The patient is morally bound only with regard to the use of medicaments and procedures of demonstrated efficacy. Applying this principle, the patient may legitimately decline a drug or procedure whose curative powers are questionable. This is not to say that a moral obligation to seek a cure exists only if the physician is in a position to guarantee with certainty that a recovery will ensue. The examples given of demonstrable efficacy, *viz.,* amputation of a limb, application of salves and bandages, certainly are not of absolute curative power. Despite the most attentive medical ministrations, some patients do not recover. However, the procedures enumerated are of known value in treating certain afflictions and hence must be pursued. Nevertheless, drugs or surgical procedures whose causal efficacy is not known with certitude may be rejected by the patient. Experimental procedures, including those which are non-hazardous in nature, certainly fall within this category.

Although there is clear dispensation to intervene in physiological processes for purposes of effecting a cure, it does not follow that a physician may subject a patient to, or that a patient may voluntarily accept, a mode of therapy which involves an element of risk. The question of the moral propriety of hazardous procedures arises in three different contexts:

1) Situations in which the existing condition is such that if the patient is left untreated he will certainly succumb as a result of his illness.

2) Situations in which the prognosis is uncertain. In such cases, the patient, if not treated, or if treated by non-hazardous procedures, may or may not survive, whereas if treated, the hazards of the illness are replaced by the hazards of the treatment.

3) Situations in which the malady is not a life-threatening one, but treatment which is hazardous in nature is indicated as a means of relieving agony, discomfort or disfigurement.

It is a principle of Jewish law that the obligation to cure and to preserve life is not limited to situations in which it may be anticipated that subsequent to therapy the patient will have a normal life-expectancy. As noted, the Talmud, *Yoma* 85a, clearly indicates that a victim trapped under the debris of a fallen wall is to be rescued even if as a result of such efforts his life will be prolonged only by a matter of moments. Not only is every human life of infinite value but every moment of human life is of infinite value. Accordingly, ritual restrictions such as Sabbath laws are suspended even for the most minimal prolongation of life.

However, when minimal duration of life (*ḥayyei sha'ah*)[101a] is weighed against the possibility of cure accompanied by normal life expectancy, Jewish teaching accepts the principle that reasonable risks may be incurred in order to effect a recovery. This is the case even if the proposed therapy is of such a nature that the drug or procedure may prove to be ineffective and the patient's life shortened thereby. This principle may be derived from the Talmudic discussion in *Avodah Zarah* 27b concerning the incident of the four leprous men described in II Kings 7:3–4. The Syrian army had besieged Samaria. In addition the region was suffering under a great famine. The lepers recognized that if they took no action they would die of hunger in a relatively short period of time. Were they, however, to cross into the Syrian lines one of two things would happen: either they would immediately be put to death as enemies or, if pitied because of their infirmity, they would be provided with food and their lives saved. Despite the danger they reasoned, "Now therefore come, and let us fall into the host of the Syrians: if they save us alive, we shall live; and if they kill us we shall but die." The Talmud views this narrative as providing scriptural sanction for assuming the risk of immediate death in an attempt to restore conditions necessary for normal life expectancy. Based upon this Talmudic discussion, R. Meir Posner, *Beit Meir, Yoreh De'ah* 339:1 and R. Jacob Reischer, *Shevut Ya'akov*, III, no. 85,[102] specifically permit use of a hazardous drug which might cause death to result "within an hour or two" on behalf of a patient who would otherwise have lived for "a day or two days." Despite the brevity of the period of time which the patient might have been expected to live without therapy, *Shevut Ya'akov* mandated consultation with "proficient medical specialists in the city" and ruled that therapy was to be instituted only if the physicians recommended it by at least a majority of two to one. He further required that the approval of the local rabbinic authority be obtained before such recommendations are acted upon.

An apparent contradiction to this position is found in *Sefer Ḥasidim,* no. 467. This source describes a folk remedy consisting of "grasses" or herbs administered by "women" in treatment of certain maladies which either cured or killed the person so treated within a period of days. *Sefer Ḥasidim* admonishes that they "will certainly be punished for they have killed a person before his time." R. Shalom Mordecai Schwadron, *Orḥot Ḥayyim, Oraḥ Ḥayyim* 328:10, resolves this contradiction by stating that the instance discussed by *Sefer Ḥasidim* involved a situation in which there was clearly a possibility for cure without hazardous intervention. According to this analysis, *Sefer Ḥasidim* sets forth the common-sense approach that hazardous procedures dare not be instituted unless conventional, non-hazardous approaches have been exhausted.

In none of these sources does one find a discussion or a consideration of the statistical probability of prolonging life versus the mortality rate or the odds of shortening life. Yet certainly, in weighing the advisability of instituting hazardous therapy, the relative possibility of achieving a cure is a factor to be considered. *Beit David,* II, no. 340, permits intervention even if there exists but one chance in a thousand that the proposed drug will be efficacious whereas there are nine hundred and ninety-nine chances that it will hasten the death of the patient. A differing view is presented by R. Joseph Hochgelehrter, *Mishnat Ḥakhamim,* who refuses to sanction hazardous therapy unless there is at least a fifty percent chance of survival.[103] He further requires, as did *Shevut Ya'akov,* that dispensation be obtained from rabbinic authorities on each occasion that such therapy is administered. However, Rabbi Moses Feinstein, a foremost contemporary authority, rules that where, in the absence of intervention, death is imminent, a hazardous procedure may be instituted as long as there is a "slim" (*safek raḥok*) chance of a cure, even though the chances of survival are "much less than even" and it is in fact almost certain that the patient will die.[104] Rabbi I. Y. Unterman, the former Chief Rabbi of Israel, maintains that medical risks are warranted "when there is hope of a cure . . . even if in most cases [the procedure] has not been successful and will shorten life."[105]

A much earlier authority, R. Moses Sofer, refused to sanction a hazardous procedure in which the chances of effecting a cure were "remote" but offers no mathematical criteria with regard to the nature of mortality risks which may be properly assumed.[106]

Tiferet Yisra'el raises a quite different question in discussing the permissibility of prophylactic innoculations which are themselves hazardous. In the situation described, the patient, at the time of treatment, is at no risk whatsoever. The fear is that he will contract a potentially fatal disease, apparently smallpox. The innoculation, however, does carry with it a certain degree of immediate risk. *Tiferet Yisra'el* justifies acceptance of this risk which he estimates as being "one in a thousand" because the statistical danger of future contagious infection is greater.[107]

At least one contemporary author differentiates between various cases on the basis of the nature of the risk involved, rather than on the basis of anticipated rates of survival. Rabbi Moshe Dov Welner[108] argues that hazardous procedures may be undertaken despite inherent risks only if the therapeutic nature of the procedure has been demonstrated. For example, a situation might present itself which calls for administration of a drug with known curative potential but which is also toxic in nature. The efficacy of the drug is known but its toxicity may, under certain conditions, kill the patient. The drug may be administered in anticipation of a cure despite the known statistical risk. The same statistical risk, argues Rabbi Welner, could not be sanctioned in administering an experimental drug whose curative powers are unknown or have heretofore not been demonstrated. This, he maintains, is why *Sefer Ḥasidim* censures the practice of administering dangerous herbs as was the custom of women in his day. According to Rabbi Welner, it was not the risk *per se* which was found to be objectionable. Use of the herbs in question was simply not accepted medical practice. Since the efficacy of such potions had not been demonstrated, risk to the life of the patient precluded their use. The same distinction is applied by Rabbi Welner with regard to surgical procedures. Surgical hazards are acceptable only when the technique is known to be effective. Experimental surgery employing untried techniques does not justify exposure to risk.

Insofar as there is disagreement between the authorities cited such disagreement is limited to the permissibility of instituting potentially hazardous therapy. Procedures which involve any significant risk factors are always discretionary rather than mandatory.

A related problem is the attitude toward hazardous therapy for alleviation of pain or other symptoms rather than for the cure of a potentially fatal illness. R. Jacob Emden adopts a somewhat ambivalent position with respect to this question.[109] This authority refers specifically to the surgical removal of gall stones, a procedure designed to correct a condition which he viewed as presenting no hazard to life or health but recognized as being excruciatingly painful. He remarks that, in the absence of danger to life, those who submit to surgery "do not act correctly" and that the procedure is "not entirely permissible." R. Emden carefully stops short of branding the procedure sinful.

The permissibility of placing one's life in danger when not afflicted by a life-threatening malady does, however, require justification. The great value placed upon preservation of life augurs against placing oneself in a risk situation. In general, Jewish law teaches that man may not expose himself to danger. An entire section of the Code of Laws (*Yoreh De'ah*, II, 116) is devoted to an enumeration of actions and situations which must be avoided because they present an element of risk. One hypothesis which may be advanced in sanctioning risks undertaken in a medical context is that the verse "and he shall cause him to be thoroughly healed" grants blanket dispensation for any sound medical practice. That such dispensation is included within the framework of this mandate may be demonstrated in the following manner: It is beyond dispute that an aggressor is liable for medical expenses even if the wound inflicted is not potentially lethal. It follows that the physician is permitted, and indeed obligated, to treat patients who suffer from afflictions which are not life-threatening. This is certainly the case when the treatment itself poses no danger. The sole question is with regard to justification of hazardous treatment of non life-threatening afflictions.

R. Moses Isserles (popularly known as Rema), the sixteenth-century author of authoritative glosses to the *Shulḥan Arukh,* appears to sanction hazardous procedures designed solely to alleviate pain. In light of the scriptural prohibition against smiting or assaulting a parent (Exodus 21:15), *Yoreh De'ah* 241:13 states that a son should not "wound" his father even for medical reasons. Thus, in treating a parent, a son is cautioned not to remove a splinter, perform blood-letting or amputate a limb. R. Moses Isserles comments that if no other physician is available and the father is "in pain" the son may perform bloodletting or an amputation on behalf of his father. A similar statement is contained in the earlier thirteenth-century commentary of Me'iri, *Sanhedrin* 84b. The phraseology employed by these sources clearly indicates that the contemplated procedures were designed to mitigate pain rather than to preserve life. There can be little question that at the time these works were composed the amputation of a limb was accompanied by a significant risk to the life of the patient. It is evident that such procedures were sanctioned despite the hazards involved.

Justification of this position may be found in statements of Naḥmanides[110] and Rabbenu Nissim Gerondi.[111] These authorities both comment that all modes of therapy are potentially dangerous. In the words of Rabbenu Nissim, "All modes of therapy are a danger for the patient for it is possible that if the physician errs with regard to a specific drug, it will kill the patient." Naḥmanides states even more explicitly, "With regard to cures there is naught but danger; what heals one kills another." Nevertheless, healing—even of non-life-threatening afflictions—is sanctioned by Scripture. Apparently then, since every therapy is fraught with danger, the hazards of treatment are specifically sanctioned when incurred in conjunction with a therapeutic protocol. Accordingly, the practice of the healing arts, despite the hazards involved, cannot be branded as sinful even if designed simply for the alleviation of pain.

Utilization of medical procedures which are ordinary and usual but which carry with them an element of risk may perhaps be justified on other grounds as well. The Talmud indicates in a variety of instances[112] that a person may engage in commonplace activities even though he places himself in a position of danger in doing so. In justifying such conduct the Talmud declares, "Since many have trodden thereon 'the Lord preserveth the simple' " (Psalms 116:6). The principle enunciated in this dictum is that man is justified in placing his trust in God provided that the risk involved is of a type which is commonly accepted as a reasonable one by society at large. It may readily be argued that any accepted therapeutic procedure may be classified in this manner.[113]

The physician may withhold otherwise mandatory treatment only when the patient has reached the state of *gesisah,* i.e., the patient has become moribund and death is imminent. Jewish laws with regard to care of the dying are spelled out with care and precision. The patient is regarded as a living person in every respect. One must not pry his jaws, anoint him, wash him, plug his orifices, remove the pillow from underneath him or place him on the ground.[114] It is also forbidden to close his eyes "for whoever closes the eyes with the onset of death is a shedder of blood."[115] Each of these acts is forbidden because the slightest movement of the patient may hasten death. As the Talmud puts it, "The matter may be compared to a flickering flame; as soon as one touches it, the light is extinguished."[116] Accordingly, any movement or manipulation of the dying person is forbidden.

5. The Moribund Patient   Although euthanasia in any form is forbidden and the hastening of death even by a matter of moments is regarded as tantamount to murder, there is one situation in which treatment may be withheld from the moribund patient in order to provide for an unimpeded death. While the death of a *goses* may not be speeded, there is no obligation to perform any action which will lengthen the life of the patient in this state. The distinction between an active and a passive act applies to a *goses* and to a *goses* only. When a patient is, as it were, actually in the clutches of the angel of death, and the death process has actually begun, there is no obligation to heal. Therefore, Rema permits the removal of "anything which constitutes a hindrance to the departure of the soul, such as a clattering noise or salt upon his tongue . . . since such acts involve no active hastening of death but only the removal of the impediment."[117] Some authorities not only sanction withholding of treatment but prohibit any action which may prolong the agony of a *goses*.[118]

It cannot be overemphasized that even acts of omission are permitted only when the patient is in a state of *gesisah*. At any earlier stage withholding of treatment is tantamount to euthanasia. What are the criteria indicative of the onset of this state? Rema defines this state as being that of the patient "close to death" who "brings up a secretion in his throat on account of the constriction of his chest."[119] Of course, if the condition is reversible there is an obligation to heal. When the condition of *gesisah* is irreversible there is no obligation to continue treatment and, according to some authorities, even a prohibition against prolonging the life of the moribund patient.

Rema's description, while a necessary criterion of *gesisah,* is certainly not a sufficient one. Were the patient to present this symptom but in the opinion of medical practitioners be capable of survival, he would clearly not be considered a *goses* and all usual obligations would remain in force. It appears that any patient who may reasonably be deemed capable of potential survival for a period of seventy-two hours cannot be considered a *goses*. If the patient is capable of surviving this length of time the death process cannot be deemed to have commenced. It would appear that Halakhah assumes axiomatically that the death process or the "act of dying" cannot be longer than seventy-two hours in duration.[120] This is evidenced by the ruling[121] that one must commence to observe the laws of mourning three days after a relative has been observed in a state of *gesisah*. Some authorities even permit a wife to remarry in the absence of witnesses testifying to the actual death of the husband provided that testimony is forthcoming to the effect that her husband was observed in a state of *gesisah*.[122] These authorities maintain that the testimony of witnesses with regard to *gesisah ipso facto* constitutes legal proof of a state of widowhood commencing three days following the onset of *gesisah*.

It appears that this state is not determined by a patient's ability to survive solely by natural means for this period unaided by drugs or medication. The implication is that a *goses* is one who cannot, under any circumstances, be maintained alive for a period of seventy-two hours. Testimony with regard to the existence of a state of *gesisah* as conclusive evidence of impending death implies that the state is not only irreversible but also not prolongable even by artificial means. Otherwise there would exist a legal suspicion that life may have been prolonged artifically by means of extraordinary medical treatment. The obvious conclusion to be drawn is that if it is medically feasible to prolong life the patient is indeed not a *goses* and, therefore, in such instances there is a concomitant obligation to preserve the life of the patient as long as possible.

It follows that a specific physiological condition may or may not correspond to a state of *gesisah* depending upon the state of medical knowledge of the day. When medicine is of no avail and the patient will expire within seventy-two hours he is deemed to be in the process of "dying." When, however, medication can prolong life such medicine, in effect, delays the onset of the death process. Accordingly, the patient who receives medical treatment enabling him to survive for a period of three days or more is not yet in the process of "dying." It follows, therefore, that those responsible for his care are not relieved of their duty to minister to his needs and to postpone the onset of death by means of medical treatment.

6. Prayer and Decision-Making The aggressiveness with which Judaism teaches that life must be preserved is not at all incompatible with the awareness that the human condition is such that there are circumstances in which man would prefer death to life. The Talmud reports[123] that Rabbi Judah the Prince, redactor of the Mishnah, was afflicted by what appears to have been an incurable intestinal disorder and as a result suffered from an apparently debilitating form of dysentery. R. Judah had a female servant who is depicted in rabbinic writings as being a woman of exemplary piety and moral character. This woman is reported to have prayed for the death of R. Judah. On the basis of this narrative, a thirteenth-century commentator, Rabbenu Nissim Gerondi,[124] states that it is permissible and even praiseworthy, to pray for the death of a patient who is gravely ill and in extreme pain. He chides those who are remiss in discharging the obligation of visiting the sick, remarking of such an individual ". . . not only does he not aid [the patient] in living but even when [the patient] would [derive] benefit from death, even that small benefit [prayer for his demise] he does not bestow upon him." The gift of life, bestowed by God, can be reclaimed only by Him. Man dare not push the divine hand, so to speak, through an overt action, but may, through prayer, presume to tell God what to do.

Contemporary rabbinic writers point out that even after R. Judah's servant expressed her feelings and conveyed information regarding her master's pain and discomfort to his disciples they not only declined to join her in prayer for his decease but did not desist from praying for prolongation of his life.[125] Although Rabbenu Nissim's comments are cited with approval by a recent codifier, R. Jehiel Michal Epstein, *Arukh ha-Shulḥan, Yoreh De'ah* 335:3, a contemporary scholar, R. Eliezer Waldenberg, draws attention to the fact that these comments were ignored by all earlier codifiers of Jewish law.[126]

There is one responsum in particular which deals with the question of prayer for termination of suffering through death but which has important implications for decision-making in general. R. Ḥayyim Palaggi, *Ḥikekei Lev,* I, *Yoreh De'ah,* no. 50, accepts the view of Rabbenu Nissim but expresses an important *caveat.* According to this authority only totally disinterested parties may, by even so innocuous a method as prayer, take any action which may lead to a premature termination of life. Husband, children, family and those charged with the care of the patient, according to R. Palaggi, may not pray for death. The considerations underlying this reservation are twofold in nature: 1) Those who are emotionally involved, if they are permitted even such non-physical methods of intervention as prayer, may be prompted to perform an overt act which would have the effect of shortening life and thus be tantamount to euthanasia; 2) Precisely because of their closeness to the situation they are psychologically incapable of reaching a detached, dispassionate and objective decision in which considerations of patient benefit are the sole controlling motives. The human psyche is such that the intrusion of emotional involvement and subjective interest preclude a totally objective and disinterested decision.

Decisions that available therapeutic methods shall not be employed because they are hazardous or of insufficiently demonstrated efficacy or a decision that the patient is already in a state of *gesisah* are also subject to unconscious bias because of the inability of the family and physician totally to transcend their personal and emotional involvement with the patient. It is entirely in keeping with these considerations that Jewish scholars have insisted that the pertinent facts be placed before a rabbinic decisor for adjudication on a case by case basis.

The Judaic Tradition and Contemporary Society

The thrust of the material which has been presented augurs in favor of aggressive treatment of terminal patients as well as defective newborns regardless of the extent of their impairment or the quality of life which may be conserved by such treatment. It is unlikely that its impact upon those physicians who, to a greater or lesser extent, practice selective non-treatment on a routine basis will be sufficiently strong to effect a dramatic *volte face*. Nevertheless, this modest effort will have achieved a modicum of success if those engaged in the practice of medicine become sensitized to the issues which have been raised and achieve an awareness of the existence of a rich theological and ethical tradition which cannot acquiesce, much less sanction, the current practice of many physicians.

When analyzing treatment versus non-treatment, informed consent, if it is to be fully informed, should entail an awareness on the part of the person granting consent not only of the medical hazards involved but also of the moral dilemmas present in such decisions. The patient or next of kin should be fully informed with regard to conflicting medical opinion and counsel; he should be equally aware of moral traditions which conflict with a course of action advocated by the medical practitioners. The physician seeking consent is bound in conscience to be absolutely certain that the patient or next of kin is fully informed, both medically and morally.

Physicians, however, are all too often not in a position to formulate moral questions on behalf of patients and their families. Medical personnel often perform their professional duties under conditions which leave them overworked, overburdened, and harried. Nor are they, for the most part, particularly competent to identify and analyze medico-moral questions. Physicians have only in rare, individual instances been the beneficiaries of extensive systematic ethical training. Moreover, the physician is hardly an objective observer. As a scientist he, quite correctly, has his own interests in research and experimentation as well as in the care and welfare of all of his patients. Nor is it easy for him to transcend his emotional involvement in the care of the individual patient, his personal and professional interest in achieving a cure or his frustration when confronted by a seeming lack of success.

The rabbinic tradition was fully cognizant of these factors in its insistence upon multiple medical consultations and in its demand that the medical data be placed before a competent rabbinic authority prior to initiation of hazardous therapy or withholding of life-supporting measures. The rabbi serves as a legal arbiter and as an ethicist, a qualified expert capable of dispassionate examination of the data and of reaching a determination based upon the legal and ethical principles of his moral tradition.

The rabbinic decisor presents a role model which might be emulated by society at large with great moral profit. A qualified and professionally trained ethicist could be an invaluable addition to the hospital staff. In a pluralistic society the ethicist would most emphatically not serve as a decisor. He would, however, be singularly qualified to analyze and interpret the medical information upon which decision-making is based so that the patient and his family would be in a position to make an informed medical decision. He would be available to analyze and discuss any moral issues which might be confronted in making such decisions. The ethicist's position would be that of analyst and discussant — not that of advisor. The information transmitted by a trained ethicist in an objective and impartial manner would enable the patient and his family to turn to their own moral and spiritual counselors, if they should desire to do so, for advice consonant with their own religious traditions. The inclusion of an ethicist as a member of the health care team would assure that the decision reached is both a medically and morally informed decision.

An important facet of the relationship between the Jewish tradition and the current state of medico-ethical practice in the general society may be illustrated by an apocryphal anecdote about an extraordinarily diligent Jewish scholar. This learned gentleman habitually spent upwards of eighteen hours a day in study and meditation. A student, fearful for his health, approached him and and asked him why he did not ease up a little, get more rest and perhaps even a bit of diversion. The scholar answered that the effect of any less intense a regimen would be catastrophic. If he were to devote less than eighteen hours a day to spiritual pursuits, then lesser scholars would follow suit and commensurately reduce the time they customarily spend in devotion to their studies. Learned laymen who were wont to spend three or four hours a day in study would devote even less time to such pursuits. This in turn would have an effect upon the simple Jew, who had heretofore been accustomed to spend but an hour or so a day reciting Psalms but would now no longer find the time for this practice in his schedule. The ultimate result could be, asserted the scholar, that Baron Rothschild would become an apostate.

Theological teachings may at times appear to be extreme and fail to achieve total acceptance. Nevertheless, an understanding and appreciation of these traditions may indeed result in the tempering of the rather extreme views currently in vogue. Hopefully, the "ripple effect" generated by an understanding of religious ethics may give rise to an element of doubt in the minds of some physicians and prompt them to rethink their positions. If doubts are raised perhaps they too will be prompted to resolve, to paraphrase the words of Judge Skelly Wright in *Application of the President and Directors of Georgetown College, Inc.,* that if they are to err, better to err on the side of life.

NOTES

1. Mohr v. Williams, 95 Minn. 263; 104 N.W. 12; ILRA (NS) 439; 111 Am. State Rep. 462; 5 An. Cases, 303 (1905).

2. Luka v. Lowrie, 171 Mich. 632; 108 N.W. 94; 7LRA (NS) 290 (1912); Mohr v. Williams, 95 Minn. 261, 104 N.W. 12, 15, (1905), King v. Commonwealth, 149 S.W. 2d 1047 (1941).

3. People v. Beardsley, 105 Mich. 206, 113 N.W. 1128 (1907).

4. It should be noted that the Supreme Court decision in Roe v. Wade, 410 U.S. 113 (1973) merely extended the right of personal privacy to include a woman's decision to terminate her pregnancy. This decision was not coupled either with an abrogation of the rights of the fetus or of the state's interest in the fetus. See 9 SUFFOLK L. REV. 1455 (1974).

5. See 27 STANFORD L. REV. 226 (1975).

6. IND. ANON. STAT. §10–113(b) (Burns Supp. 1973); ME. REV. STAT. ANON. tit. 22 §§1575–76 (Supp. 1973); see also N.Y. PUB. HEALTH LAW §4164 (McKinney Supp. 1974); and 27 STANFORD L. REV. 219, n. 36 (1975).

7. John A. Robertson, 27 STANFORD L. REV. 227–230 (1975).

8. People v. Beardsley, *supra,* note 3, at 206.

9. 331 F. 2d 1000, 1009 18 (Wash. D.C., 1964).

9a. Of course, the effect of the California Natural Death Act, which became effective on January 1, 1977, and that of any similar legislation which may be enacted by other states, is to nullify the principle that a waiver signed by a patient has no effect upon criminal culpability. The Natural Death Act binds the physician to follow the directive of his patient in withdrawing life-sustaining procedures under certain circumstances in the event that death becomes imminent and relieves medical personnel of both civil and criminal liability when acting in accordance with provisions of the patient's "living will."

10. See Jacobson v. Mass., 197 U.S. 11 (1904); People v. Pierson, 176 N.Y. 201, 68 N.E. 243 (1903); In re Brooks' Estate, 32 Ill. 2d 361, 205 N.E. 2d 435 (1965).

11. People ex rel. Wallace v. Labrenz, 411 Ill. 618, 104 N.E. 2d 769, cert. denied, 344 U.S. 824, 73 S. Ct. 24, 97 L. Ed. 642 (1952); Morrison v. State, Mo. App., 252 S.W. 2d 97 (1952); Mitchell v. Davis, Tex. Civ. App., 205 S.W. 2d 812 (1947).

12. Application of the President and Directors of Georgetown College, Inc., 331 F. 2d 1000., 1008 (Wash. D.C. 1964).

13. 44 Misc. 2d 27, 28, 252 N.Y.S. 2d 705, 706 (Sup. Ct. Nassau County, 1962).

14. Application of the President and Directors of Georgetown College, Inc., 331 F 2d 1000, 1008 (Wash. D.C. 1964).

15. *Id.* at 1008–1009. The Supreme Court of New Jersey, in ruling that in certain limited circumstances the constitutional right to privacy may be invoked by a patient or the patient's guardian in directing that life-support systems be withdrawn, ruled that exercise of this right, where it exists, is protected from criminal persecution. Accordingly, an individual terminating medical treatment pursuant to his right of privacy is protected from criminal persecution for attempted suicide; similarly, other persons cannot be charged as accessories to an act which could not be a crime. See In re Quinlan, 70 N.J. 10, 51–52, 355, A 2d647, (1976).

16. *Id.* at 1009.

17. 239 Federal Supplement 752, 754 (1965).

18. *Id.* at 754. Cf. Superintendent of Belchertown State School et al. v. Saikewicz, Mass., 370 N.E. 2d 417 (1977), in which the Massachusetts Supreme Judicial Court stated that this interest is lessened by prevailing medical ethical standards which do not demand that all efforts be made toward life prolongation in all circumstances, e.g. prolongation of the life of the terminally ill with accompanying physical and emotional anguish.

19. 58 N.J. 576, 279 A. 2d 670 (1971).

20. *Id.* at 672.

21. *Id.* at 673.

22. In another, somewhat similar case, Raleigh Fitkin-Paul Morgan Memorial Hospital v. Anderson, 42 N.J. 421, 201 A. 2d 573 (1964), cert. denied 377 U.S. 984 (1964), the New Jersey Supreme Court held: "The blood transfusions (including transfusion made necessary by the delivery) may be administered if necessary to save her life or the life of her child, as the physician in charge at the time may determine." Some doubt exists as to whether the court meant to authorize transfusion only for the purpose of saving the life of the child or whether the authorization included, as well, transfusions designed only to save the life of the mother. The physicians involved understood the court order as authorizing treatment designed purely to save the mother's life and apparently gave the mother transfusions after the child was delivered. See 40 NOTRE DAME LAW, 126 n. 3 (1964).

23. John F. Kennedy Memorial Hospital v. Heston, *supra,* note 19, at 673.

24. 98 U.S. 145, 25 L. Ed. 244 (1878).

25. 32 Ill. 3d 361, 205 N.E. 2d 435 (Sup. Ct. 1965).

26. In a related decision the Supreme Court of Tennessee overruled a lower court decision and declared that the handling of poisonous snakes pursuant to religious beliefs could be enjoined constitutionally by the State. The court found that the States have a "compelling interest" in "a strong, healthy, robust, taxpaying

citizenry" and hence has "a right to protect a person from himself and to demand that he protect his own life." State ex rel. Swann v. Pack, Tenn., 527 S.W. 2d 99, 113 (1975).

27. It should be noted that a New York court invoked *Georgetown* in emphasizing that when a life-saving emergency exists a hospital may act without need for judicial authority even against the express desire of the patient and may amputate the gangrenous legs of the patient. See Matter of Roosevelt Hospital, *New York Law Journal,* Jan. 13, 1977, p. 7, col. 3 and p. 10, col. 3. In this case the court held the principle expressed in *Georgetown* to be applicable despite the obviously crippling nature of the procedure necessary to preserve life.

28. Mass., 370 N.E. 3d 417, Mass. Adv. Sh. 2461 (1977).

29. In re Quinlan, 70 N.J. 10, 355 A. 2d 647 (1976).

30. *Id.* at 41.

31. The bodily invasion of Karen Quinlan is described as "very great—she requires 24 hour intensive nursing care, antibiotics, the assistance of a respirator, a catheter and feeding tube"; in contradistinction a transfusion is described as "a minimal bodily invasion." *Id.* at 41.

32. *Id.* at 54, n. 10.

33. 156 N.J. Super. 282 (1978).

34. *Id.* at 290. The finding in this case is obviously at variance with the earlier post-*Quinlan* view of the New York Court expressed in Matter of Roosevelt Hospital. See above, n. 27.

35. The court declined to rely upon a finding that possible lifetime confinement to a wheelchair or, alternatively, dependence upon artificial legs and prosthetic devices and confinement to a nursing home for his remaining years would constitute "dim prognosis." *Id.* at 290, n. 2.

36. *Summa Theologica,* Pt. II-II, *Q.* 25, Art 5.

37. "The Prolongation of Life," *The Pope Speaks,* IV, 395.

38. *Ethical and Religious Directives for Catholic Hospitals* (St. Louis, 1949), p. 5.

39. See Gerald Kelly, S.J., "The Duty of Using Artificial Means of Preserving Life," *Theological Studies,* 11 (1950), 207.

40. Thomas J. O'Donnell, S.J., *Morals in Medicine* (Westminister, 1957), pp. 67–68; Kelly, *op. cit.,* p. 218; Charles J. McFadden, O.S.A., *Medical Ethics* (Philadelphia, 1967), p. 245; Joseph V. Sullivan, *Catholic Teaching on the Morality of Euthanasia,* p. 72.

41. O'Donnell, *loc. cit.*

42. Kelly, *op. cit.,* p. 205.

43. O'Donnell, *op. cit.,* pp. 57–61. Indeed, O'Donnell argues that it is the pain associated with amputation rather than the amputation *per se* which renders the procedure extraordinary. Cf., however, H. Noldin, S.J., *Summa Theologicae Moralis* (14th ed., 1922), Vol. II, n. 326, who states ". . . the obligation [of undergoing amputation] is not to be imposed both because many have a great horror of it and . . . because it is a grave inconvenience to live with a mutilated body." O'Donnell asserts that in light of present day surgical techniques and the perfection of artificial limbs these considerations do not ordinarily apply.

44. See Edwin F. Healy, S.J., *Medical Ethics* (Chicago, 1956), pp. 72–74. Healy recognizes that it is difficult to express mathematically the degree of estimated danger which would render a particular procedure extraordinary. He nevertheless opines that surgery involving a mortality rate of "between 15 and 20 percent or higher" must be classified as extraordinary. Any percentage between these two norms is classified by Healy as "doubtfully ordinary" and therefore not obligatory.

45. See Kelly, *op. cit.,* p. 205.

46. Edwin F. Healy, S.J., *Moral Guidance* (Chicago, 1949), p. 162.
47. *Catholic Teaching on the Morality of Euthanasia* (Washington, D.C., 1949), p. 64.
48. *Medical Ethics,* p. 68.
49. *Medical Ethics* (Philadelphia, 1967), p. 261.
50. *Loc. cit.*
51. *Medical Ethics,* p. 84.
52. *De Justitia et Jure,* Disp. 10, n. 30.
53. *Op. cit.,* p. 254.
54. *Medical Ethics,* p. 76.
55. *Ibid.,* pp. 70–71. Cf. *infra* note 101a.
56. Joseph McAllister, *Ethics* (Philadelphia, 1955), p. 175. See also Augustine Lehukull, S.J., *Theologia Moralis* 19th ed., (1902), Vol. I, nn. 571–572 and Heribert Jone, *Moral Theology,* trans. and adapted by Urban Adelman (Westminster, 1953), n. 210.
57. This position is based upon De Lugo, *op. cit.,* Disp. 16, n. 152, where the terms "common" and "which men commonly use" are juxtaposed with "ordinary." See O'Donnell, *op. cit.,* p. 63.
58. *Op. cit.,* pp. 65–67.
59. *Homiletic and Pastoral Review,* XLIX (August, 1944), 904. Sullivan, *op. cit.,* p. 72, sanctions withdrawal of intravenous feeding if the patient is beyond all hope of recovery and is suffering obvious pain. Kelly, *op. cit., p. 218,* is substantially in agreement with Sullivan but expresses hesitation because of possible misapplication of the principle in other cases. McFadden, *op. cit.,* p. 245, agrees in theory that the means are extraordinary because they are both artificial and useless. The treatment is deemed "useless" because of the absence of any "permanent beneficial result." In practice, however, McFadden hesitates to sanction withdrawal.
60. *Medical Ethics,* p. 66.
61. *Ibid.,* p. 67.
62. *Irish Ecclesiastical Record,* LVIII (1941), 552–554.
63. This position is endorsed by John C. Ford, S.J., *Theological Studies,* III (1942), 591 and apparently by Kelly, *op. cit.,* p. 209, as well.
64. Quoted by Kelly, *op. cit.,* p. 212.
65. *Medical Ethics,* p. 89.
66. "To Save or Let Die," *Journal of the American Medical Association,* Vol. 229, no. 2 (July 7, 1974), 172–176.
67. *Sanhedrin* 37a.
68. See also *Tosafot Yom Tov, Sotah* 1:9 and R. Eliezer Waldenberg, *Assia,* Nisan 5728, pp. 18–19.
69. See R. Eliezer Waldenberg, *Ziz Eli'ezer,* IX, no. 47, sec. 5, who declares that despite the presence of pain everything possible must be done, even on the Sabbath, to prolong life "even the patient himself cries, 'Let me be and do not give me any aid because for me death is preferable.' " See also R. Jehiel Michal Tucatzinsky, *Ha-Torah ve-ha-Medinah,* IV (1952), 39.
70. Commentary on *Mishneh Torah, Hilkhot Sanhedrin* 18:6.
71. See Ezekiel 18:4: "Indeed all the lives, they are thine . . ."
72. See also *Shulḥan Arukh ha-Rav,* VI, *Hilkhot Nizkei Guf,* 4.
73. *Yoreh De'ah* 157:1.
74. *Oraḥ Ḥayyim* 329:3.
75. See R. Jehiel Michael Tucatzinsky, *Ha-Torah ve-ha-Medinah,* IV (1952), 34 and V-VI (1953–54), 331–334.
76. *Oraḥ Ḥayyim* 329:4.

77. See J. Hamburger, *Real-Encyclopaedie für Bibel und Talmud,* Supplement II (Leipzig, 1901), p. 37; H. J. Zimmels, *Magicians, Theologians and Doctors* (London, 1952), p. 172, n. 72.

78. It is of interest to compare this view with that of Martin Luther who refused to baptize deformed children and who declared that they ought to be drowned because they have no soul. See D. McKenzie, *The Infancy of Medicine: An Enquiry into the Influence of Folk-lore upon the Evolution of Scientific Medicine* (London, 1927), p. 313.

79. See R. Eliezer Waldenberg, *Ziz Eli'ezer,* XIII, no. 88, who rules unequivocally that defective newborns must be given the same medical treatment as normal children; therapeutic and surgical procedures designed to correct life-threatening abnormalities must be instituted without consideration of the quality of life preserved thereby.

80. *Sanhedrin* 73a.

81. See T. C. Allbutt, *Greek Medicine in Rome* (New York, 1921), p. 402.

82. See Abraham ibn Ezra, *Commentary on the Bible, ad locum.*

83. See A. Harkavy, *Likkutei Kadmoniyot* (St. Petersburg, 1903), II, 148 and Harry Friedenwald, *The Jews and Medicine* (Baltimore, 1944), p. 9.

84. See commentaries of *Tosafot* and *Rashba, ad. locum.*

85. *Midrash Temurah,* ed. J. D. Eisenstein, *Ozar Midrashim* (New York, 1915), II, 580–581.

86. *Commentary on the Mishnah, Nedarim* 4:4; cf. Maimonides, *Mishneh Torah, Hilkhot Nedarim* 6:8.

87. Cf., Rabbi Baruch ha-Levi Epstein, *Torah Temimah,* Exodus 21:19 and Deuteronomy 22:2. This explanation of Maimonides' apparent contradiction of the Talmudic text as well as the comments of *Torah Temimah* contradict Jakobovits' statement to the effect that Maimonides' system does not require Biblical sanction for the practice of medicine. See Immanuel Jakobovits' *Jewish Medical Ethics* (New York, 1959), p. 260, n. 8. See *infra,* note 101.

88. *Yoreh De'ah,* 336:1. See R. Eliezer Waldenberg, *Ramat Rahel* no. 21 and *idem, Ziz Eli'ezer,* X, no. 25, ch. 7. See *infra* note 96.

89. *Torat ha-Adam, Kitvei Ramban,* ed. Bernard Chavel (Jerusalem, 5724), II, 43.

90. See R. Eliezer Waldenberg, *Ramat Rahel,* no. 21.

91. *Commentary on the Bible,* Exodus 21:19.

92. See R. Solomon ben Adret, *Teshuvot ha-Rashba,* I, no. 413.

93. See also Bahya ibn Paquda, *Hovot ha-Levavot,* trans. Moses Hyamson (Jerusalem, 1965), *Sha'ar ha-Bittahon,* ch. 3, p. 309.

94. *Teshuvot Tashbez,* I, no. 51 cited by R. Ovadiah Yosef, *Yabbi'a Omer,* IV, *Hoshen Mishpat,* no. 6, sec. 4. Nevertheless Ibn Ezra's interpretation of Exodus 21:19 is followed by the 14th-century biblical exegete, Rabbenu Bahya, in his commentary on that passage and by R. Jonathan Eybeschuetz, *Kereti u-Feleti, Tiferet Yisra'el, Yoreh De'ah* 188:5. See also R. Elijah of Vilna, *Aderet Eliyahu,* Exodus 21:19.

95. *Kitvei Ramban,* II, 42–43.

96. *Ibid,* 42. It has been suggested that the term *reshut* in the dictum, "From here [it is derived] that the physician is granted *permission* to cure" should properly be rendered "authority" rather than permission. The term *reshut* is used in the sense of "authority" in *Avot* 1:10: *ve-al titvada la-rashut,* "and do not be intimate with the ruling authorities." If *reshut* is translated as "authority," Nahmanides' comment to the effect that exercise of this "authority" is obligatory is quite congruous with the text itself.

97. This opinion is published in the responsa collection of his son, R. Abraham

Bornstein, *Avnei Nezer, Hoshen Mishpat,* no. 193. R. Eleazar Fleckeles, *Teshuvah me-Ahavah,* III, no. 408 (*Yoreh De'ah* 336), opines that permission to utilize therapeutic measures in the treatment of internal maladies and disorders is the subject of dispute between Rav Aḥa and Abayye, *Berakhot* 60a.

98. *Guide of the Perplexed,* III, chaps. 17–18.

99. This appears to be the manner in which Naḥmanides was interpreted by R. David ben Samuel ha-Levi, *Taz, Yoreh De'ah* 336:1; see also R. Eliyahu Dessler, *Mikhtav me-Eliyahu* (Bene-Berak, 5725), III, 170–175 and R. Eliezer Waldenberg, *Ramat Raḥel,* no. 20, sec. 3. Cf. R. Abraham Isaiah Karelitz, *Emunah Bittaḥon ve-Od* (Jerusalem, 5714), pp. 65–66.

100. See Baḥya ibn Paquda, *Hovot ha-Levavot, Sha'ar ha-Bittaḥon,* chapter 4; R. Simeon ben Ẓemaḥ Duran, *Teshuvot Tashbeẓ,* III, no. 82; R. Joel Sirkes, *Bayit Ḥadash, Yoreh De'ah* 336; R. Abraham Gumbiner, *Magen Avraham, Oraḥ Hayyim* 328:6; R. Moses Sofer, *Teshuvot Ḥatam Sofer, Oraḥ Ḥayyim,* no. 176; *Besamim Rosh,* no. 386; R. Jacob Ettlinger, *Binyan Ẓiyyon,* no. 111; R. Shlomo Ganzfried, *Kiẓur Shulḥan Arukh* 193:3; R. Nissim Abraham Ashkenazi, *Ma'aseh Avraham, Yoreh De'ah,* no. 55; R. Nathan Landau, *Kenaf Ra'anannah, Oraḥ Hayyim,* no. 60; R. Ovadiah Yosef, *Yabbi'a Omer,* IV, *Hoshen Mishpat,* no. 6, sec. 4; R. Moses ben Abraham Mat, *Matteh Moshe,* IV, chap. 3; R. Samson Morpugo, *Shemesh Ẓedakah, Yoreh De'ah,* no. 29; R. Hayyim Joseph David Azulai, *Birkei Yosef, Yoreh De'ah,* 336:2; R. Yehudah Eyash, *Shivtei Yehudah* no. 336; R. Eliezer Waldenberg, *Ramat Raḥel,* no. 20; *idem., Ẓiẓ Eli'ezer,* VIII, no. 15, chap. 17, *siyyum;* IX, no. 17, chap. 6, sec. 17; X, no. 25, chaps. 19 and 20; XI, no. 41, R. Jacob Prager, *She'elot Ya'akov,* no. 5; *Mishnah Berurah, Oraḥ Hayyim* 128:6; and R. Joshua Neuwirth, *Shemirat Shabbat ke-Hilkhatah* 19:2.

101. See R. Abraham Danzig, *Hokhmat Adam* 151:25.

101a. See R. Abraham I. Kook, *Mishpat Kohen,* no. 143, who, without adducing vigorous support for his position, opines that *ḥayyei sha'ah* is to be defined as a period of up to twelve months. A similar definition of *ḥayyei sha'ah* is developed in greater detail by R. Shelomo Kluger, *Hokhmat Shelomoh, Yoreh De'ah* 155:1, also cited in *Darkhei Teshuvah* 155:6.

102. See also R. Jacob Ettlinger, *Binyan Ẓiyyon,* no. 111; R. Eliezer Waldenberg, *Ẓiẓ Eli'ezer,* IV, no. 13; R. Israel Lipshitz, *Tiferet Yisra'el, Yoma,* 8:41; R. Solomon Eger, *Gilyon Maharsha, Yoreh De'ah* 155:1.

103. This is also the position of R. Eliezer Waldenberg, *Ẓiẓ Eli'ezer,* X, no. 25, chap. 5, sec. 5. Cf. R. Hayyim Ozer Grodzinski, *Teshuvot Aḥi'ezer,* II, *Yoreh De'ah,* no. 16, sec. 8.

104. *Iggerot Moshe, Yoreh De'ah,* II, no. 58.

105. *No'am,* XIII (5730), 5. See also R. Shalom Mordecai Schwadron, *Da'at Torah, Oraḥ Hayyim* 328:10.

106. *Teshuvot Ḥatam Sofer, Yoreh De'ah,* no. 76.

107. *Bo'az, Yoma* 8:3.

108. *Ha-Torah ve-ha-Medinah,* VII-VIII (1956–57), 314.

109. *Mor u-Keẓi'ah, Oraḥ Hayyim,* 328.

110. *Torat ha-Adam, Kitvei Ramban,* II, 43.

111. Commentary to *Sanhedrin,* 84b.

112. *Shabbat* 129b; *Avodah Zarah* 30b; *Niddah* 31a; and *Yevamot* 72a.

113. Cf., R. Jacob Breisch, *Helkat Ya'akov,* III, no. 11.

114. *Yoreh De'ah* 339:1.

115. *Ibid.*

116. *Shabbat* 151b; and *Semaḥot* 1:4.

117. *Yoreh De'ah* 339:1.

118. *Teshuvot Beit Ya'akov,* no. 59; *Iggerot Moshe, Yoreh De'ah,* II, no. 174;

cf. also R. Moses Isserles, *Darkei Moshe, Yoreh De'ah* 339. However, *Shevut Ya'akov,* I, no. 13; *Teshuvot Hatam Sofer, Yoreh De'ah,* no. 338; *Bi'ur Halakhah, Orah Hayyim* 329:2; R. Eliezer Waldenberg, *Ramat Rahel,* no. 28; *idem, Ziz Eliezer,* VIII, no. 15, chap. 3, sec. 16; IX, no. 47; and *idem, Assia,* Nisan 5738, pp. 17–18 see no prohibition against prolonging the life of a *goses.* The latter two authorities view prolongation by means of accepted medical treatment as obligatory. This is also the position of R. Nathan Zevi Freeman, *Nezer Mata'ai,* no. 30.

119. *Even ha-Ezer* 121:7 and *Hoshen Mishpat* 211:2.

120. See *Perishah, Tur Yoreh De'ah,* 339:5 who writes, "It appears from this that it is the nature of *gesisah* to be three days." Since it is simply not possible to understand this authority as asserting that *gesisah* must *always* extend for a period of three days, his comment must be understood as stating that the period of *gesisah* extends no longer than three days. See also R. Isaac Liebes, *Teshuvot Beit Avi,* II, no. 153 and G. B. Halibard, "Euthanasia," in *The Jewish Law Annual,* I (1978), 198, n. 2.

121. *Yoreh De'ah* 339:2.

122. *Beit Shemu'el, Even ha-Ezer* 17:18 and 17:94. Cf., However, R. Ezekiel Landau, *Dagul me-Revavah, Even ha-Ezer* 17:94; *Pithei Teshuvah, Even ha-Ezer* 17:131; *idem, Yoreh De'ah* 339:3; and *Gilyon Maharsha, Yoreh De'ah* 339:2.

123. *Ketubbot* 104a.

124. Commentary to *Nedarim* 40a.

125. Cf., however, *Bava Mezia* 84a which reports that the Sages prayed for the demise of R. Yohanan. See also R. Eliezer Waldenberg, *Ramat Rahel,* no. 5., sec. 3.

126. *Ziz Eli'ezer,* IX, no. 47; *Ramat Rahel,* no. 5.

2

The Physician and the Patient in Jewish Law

FRED ROSNER

Introduction

Does man have a part in shaping his future? Is man's lifespan on this earth predetermined or can man alter the course of events during his stay in this world? The predetermination of a person's lifespan, or lack thereof, has been discussed at length by philosophers and theologians including Jewish savants such as Rav Hai Gaon[1], Rav Saadiah Gaon[2] and Moses Maimonides[3] with most scholars concluding that the duration of life is not predetermined. What can man do, then, to lengthen his life? One way is to behave in the manner prescribed by God and receive as a reward "added years." Another way is to improve one's health so as to live longer. These alternatives pose the following questions: Does a sick person have the right to secure healing of his body or should the illness run its course without interference? Should a person rely solely on Divine providence for his physical as well as spiritual healing? These questions pertain to the patient. From the physician's standpoint, a similar series of questions can be raised. Is a mortal allowed by Jewish law to become a physician and practice medicine or does such an act constitute "interference with the deliberate designs of Providence?"[4] Does a physician play God when he practices medicine? Part I of this paper deals with the duties of the physician; Part II discusses the role of the patient.

In a Midrashic story[5] Rabbi Ishmael and Rabbi Akiva were walking through the streets of Jerusalem and met a sick man. The ill person asked: "Masters, tell me how I can be cured?" They answered: "Do thus and thus until you are cured." He said to them: "And who afflicted me?" "The

Holy One, Blessed be He," they replied. He said: "And you interfered in a matter which is not your concern. God afflicted and you wish to heal?" The rabbis asked: "What is your vocation?" He responded: "I am a tiller of the soil. Here is the vine-cutter in my hand." They queried: "But who created the vineyard?" "The Holy One, Blessed be He," he answered. "You interfered in this vineyard which is not yours? He created it and you cut away its fruits?" they asked. "Do you not see the vine-cutter in my hands? Were I not to go out and plow and till and fertilize and weed, the vineyard would not produce any fruit," he explained. They said: "Fool, from your own work you have not learned what is written (Psalms 103:15): *'As for man his days are as grass.'* Just as the tree, if not weeded, fertilized and ploughed will not grow and bring forth its fruits . . . so it is with the human body. The fertilizer is the medicine and the healing means, and the tiller of the earth is the physician."

I

"For I am the Lord that healeth thee" (Exodus 16:26.)

The extreme viewpoint, namely, total rejection of the permissibility of human healing, was espoused by the Karaites who vehemently objected to medicine and physicians. They relied entirely on prayer for their healing as (*Shabbat* 32a):

> Man must ever pray not to become ill for if he becomes so, it is demanded of him to show merit in order to be healed.

The Karaites must further have adhered to the literal interpretation of the following Biblical phrase (Exodus 16:26):

> And he said: if thou wilt diligently hearken to the voice of the Lord, thy God and wilt do that which is right in His eyes, and wilt give ear to His commandments and keep all His statutes, I will put none of the diseases upon thee, which I have put upon the Egyptians, for I am the Lord that healeth thee.

The last phrase "for I am the Lord that healeth thee" literally translated from the original Hebrew means *for I am the Lord thy physician.* In fact, Rabbi Abraham Ibn Ezra, in his commentary, states that just as God "healed" the undrinkable waters at Marah for the Israelites, so too God will remove or heal all plagues on the earth and there will be no need for physicians. This perhaps is the basis for the Karaitic objection to human healing and medicine.

Alternate interpretations of the above scriptural verse are possible. The

Talmud (*Sanhedrin* 101a) asks if we are told that God "will put none of the diseases upon thee," what need is there for a cure? Rabbi Yoḥanan answers that the verse means as follows: "If thou wilt harken (to the voice of the Lord), I will not bring disease upon thee, but if thou wilt not, I will; yet even so, *I am the Lord that healeth thee.*" Rabbi Baruch ha-Levi Epstein in his *Torah Temimah* explains that the intent of this Biblical phrase is to show that the illness of the Egyptians was incurable as it is written (Deut. 28:27): "the boil of Egypt . . . wherefrom one cannot be healed." However, afflictions of the Israelites can be healed by God.

The father of all Biblical commentators, Rashi, explains "for I am the Lord that healeth thee" to mean that God teaches the laws of the Torah in order to save man from these diseases. Rashi uses the analogy of a physician who says to his patient not to eat such and such a food lest it bring him into danger from disease. So too is it stated, continues Rashi, obedience to God "will be health to thy body and marrow to thy bones" (Prov. 3:8). In a similar vein, the extra Talmudic collection of Biblical interpretation known as the *Mekhilta* asserts that the words of Torah are life as well as health as it is written (Prov. 4:22): "For they are life unto those that find them and health to all their flesh." Other commentators (*Siftei Ḥakhamim,* and Rabbi Samson Raphael Hirsch among them) extend this thought by propounding that the Divine Law restores health, and certainly prevents illness from occurring, thus serving as preventive medicine against all physical and social evil.

Rabbi Jacob ben Asher *(Ba'al Haturim),* states that heavenly cure comes easily whereas earthly or man-made cures come with difficulty. Finally, Rabbi Meir Loeb ben Jehiel Michael *(Malbim),* in his commentary on the phrase "for I am the Lord that healeth thee" speaks of mental illness. He asserts that the Laws of the Torah were given by God to Israel not like a master ordering his slave but like a physician ordering his patient. In the former case, the master benefits, not the slave. In the latter case, the patient and not the physician is healed from illness. Similarly, God's statutes are for our benefit, not His.

The multitude of interpretations of the scriptural phrase "for I am the Lord that healeth thee" indicates that this verse is not to be understood literally. There is no prohibition inherent in this verse against a mortal becoming a physician and healing the sick. In fact, specific permissibility and sanction for the physician to practice medicine is given in the Torah as described below. The physician, however, must always recognize that God is the true healer of the sick and that a doctor is only an instrument of God in the ministrations to the sick.

"And heal he shall heal" (Exodus 21:19).

Compensation for personal injuries is described in the Bible in the following verses (Exodus 21: 19-20):

And if men quarrel and one smiteth the other with a stone or with his fist and he die not, but has to keep in bed . . . he must pay the loss entailed by absence from work and cause him to be thoroughly healed.

The last phrase translated literally reads "and heal he shall heal." The Talmud (*Bava Kamma* 85a) interprets this duplicate mention of healing as intended to teach us that authorization was granted by God to the physician to heal. Rashi extends the words of the Talmud when he asserts "lest it be said that God smites and man heals." Thus he implies that a need exists for specific Biblical sanctioning of human healing.

Many Biblical commentators including Rabbi Samson Raphael Hirsch and Rabbi Baruch ha-Levi Epstein *(Torah Temimah)* echo the above Talmudic teaching. That is, by the insistence or emphasis expressed in the double wording, the Torah uses the opportunity to oppose the erroneous idea that having recourse to medical aid shows lack of trust and confidence in Divine assistance. The Torah takes it for granted that medical therapy is used and actually demands it.

Other commentaries on the scriptural phrase "and heal he shall heal," including those of the *Mekhilta* and *Malbim,* explain that the repetition of the word "heal" means that the patient must be repeatedly healed if the illness or injury recurred or became aggravated. In discussing the above case concerning personal injury, the Talmud (*Bava Kamma* 85a) also requires that where ulcers have grown on account of the wound and the wound breaks open again, the offender would still be liable to heal it (*i.e.,* pay the medical expenses) even repeatedly.

The most popular interpretation of "and heal he shall heal" (Rashi, *Targum Onkelos,* Talmud *Bava Kamma* 85a and others) is that compensation for the injury must be paid by the offender. Such compensation consists of five items: the physician's fees and medical bills, payment for loss of time from work, the shame incurred by disfigurement, the pain suffered, and the physical damage produced. All agree, however, that human healing is sanctioned by this phrase of the Bible, if not explicitly, at least implicitly.

Rabbi Abraham ibn Ezra seems to place a restriction on the permissibility for a physician to heal when he states that only external wounds can be healed by man. Internal wounds or ailments should be left to God. However, there is nearly universal acceptance that the sanctioning to the physician to heal is all inclusive, encompassing all internal and external physical and mental illness. In fact, a commentary on the Talmud by *Tosafot* specifically states (*Bava Kamma* 85a) that not only is it permitted to heal man-induced wounds but even heavenly-induced sicknesses and afflictions, *i.e.,* all illnesses.

"And thou shalt restore it to him" (Deut. 22:2).

The above scriptural phrase refers to the restoration of lost property.

Moses Maimonides says that this law also includes the restoration of the health of one's fellow man, if he has lost it. Thus, Maimonides derives the Biblical sanction for human healing from a different phrase in the Scriptures than most other Jewish savants. *Torah Temimah* in two separate places (Deut. 22:2 and Exodus 21:19) asks why Maimonides totally omits the phrase "and heal he shall heal" as a warrant for the physician to heal. Epstein offers an answer to his own question when he states that the verse in Exodus only grants permission for a physician to heal whereas "and thou shalt restore it to him" makes it obligatory.

Maimonides' reasoning is probably based upon a key passage in the Talmud (*Sanhedrin* 73a) where it states: "Whence do we know that one must save his neighbor from the loss of himself? From the verse 'and thou shalt restore it to him'." Thus, not only if one is sick is a physician required but also if someone is attempting suicide, one must provide psychiatric or other competent assistance to save the person's life and health. Maimonides' major pronouncement on this matter is found in his commentary on the Mishnah (*Nedarim* 4:4). He states:

> It is obligatory from the Torah for the physician to heal the sick and this is included in the explanation of the Scriptural phrase "and thou shalt restore it to him," meaning to heal his body.

"Neither shalt thou stand idly by the blood of thy neighbor" (Levit. 19:16).

Duties toward our fellowmen are described in Leviticus 19:11–16. According to Hertz,[6] these precepts restate the fundamental rules of life in human society that are contained in the second tablet of the Decalogue. These moral principles were expounded by the Sages and applied to every phase of civil and criminal law. One example, cited in the Talmud (*Sanhedrin* 73a) is:

> Whence do we know that if a man sees his neighbor drowning or mauled by beasts or attacked by robbers, that he is bound to save him? From the verse "thou shalt not stand idly by the blood of thy neighbor."

Maimonides codifies the above Talmudic passage in his *Mishneh Torah* (*Hilkhot Roẓe'aḥ* 1:14) where he states:

> Whoever is able to save another and does not save him transgresses the commandment "neither shalt thou stand idly by the blood of thy neighbor" (Levit. 19:16). Similarly, if one sees another drowning in the sea, or being attacked by bandits or being attacked by a wild animal and is able to rescue him . . . and does not rescue him . . . he transgresses the injunction "neither shalt thou stand idly by the blood of thy neighbor."

Such a case of drowning in the sea is considered as loss of one's body and therefore, if one is obligated to save a whole body, one must certainly cure disease which usually afflicts only one part of the body.

Code of Jewish Law and Medical Practice

From the discussion so far, it seems evident that permission for the physician to heal is granted in the Torah from the phrase "and heal he shall heal." Some scholars, notably Maimonides, claim that healing the sick is not only allowed but is actually obligatory. Rabbi Joseph Caro, in his code of Jewish law (*Shulḥan Arukh, Yoreh De'ah* no. 336) combines both thoughts.

> The Torah gave permission to the physician to heal; moreover this is a religious precept and it is included in the category of saving life; and if he withholds his services, it is considered as shedding blood.

Rabbi David ben Samuel ha-Levi *(Taz)* asks: If it is a religious precept to heal, why did the Torah have to grant specific permission for the physician to do so? His answer is that true healing lies only with God, but God gives the physician the wherewithal to heal by earthly or natural means. Once permission has been granted, then it is a commandment on the physician to heal. A similar thought is expressed by Rabbi Abraham Maskil le-Eitan *(Yad Avraham),* who states that permission is only granted if the physician heals with his heart toward heaven.

Rabbi Shabbetai ben Meir ha-Kohen *(Siftei Kohen),* offers an alternate reason for the Torah granting permission to heal — that is in order to avoid the physician saying "who needs this anguish? If I err, I will be considered as having spilled blood unintentionally." In a similar vein, Caro, in his *Beit Yosef* commentary on Jacob ben Asher's code of Jewish law called the *Tur* (*Yoreh De'ah,* no. 336), quotes Naḥmanides, himself a physician, who says that without the warrant to treat, physicians might hesitate to treat patients for fear of fatal consequences "in that there is an element of danger in every medical procedure; that which heals one may kill another."

The Jewish attitude toward the physician and his medical art, as well as the patient's responsibility to seek medical aid is beautifully depicted by Ben Sira (Ecclus. 38) who perceived in the physician an instrument of Providence as he expresses it:[7]

Honor a physician before need of him
Him also hath God apportioned.
From God a physician getteth wisdom
And from a king he shall receive gifts.
The skill of a physician shall lift up his head

And he shall stand before nobles
God bringeth out medicines from the earth
And let a prudent man not refuse them.
Was not water made sweet with wood
For to acquaint every man with His power?
And He gave man understanding
To glory in His might.
By them doth the physician assuage pain
And likewise the apothecary maketh a confection,
That His work may not fail
Nor health from among the sons of men.
My son, in sickness be not negligent
Pray unto God, for He will heal.
Free from iniquity, and from respect of persons
And from all transgressions cleanse thy heart.
Offer a sweet savor as a memorial
And fatness estimated according to thy substance.
And to the physician also give a place
And he shall not remove, for there is need of him likewise,
For there is a time when in his hand is good success.
For he too will supplicate unto God
That He will prosper to him the treatment
And the healing, for the sake of his living.
He that sinneth against his Maker
Will behave himself proudly against a physician.

II

From the three Biblical citations cited and from Part I, it is perfectly clear that the Torah gave specific sanction to the physician to heal and, according to some authorities, made it obligatory upon him to provide his medical skills to cure disease. It is not evident from the above, however, that the patient is permitted by Jewish law to seek human healing. Is an individual who asks a physician to treat him denying Divine Providence? Is such an individual transgressing the Biblical teaching "For I am the Lord that healeth thee" (Exodus 15:26)? Is a person's illness an affliction by God that serves as punishment for wrongdoing? And does such a person remove his atonement for sin by not accepting the suffering imposed by Divine judgment? Should there be, or is there a distinction between heavenly afflictions and man-induced sickness in regard to the patient seeking medical aid? How does one define heavenly illness? What is cancer—God induced (*i.e.,* genetic) or man induced (*i.e.,* drugs, viruses, irradiation), or both? The number of such questions is endless and lengthy prose could be written attempting to analyze them.

The two sides of the question are illustrated in the Talmud (*Berakhot* 60a) where it states that on going to be phlebotomized, a person should recite the following prayer:

> May it be Thy will, O Lord my God, that this operation may be a cure for me and mayest Thou heal me for Thou art a faithful healing God and Thy healing is sure since men have no power to heal but this is a habit with them.

From this passage it would appear that conflicting viewpoints could emerge. The fact that the Talmud describes a patient going to a physician for an operative procedure can be interpreted to mean that certainly this is permissible. The only requirement is for the patient to recognize that the physician is acting as an agent of the Divine healer. In fact, Rashi explains the Talmudic passage to mean that the afflicted person should have prayed for Heavenly intervention rather than human healing and perhaps the bloodletting might not have been necessary.

On the other hand, the Talmudic statement continues with an assertion by Abbaye to the effect that a patient should not utter such a prayer because, in fact, the Torah gave specific consent for human healing in the phrase "and heal he shall heal." Therefore, says Abbaye, a patient should seek the help of a physician. A similar but not identical prayer is found in the codes of Jewish law of Maimonides (*Hilkhot Berakhot* 10:21) and Rabbi Joseph Caro (*Shulḥan Arukh, Oraḥ Ḥayyim,* no. 230:4).

A rather negative attitude to the question of the patient obtaining medical assistance is taken by Naḥmanides who, in his commentary on the scriptural phrase "and My soul shall not abhor you" (Levit. 26:11), states that God will remove sickness from among the Israelites as he promised "for I am the Lord that healeth thee" (Exodus 15:26). The righteous, continues Naḥmanides, during the epochs of prophethood, even if they sinned and became ill, did not seek out physicians, only prophets. What therefore is the need for physicians if God promised to remove all sickness from man? To advise which foods and beverages to avoid in order not to get sick, answers Naḥmanides, himself a physician. He explains the phrase "and heal he shall heal" to mean that the physician is allowed to practice medicine but the patient may not seek his healing but must turn to Divine Providence. Only people who do not believe in the healing powers of God turn to physicians for their cure, and for such individuals the Torah sanctions the physician to heal. The latter should not withhold his healing skills for fear lest the patient die under his care nor should he say that God alone heals.

Other than the Karaites who strongly objected to physicians and medicines, Naḥmanides seems to stand alone in his apparent prohibition for patients to seek medical aid. It is possible that he refers only to the righteous who are free of illness because of their piety and who do not require human healing. Perhaps the general populace, however, even devout believers in God, are allowed to seek human healing. Such an interpretation of Nahmanides' discussion is found in the commentary of Rabbi David ben Samuel ha-Levi on Caro's code (*Yoreh De'ah* no. 336:1). It may also be that Nahmanides refers only to heavenly illnesses, but for man-induced wounds and sicknesses healing may be sought.

Caro does not seem to make such a distinction when he states (*Orah Hayyim* no. 571) that

> He who fasts and is able to tolerate the fast is called holy; but if not, such as if he is not healthy and strong, he is called a sinner.

It appears evident from this quote that it is an obligation upon man to take all possible action to insure a healthy body, and this includes the services of a physician. A less likely interpretation of Caro's statement is that if a person is able to tolerate sickness or pain, just as in the case of the fast, he should do so and not seek medical aid.

Another source that can be interpreted either in support or against the permissibility for a patient to obtain human healing is the following story related in the Talmud (*Berakhot* 5b). Rabbi Yohanan once fell ill and Rabbi Hanina went to visit him saying, "Are your sufferings welcome to you?" Rabbi Yohanan replied, "Neither they nor their reward," implying that one who lovingly accepts sufferings in this world will be greatly compensated in the world to come. Rabbi Hanina then said "Give me your hand" which Rabbi Yohanan did, and he cured him. Why could not R. Yohanan cure himself, asks the Talmud? The reply is "Because the prisoner cannot free himself from jail," meaning the patient cannot cure himself. On the one hand, we see that R. Yohanan required healing from R. Hanina. On the other hand, R. Hanina did not use human healing as he cured R. Yohanan by touching the latter's hand. Perhaps no "natural" cure was available.

The strongest evidence from Jewish sources that gives the patient permission to seek treatment from a physician is found in Maimonides' *Mishneh Torah*. He states (*Hilkhot Deot* 3.3) that a person should

> set his heart that his body be healthy and strong in order that his soul be upright to know the Lord. For it is impossible for man to understand and comprehend the wisdoms (of the world) if he is hungry and ailing or if one of his limbs is aching . . .

He also recommends (*ibid.,* 4:23), as does the Talmud (*Sanhedrin* 17b), that no wise person should reside in a city that does not possess a physician. Maimonides' position is further stated (*ibid.,* 4:1) as follows:

Since when the body is healthy and sound (one treads in) the ways of the
Lord, it being impossible to understand or know anything of the
knowledge of the Creator when one is sick, it is obligatory upon man to
avoid things which are detrimental to the body and acclimate himself to
things which heal and fortify it.

An English translation of this entire chapter in Maimonides' code that deals
with hygienic principles is available for the interested reader (*Journal of the
American Medical Association,* vol. 194: 1352–1354, Dec. 27, 1965).

There are numerous Talmudic citations which support the position that
not only allows but requires the patient to seek medical aid when sick. We
are told (*Bava Kamma* 46b) that he who is in pain should go to a physician.
Further (*Yoma* 83b), if one is bitten by a snake, one may call a physician
even if it means desecrating the Sabbath because all restrictions are set aside
in case of possible danger to human life. Similarly (*Avodah Zarah,*
28b), if one's eye becomes afflicted on the Sabbath, one may prepare and
apply medication thereto, even on the Sabbath. When Rabbi Judah the
Prince, compiler of the Mishnah, contracted an eye disease, his physician
Samuel Yarhina'ah cured it by placing a vial of chemicals under the Rabbi's
pillow so that the powerful vapors would penetrate the eye (*Bava Mezia*
85b). The Talmud also speaks (*Ketubbot* 75a) of another physician curing a
patient. Finally (*Bava Kamma* 85a), in a case of bodily injury where the
offender says to the victim that he will bring a physician who will heal for
no fee, the victim can object and say "a physician who heals for nothing is
worth nothing." If the offender offers to bring a physician from far away,
the victim may say "my eye will be blind before he arrives." If the injured
person says to the offender "Give me the money and I will cure myself" the
later can retort "you might neglect yourself and remain a cripple." From
these and other Talmudic passages, it seems evident that an individual is
undoubtedly permitted and probably required to seek medical attention
when he is ill.

Further support for this contention is mentioned by the present Chief
Rabbi of Great Britain, Immanuel Jakobovits, who cites the 15th century
philosopher Isaac Arama's work *Akedat Yizhak.* Rabbi Arama proves
from Biblical narratives such as the Patriarchs' efforts to save themselves
when in danger, and legislation such as the duty to construct parapets
around roofs (Deut. 22:8) for the prevention of accidents, that man must
not rely on miracles or Providence alone, but must himself do whatever he
can to maintain his life and health.

Rabbi Hayyim Azulai, an 18th century commentator on Caro's code,
writing under the pen name of *Birkei Yosef,* summarized Jewish thought
and practice relating to our questions. His views are cited by Rabbi
Jakobovits as follows:

Nowadays one must not rely on miracles, and the sick man is in duty bound to conduct himself in accordance with the natural order by calling on a physician to heal him. In fact, to depart from the general practice by claiming greater merit than the many saints (in previous) generations, who were cured by physicians, is almost sinful on account of both the implied arrogance and the reliance on miracles when there is danger to life . . . Hence, one should adopt the ways of all men and be healed by physicians . . .

One might arrive at the same conclusion if one were to literally interpret the Pentateuchal admonition "Take ye therefore good heed unto yourselves" (Deut. 4:15).

NOTES

1. Kaufmann, D., "Ein Responsum des Gaons R. Haya uber Gottes Voherwissen und die Dauer des Menschlichen Lebens," Leipzig. *Zeitschr. Deutsche Morgenländische Gesellschaft,* D9:73–84, 1895.

2. Weil, G., *Maimonides Uber die Lebensdauer.* Basel, S. Karger, 1953, 59 pp.

3. Rosner, F., "Moses Maimonides' Responsum on Longevity," *Geriatrics* 23:170–178, 1968.

4. Jakobovits, I., *Jewish Medical Ethics.* New York, Bloch Publishers, 1959, pp. 2–6.

5. Eisenstein, J. D., *Ozar Midrashim.* New York, 1915, Vol. 2, pp. 580–581.

6. Hertz, J. H., *The Pentateuch and Haftorahs.* London, Soncino Press, 2nd edit., 1962, pp. 499–501.

7. Friedenwald, H., *The Jews and Medicine.* Baltimore, Johns Hopkins Press, 1944, Vol. 1, pp. 6–7.

Sexuality and Procreation

3

Be Fruitful
and Multiply

DAVID S. SHAPIRO

I.

On the fifth day of creation, God commanded the waters to teem with swarms of living creatures. On this day the fish and birds were created. For the first time the Creator conferred a blessing on His handiwork:

> God blessed them saying: "Be fruitful and multiply, and fill the waters in the seas, and let the birds multiply in the earth."[1]

In this passage, the Hebrew root for blessing—*barekh*—a key-word in Genesis, appears for the first time.

On the sixth day, the earth was commanded to bring forth living creatures, cattle, creeping things, and beasts of the earth. God saw that what He had made was good. He, therefore, decided to create man in His own image. Man was to have dominion over all that moves in the seas, in the air, and on the face of the earth. The blessing which the Creator had pronounced on the creatures of the fifth day was now repeated in behalf of the last and choicest of His creatures—Man. God created man male and female.

> God blessed them, and said unto them: "Be fruitful, and multiply, and replenish the earth, and subdue it; and have dominion over the fish of the sea, and over the fowl of the air, and over every living thing that moves upon the earth."[2]

The Creator, who endowed all forms of life with the capacity to grow and propagate, who made "fruit trees of every kind on earth that bear fruit with

Reprinted from David S. Shapiro, *Studies in Jewish Thought,* Yeshiva University Press, 1975. Copyright © 1975 by David S. Shapiro.

59

the seed in it'',[3] did not bless the vegetable kingdom. This denial was not the result of the inability of the earth or vegetation to accept the Divine blessing. If the earth may be cursed,[4] it may also be blessed. Moreover, it is clearly stated in Deuteronomy:

> Look down from Your holy abode, from heaven, and bless Your people Israel and the soil You have given us.[5]

The earth as well as the fruit of the earth have the capacity for blessing:

> Blessed shall be . . . the fruit of your land;[6] He will bless your bread and your water.[7]

Why was there no blessing extended? Obviously a blessing directed toward inanimate nature would be meaningless, since it has no *raison d'être* for independent existence. Once animate life emerged, the Divine blessing could become operative and meaningful. Vegetation was to serve as food for both man and beast. The blessings bestowed upon the latter would ultimately redound to plant life which was to function as the means of sustenance for all living creatures.[8]

According to Genesis, God's blessing was extended to the fish and birds and finally to man. Why were the higher animals not blessed? This question has been variously answered in ancient and medieval sources.[9] It appears, however, to this writer that the blessing is all-inclusive and comprises all gradations of life, beginning with the fish and culminating in the highest form of created being—Man. The Scriptures cite only the two extremes of animate life, implying thereby that all intermediate levels were included. There may also be another reason for this exclusion. The blessing of endless propagation was conferred on the fish and the fowl who live in areas uninhabitable by men. Their fruitfulness cannot conflict with the welfare of human beings. However, the prolificacy of animals who occupy the dry land would make clashes with the human race inevitable. The blessing of fruitfulness was therefore extended only to man and not to the other creatures who dwell on the dry land.[10]

The Bible tells us that after the Flood, the blessing of fruitfulness was once more conferred upon man. This time the animals were not included in the blessing. They were, however, included in the covenant which protected them from extinction.[11] The blessing of fertility was later extended to Abraham and Sarah,[12] with Ishmael included.[13] Through Isaac, Abraham was to be blessed with seed as numerous as the stars on high and as the sand by the seashore.[14] This blessing was likewise repeated to Jacob[15] in the earlier days of his life and also later.[16] The blessing that out of their seed a great nation would arise, great in spirit as well as in numbers, was invoked upon both Abraham[17] and Jacob.[18] The blessing that Biblical personalities confer on their children or grandchildren is chiefly that of fertility. Thus, the members of Rebekah's family, before sending her off with Eliezer to be given in betrothal to Isaac, give her their blessings: "Our sister, may you grow into thousands of myriads."[19] Isaac blessed Jacob similarly,[20] and Jacob similarly, his grandchildren Manasseh and Ephraim.[21] The blessing given to Joseph[22] is also of the same character.

Like the blessing that was granted to man originally: "Be fruitful and multiply and fill the earth," so the children of Israel received Heaven's blessing when they came down to Egypt: "The children of Israel were fruitful and prolific, they multiplied and increased very greatly, so that the land was filled with them."[23] The fulfillment of the Divine promise aroused the envy of the Egyptians, who sought ways and means of reducing the numbers of the children of Israel. When God became angry with the children of Israel and was determined to destroy them, He promised Moses that He would make of him a great nation. Moses appeals to God in the name of the Patriarchs, citing the oath sworn to them to multiply their seed like the stars above.[24] Balaam in his oracles calls attention to the fulfillment of the promise to the forefathers.[25] In his last address to Israel, Moses refers to the fulfillment of the blessing which has multiplied Israel like the stars of the heaven, to which the lawgiver adds his own benediction:

> May the Lord, the God of your fathers, increase your numbers a thousandfold, and bless you as He promised you.[26]

The reward of obedience to the commandments of God would be prevention of miscarriage.[27] God will multiply Israel, so that there will be no barren one among them, neither male nor female.[28] The reverse will happen if God's commandments will be disregarded:

> You shall be left few in number, after having been as numerous as the stars in heaven.[29]

The great blessing, then, for the human species is fertility—not because more hands were needed to operate farms or to engage in defense. That the blessing of fertility included all animate beings (particularly those whose usefulness to man is less obvious) precludes its having a utilitarian purpose. The first chapter of Genesis does not conceive of the blessing of fertility as associated with labor, aggression, or defense. In this chapter, God has designated grass and fruit-trees to serve as food for both men and animals. The hard labor to which man was subjected and the need for many hands to assist him in his back-breaking work was not contemplated in the original plan of creation. Genesis pictures a pacific world in which there is no conflict between man and man or between man and other creatures. Neither does it envision internecine warfare within the animal kingdom.[30] The blessing of fertility would appear to have emanated from the great delight experienced by God in creating the world and its inhabitants. "May the glory of the Lord endure forever; let the Lord rejoice in His works."[31]

According to the Aggadah, these words constituted the song of the universe when creation was completed.[32] The joy of God in His work was reflected in the response of His creatures, who broke forth in a universal paean. "God saw all that He had made and behold it was very good."[33] God loved the world, its living creatures, and man above all, so that He poured forth upon them with the greatest abundance the blessing of creativity that enables every species to reproduce life according to its kind. The blessing of fertility is associated with God's vision of the world and life as good, as we read in Genesis 1:21–22:

> God created the mighty sea-creatures and every living thing that creeps, which the waters brought forth in swarms; and all the winged birds of every kind; God saw how good this was; God blessed them, saying: "Be fruitful and multiply, fill the waters in the seas, and let the birds increase on the earth."

The vision of the goodness of life preceded the blessing and motivated it. The creation of man in God's image likewise motivated the blessing of fertility for man.[34]

II.

God's blessing can be converted into a commandment; just as to "be a blessing" is a benediction as well as a commandment.[35] Commandments can be issued to man alone. Other creatures procreate instinctively. Man can organize and discipline his procreative activity. He can consciously limit it; he can destroy it; he can use it indiscriminately, perversely, and self-destructively. Other creatures mate seasonally. For man, mating knows no limitations.

More than in any other, it seems that the universe has run riot in the area of reproduction. The teeming seas, the jungles luxuriant with an infinite variety of vegetation and endlessly spreading foliage, are evidence of a heavenly blessing upon which no limits have been placed. The procreational drive in man, that area which is the least disciplined and the least amenable to control, that which seeks an outlet for itself in normal and abnormal patterns of behavior, that which has often been thought of, rightly or wrongly, as the source of man's sublime aspirations, as well as source of his degeneration, the all encompassing libido, is very likely what it is, so fierce and uncontrollable in its demands, so expansive and unyielding to limitations, just because it is the product not only of Divine creativity, but of a Divine blessing. In the case of man, the blessing has been hedged about by a Divine imperative.

The Biblical text reads:

God blessed them, and God said unto them: "Be fruitful and multiply."[36]

The subject *God* is repeated twice. The blessing extended to other creatures has but one subject: "God blessed them saying: 'Be fruitful and multiply'."[37] The two phrases in the case of man imply a commandment in addition to the blessing.[38]

Likewise, in the ninth chapter of Genesis, which recounts the blessing that God bestowed upon man after the Flood, we read:

> And God blessed Noah and his sons and said to them: "Be fruitful and multiply and fill the earth."[39]

There is here also a doubling of the phrase as found in the first chapter of Genesis, without the repetition of that subject *God*. However, in order to insure against any possibility of error, the phrase was repeated immediately after the prohibition of bloodshed:

> As for you, be fruitful and multiply; abound on the earth and increase on it.[40]

In the light of the above, the Oral Tradition has declared procreation a religious duty, an imperative placed upon man by the Divine Law, a commandment whose purpose is to channelize a wild instinct and subject it to the conscious control of man's intelligence, for the purpose of perpetuating the human species.

The commandment is thus formulated in the Book of the Commandments of Maimonides:[41]

> God has commanded us to be fruitful and multiply with the intention of preserving the human species, and this is what the Scriptures state: "As for you, be fruitful and multiply."

The Book of Training[42] likewise cites procreation as a positive commandment, the first of the commandments, the first chapter of Genesis serving as his proof-text.

The problem may be raised as to what Maimonides meant by the statement that the commandment to be fruitful is to be guided by intention. If literally interpreted we would be led into the difficult and endless argumentation as to whether the performance of any commandment must be accompanied by intention or not—a moot halakhic question.[43] Very likely the requirement of intention does not apply in the case of a commandment involving action and resulting in positive achievement.[44] Of course, one should have in mind the fulfillment of God's will, but lack of intention does not necessarily invalidate a religious act.[45] Maimonides may have meant rather to define the limits of the commandment. It is binding only insofar as it contributes to the preservation of the species, in accordance with the demands of the law.[46] Once one has done his share towards this goal, he is no longer obligated.

III.

Two specific halakhic problems emerge at this juncture. Is the duty of procreation binding on women or only on men? Is it a universal obligation or does it apply only to those who received the Torah at Sinai? In other words, are women and non-Jews under obligation to marry?

The answer to the first question is given in an ancient Mishnah:[47]

> A man is commanded concerning fruitfulness and multiplication, but not a woman; Rabbi Yoḥanan ben Beroka said, "Concerning both of them it is said: 'Male and female He created them; God blessed them, and God said to them, Be fruitful and multiply, fill the earth and master it.' "[48]

The Gemara immediately raises the question: How do the Sages (who disagree with Rabbi Yoḥanan ben Beroka) cope with the text in Genesis which seems to imply that the commandment to be fruitful applies to male and female alike? The answer given is that the Sages hold that the duty of procreation applies to the male sex, because the Biblical text is speaking of activities that require boldness and aggressiveness. Mastering the earth is a masculine activity, since it involves prowess and relentless expenditure of physical energy. All activities included in the text are associated with mastery of the earth. Hence, they are regarded as functions of masculinity. The opinion of the Sages is based on the view generally accepted in civilized societies that it is man who seeks out the woman and not vice versa. Some degree of aggressiveness is required in seeking out a mate, a quality that is not in harmony with the essential or ideal character of woman.[49] The Talmud phrases it in a somewhat different manner:

> Why is it written: "When a man will take a wife," and not vice versa: "When a woman will be taken by a man"? Because normally a man seeks after a wife and it is not normal for a woman to seek after a husband; whoever loses an article goes out in search for it.[50]

Another reason given by the rabbis in the Talmud is that in the case of Jacob the commandment is couched in the masculine singular, implying that the male alone is enjoined. The plural form in Genesis 1:28 and 9:1, 7 must, consequently, be understood as referring to the blessing as well as the commandment, the blessing for both, the command for one.[51] A rationale for the exemption of women from the obligation of procreation is given by the great Gaon of this century, Rabbi Meir Simḥah ha-Kohen of Dvinsk, in his Biblical commentary.[52] He writes:

> It is not amiss to assume that the reason why women are exempt from the obligation of procreation is grounded in the reasonableness of the judgments of the Lord and His ways. The Torah did not impose upon Israel burdens too difficult for a person to bear . . . Women whose lives are jeopardized by conception and birth were not enjoined . . .

However, some of the medieval sages maintained that, although women were not included in the specific commandment of propagation, they are, nevertheless, obligated by the commandment implied in Isaiah.[53]

> For thus says the Lord, the Creator of the heavens, He is God, He fashioned the earth and He made it, He has established it; He did not create it to be waste, He has fashioned it so that it will be inhabited.

The question arises whether the passage of Isaiah is merely a paraphrase of the blessing or commandment contained in Genesis, or whether it contains an additional injunction. The basis for this query is the fact that the Mishnah quotes the passage from Isaiah rather than the standard "Be fruitful and multiply" of Genesis.[54] A prophetic statement is generally assumed to be of a status secondary to a Pentateuchal injunction in its legally binding character.[55] The Tosafists, nevertheless, regard the passage from Isaiah: "He has fashioned it so that it will be inhabited", as entailing a comprehensive imperative obligating everybody, without exception. Even where the Pentateuchal commandment does not apply, the Isaianic principle is operative. Consequently, according to the Tosafists, women have an obligation to participate in the fulfillment of the Divine plan for mankind, so that the earth will be inhabited and not remain desolate.[56]

While for the Tosafists the passage from Isaiah possesses the character of a principle, an *a priori* imperative, because of which a world exists in which the Torah and its commandments can play a central role and in which the sovereignty of the Creator will be recognized, for other sages, Isaiah's words simply paraphrase Genesis. Thus, Maimonides in his Code does not cite the verse from Isaiah. In his Code he rules that it is permissible for a woman to remain unmarried—or even for a man to marry a woman who is barren[57]—although she should marry to avoid suspicion of unsavory behavior.[58]

Maimonides' view seems to be substantiated by the Tosefta:

> A man is not permitted to live without a wife, but a woman may live without a husband; a man is not allowed to drink a root-drink for the purpose of rendering himself impotent; a woman may drink a root-drink to render herself sterile; a man may not marry a woman who is barren,

old, or wombless, or one who is too young or incapable of bearing children; but a woman may marry even a eunuch; the castration of a male involves specific Biblical penalties; the sterilization of a female does not involve specific Biblical penalties.

The opinion of the Tosafists might be reconciled with the rulings of the Tosefta only if we are to assume that a woman may remain unmarried after she has already fulfilled her procreative obligations in accordance with the Isaianic principle. This explanation would also apply to other items included in the Tosefta.

Other passages in the Talmud seemingly confirm the Maimonidean view. A woman who demanded a divorce from her husband on the grounds of childlessness was granted her request only when she supported her claim with the need for a child to sustain her in old age. She is under no obligation to bear children and the desire to fulfill the first commandment may not serve as grounds for divorce. Judith, the wife of Rabbi Ḥiyya, suffered greatly in childbirth and drank a potion to sterilize her, because her husband told her that a woman is not bound by the commandment pertaining to fruitfulness.[59]

The point-of-view of the Tosafists, in respect to the above-cited cases, may be understood in the light of the following. Specific commandments directed at individuals are compulsory. It is the duty of the courts to see that they are enforced.[60] The statement of Isaiah is not apodictic. It is not a direct commandment, but a statement of purpose. A statement of purpose imposes a moral obligation but is not legally enforceable. Moreover, a specific commandment may not be modified, except where explicit conditions are stipulated for such modifications. General directives are handed over to the discretion of the Sages, who determine the prerequisites for its implementation.[61] Thus, women would be exempt from bearing children whenever their health was jeopardized, even if their lives were not endangered. Perhaps Maimonides' understanding of the Isaianic principle is not too far removed from that of the Tosafists.

An additional rationale for the exemption of women from the commandment to be fruitful has been suggested by Rabbi Meir Simḥah ha-Kohen.[62] "It is impossible," he states, "that the reason why the Torah has exempted women from the obligation of procreation is that the natural desire for marriage is stronger in women than in men. According to the Talmud, a woman prefers, under all circumstances, to marry rather than remain single, a disposition nature has implanted in woman that is stronger than any legal injunction.[63] The observance of this commandment may lead to the possibility that a man who has no children might marry another woman who can bear him children. The Torah does not in any way contravene nature. To compel a woman who cannot have children with her husband to leave him and seek another husband is contrary to nature. She cannot be required to leave the husband whom she loves and accept another man whom she does not love. Only in the case of a man, who may legally marry a wife in addition to his present one,[64] may this rule apply.''

Relative to our earlier remarks that the commandment of propagation was intended (in addition to its obvious purpose) as a means of subduing and channelizing man's most powerful impulse, it might be said that the need to conquer this drive is not as imperative for woman as it is for man. Woman has a stronger urge for domesticity than man, but she is not consumed by the sexual impulse to the same extent as he is. She is more chaste and reserved, for psychological, as well as biological, reasons.[65]

IV.

A view has been expressed that, even if there is no obligation on the part of woman to bear children, she is, nevertheless, unavoidably involved in the *mitzvah*. In this respect, marriage is a *mitzvah* for woman as well as for man.[66] Rabbi Nissim ben Reuben[67] and also Meiri[68] adopt this opinion. In citing the ruling on the basis of which the latter sages draw their conclusions, Maimonides likewise employs the term *mitzvah:*

> It is the duty of a woman to become betrothed in person rather than by proxy.[69]

It seems that Maimonides understands the *mitzvah* in this context in the same manner as Rabbi Nissim and Meiri. In the light of our comments above on the Isaianic principle, the opinion of these sages on this matter may be more readily comprehensible.[70]

Another perspective on this problem is suggested by a passage in the Book of Jeremiah:[71]

> Take wives and give birth to sons and daughters, and take wives for your sons, and your daughters give to husbands, so that they may bear sons and daughters and multiply there and do not decrease.

From Jeremiah's message of encouragement to the exiles in Babylonia, the Talmud derives the ruling that it is the duty of a father to facilitate the marriage of his daughter by providing her trousseau. This duty is considered Biblically binding.[72] An early rabbinic work, *She'eltot,* cites this passage as one of the proof-texts making marriage and procreation a religious obligation.[73] Maimonides, however, in line with his view that there is no commandment of procreation for woman, regards Jeremiah's injunction—that the father make provisions for his daughter to enable her to marry—not as Biblical law but as a rabbinic enactment.[74] It is possible that Maimonides also related the injunction of Jeremiah, in addition to the above considerations, to another rule expounded in the Talmud,[75] which reads thus in Maimonides' paraphrase: ''The sages have instructed a person to marry off his sons and daughters as soon as they mature, for, if allowed to remain unmarried, they will fall into a life of sinfulness or preoccupation with sinful fancies."[76] The duty of the father to marry off his daughters would not necessarily, on this basis, be included in the category of the laws of procreation, but would rather be regarded as a derivative of the Biblical law: "Do not profane your daughter to lead her into harlotry, so that the land will not fall into harlotry, and the land filled with lewdness."[77]

It appears that the Palestinian Talmud[78] is inclined to accept the opinion of Rabbi Yoḥanan ben Beroka that would make propagation a religious obligation for women. The Babylonian Talmud favors the reverse view. The *Posekim* (codifiers), for whom the Babylonian Talmud generally carries greater weight, gave preference to the opinion of the latter. What the ideological differences were that gave rise to the divergent views of the Palestinians and Babylonians is not clearly discernible. Perhaps the urgent need to maintain a Jewish community in the Holy Land was the basic factor in giving preference to the view of Rabbi Yoḥanan ben Beroka.

The opinion that though a woman is not commanded, yet, for her, participation in the fulfillment of procreation constitutes a religious duty is expressed in the Midrash *Tanḥuma*[79] and the medieval *Lekaḥ Tov*.[80] In these texts it is stated that man is more obligated than woman. Possibly what is implied is that in the case of woman the fulfillment of the religious obligation is altogether voluntary and cannot be enforced by religious courts.

V.

The prevailing halakhic view that woman is not obligated to fulfill the commandment to "be fruitful and multiply," at least not in the same sense or to the same extent as man, is, as pointed out, motivated by a rationale which appears paradoxical, but is not actually so. Woman may not be compelled to build a family, because essentially she is not the one to seek out a mate, as she does not possess the aggressiveness necessary to initiate those processes that lead to the establishment of a family. On the other hand, the lack of aggressiveness makes a commandment superfluous, since woman is innately endowed with those subtleties and subconscious stratagems which enable her to gain the end that nature intended for her. These stratagems cannot be activated by a fiat. Again, woman's very life is at stake in the process of labor. She cannot be ordered to place herself in so hazardous a position, although she is, of course, not forbidden to seek marriage and children, since these activities are part of the natural order. It would also be unnatural to compel her to seek another husband if her first was infertile. Nor is the commandment leading to marriage necessary in her case as an instrument for subduing or tempering a tempestuous passion. The prevailing halakhic rulings appear to be grounded in profound insights into the nature and behavior of the sexes under normal circumstances.

However, there may be an even more profound significance to the exclusion of woman from the formal halakhic obligation of procreation, whether as a motive or a by-product. A quotation from a recent publication on the revolt of women in modern Islam may shed some light on this subject:

> Motherhood was the main role conferred on woman by tradition, which considered them lacking in physical and mental qualifications, especially for the two highest roles in Islam, warrior and religious man. Self-preservation of the society also put a premium on having children . . . The childless wife is an object of contempt, often said to be cursed by God, and she is the common victim of divorce. One Cairo working mother summed up the attitude by saying that "a woman is not considered a woman unless she has had children."[81]

The release of the Jewish woman from the commandment of procreation has made possible the evolvement of a concept of woman as a personality and not as a child-bearing machine. Certainly woman is involved in the commandment to preserve the race, but it is her privilege to determine whether she becomes involved or not. The rabbinic opinion on this subject and its formulation in Jewish law may have been the first stage in the full emancipation of woman.

The freedom of woman from the obligation to propagate may be viewed also from another vantage-point. Woman has from time immemorial been regarded in all ancient religions as the fertility symbol *par excellence*. The orgiastic rites and the institution of sacred prostitution in the worship of the goddesses of fertility, whether Astarte, Aphrodite, or Venus, were accepted as an integral part of man's religion. The liberation of woman from the obligation of procreation would tend to disassociate her from serving as a symbol of fertility. The props would thus be removed from under one of the oldest pagan rites known to man.

That the exception of women from the commandment of procreation is not contrary to the literal meaning of the Biblical text is confirmed by Genesis 2:24:

> Therefore shall a man forsake his father and mother and cling to his wife.

It is man who abandons his parents' home to seek a wife and not vice versa. The comment of Philo on this passage is in harmony with our remarks above:

> And most excellent and careful was it not to say that the woman should leave her parents and be joined to her husband—for the audacity of man is

bolder than the nature of woman . . . but that for the sake of woman man is to do this.[82]

VI.

Is the commandment of procreation applicable to non-Jews as well as Jews? On the surface it would seem obvious that the obligation devolves upon them as well, for was this commandment not given to Adam and Noah, the fathers of the human race? Thus, one of the great codifiers of early times, Rav Ahai of Shabha, [83] explicitly states that the commandment is of universal scope. However, most of the codifiers have maintained that a non-Jew may remain celibate and not thereby evade the fulfillment of the Divine commandment.

The ground for the exclusion of Gentiles from this commandment is to be found in the Talmud,[84] which states:

> Every commandment that was given to the sons of Noah and repeated at Sinai applies to both Israel and the sons of Noah; a commandment that was given to the sons of Noah and was not repeated at Sinai is intended only for the sons of Israel and not for the sons of Noah.

This declaration implies that the Sinaitic revelation is the source of the commandments that bind both Israel and the nations. The Noachide revelation as such is no longer a living tradition among the nations of the world[85] and is known only through the Torah given at Sinai. Hence, the acceptance of the Noachide commandments must be based upon the Written and Oral Law which alone have preserved the record of the Noachide revelation. One who observes these commandments because of their reasonableness is regarded as a wise, but not as a God-revering, man.[86] Whatever was repeated at Sinai from the original revelation was directed both to Israel and humanity at large. What was not repeated was removed from its former area of application and limited to Israel.[87] The commandment of procreation was not repeated at Sinai. Therefore, it no longer applies to the Noachides.[88]

The question, of course, arises as to the reason for the exclusion of Noachides from the obligation to propagate. Perhaps the fact that the sexual instinct had been used perversely by the Generation of the Flood and had been elevated to a divine status[89] was responsible for its removal from the sphere of Divine commandments. The preservation of the species would be assured by the very dint of a most powerful human drive.[90] It may, moreover, be possible that once the earth was replenished with human beings, the commandment was removed from the Noachides and transferred to the children of Israel, who were few in number,[91] to ensure their physical survival, so that their covenant with God will be continued throughout the generations.

VII.

How large a family need one raise to fulfill his obligation? The answer is contained in the Mishnah:

A man shall not abstain from the performance of the duty of the propagation of the race unless he already has children. As to the number, Bet Shammai ruled: two males, and Bet Hillel ruled: a male and female, for it is stated in Scripture, male and female created He them.[92]

According to the Talmud, for Bet Shammai, Moses, who had two sons before he separated from his wife,[93] provides the example for the sufficiency of two sons. Another version of the dispute between the two schools is cited by the Talmud in the name of Rabbi Nathan, according to which, the school of Shammai requires a minimum of two sons and two daughters, whereas Bet Hillel requires a son and daughter. The case of Cain and Abel and their twins provide Bet Shammai with evidence for their view. A third opinion maintains that for the school of Shammai the minimum is a son and daughter and for the school of Hillel a daughter or a son. The opinion of the Hillelites is based, according to Rava, on the grounds that, since the reason for the commandment to propagate is to assure the survival of mankind, the birth of one child is to be considered as helping to fulfill that goal.[94]

Bet Shammai's view that the commandment of procreation is fulfilled in the birth of sons (regarded as the authentic tradition by the Mishnah) reflects the more aggressive and militant outlook, as well as intense zeal for the centrality of the study of Torah in Israel. The strength of the Jewish people and its survival depend on its men who study Torah, who defend the borders of its homeland, who till its soil, and who carry the word of God to the farthest ends of the earth. The disciples of Hillel are more tolerant and universalistic in their religious orientation. The very beginnings of human history serve as their model. The Shammaites take Moses, the builder of the Jewish people, as their paragon, especially since, according to tradition, he was close to their school's emphasis on the quality of justice.[95] The prevailing halakhic opinion is, of course, that of Bet Hillel.[96]

VIII.

The significance of the commandment of procreation is brought out in a number of aggadic passages.

Rabbi Eliezer stated: "He who does not engage in the propagation of the race is as though he sheds blood; for it is said, 'Whoso sheddeth man's blood, by man shall his blood be shed,' and this is immediately followed by the text, 'And you, be ye fruitful and multiply.' '' Rabbi Jacob said: ''As though he has diminished the Divine image; since it is said, 'For in the image of God made He man,' and this is immediately followed by, 'And you be fruitful.' '' Ben Azzai said: ''As though he sheds blood and diminishes the Divine image; since it is said, 'And you, be ye fruitful and multiply.' ''

In another passage we read:

Our rabbis taught: '' 'And when it rested, he said: Return O Lord unto the ten thousands and thousands of Israel,' teaches that the Divine Presence does not rest on less than two thousand and two myriads of Israelites. Should the number of Israelites happen to be two thousand and two myriads less one, and any particular person has not engaged in the propagation of the race, does he not thereby cause the Divine Presence to depart from Israel!'' Abba Ḥanan said in the name of Rabbi Eliezer: ''He deserves the penalty of death; for it is said, 'And they had no children,' but if they had children they would not have died.'' Others say: ''He causes the Divine Presence to depart from Israel; for it is said: 'To be a God unto thee and to thy seed after thee'; where there exists 'seed after thee', the Divine Presence dwells among them; but where no 'seed after thee' exists, among whom should it dwell! Among the trees or among the stones?''[97]

The duty of procreation is in these aggadic passages viewed from three perspectives. Firstly, human life is envisaged as a value *per se*. Shedding man's blood is the most heinous of crimes. Failure to perpetuate the species (to the extent that one has the obligation to do so) is tantamount to diminution of human life and, hence, is morally equivalent to murder. Secondly, man is the image of God on earth. By failing to reproduce himself he deprives the world of the quality of Divinity, which reflects itself in each new life. Thirdly, a life dedicated to the service of God is specially precious because it helps to bring about the fulfillment of the goal of creation— God's dwelling among the children of men.[98]

Another motivation for procreation is contained in the statement of Rav Assi:

The Son of David will not come before all the souls in their storehouse will have been disposed of.[99]

According to this opinion, procreation is a process whereby homes are being prepared for souls upon the earth, and the fulfillment of this process will accelerate the Messianic redemption. Souls are sent down to perform a task. When these souls shall have completed their task, the Messiah will appear.

IX.

In the mystical literature of Judaism, the duty of propagation occupies a very significant place. Thus, in the Zoharic register of the major commandments of the Torah, we read as follows:

> The sixth precept is to be fruitful and multiply. For he who performs this precept causes the stream (of Divine influence) to be perennially flowing, so that its waters never fail, and the sea is full on every side, and new souls are created and emerge from that tree,[100] and the celestial hosts are increased in company with those souls . . . He who refrains from propagating his kind derogates, if one might say so, from the general form in which all individual forms are comprehended, and causes that river to cease its flow and impairs the holy covenant on all sides . . . As for his soul, she will not enter at all behind the curtain, and he will be banished from the next world.[101]

The basic concept of the Zohar is that all of man's actions affect those realms on high from which all existence derives and is sustained. The constructive actions of man (particularly those of a son or daughter of Israel) stimulate the flow of Divine energy through the medium of the Ten *Sefirot,* thereby enriching the cosmos with its blessing and hastening the process of redemption and the unification of all worlds. Actions which are contrary to the will of God bring about a stoppage of the flow of heavenly abundance and deflect Divine energy into the demonic realm, where it gives nourishment to universal evil forces, which derive their potency from the quality of Divine Judgment. The commandment of procreation, like all other commandments, brings its influence to bear on all dimensions of existence, both earthly and heavenly, especially since the universe is enriched, through the fulfillment of this commandment, with the beneficent acts of newly created souls.

In the light of the Lurianic Kabbalah as expounded by the famed Rabbi Isaiah Horowitz,[102] the object of propagation is the reproduction in physical form of that configuration of the Divine potencies on their highest level — the Supernal Man of the World of Emanation. The *Sefirot,* endowed with Divine power, are both active and passive, or, in the symbolic language of the Kabbalah, male and female.[103] The four major aspects of the Supernal Man, which correspond to the Tetragrammaton, are Wisdom (*Hokhmah,* J), Understanding (*Binah,* H), Harmony (*Tiferet,* W), and Sovereignty (*Malkhut,* H). Wisdom represents insightful, intuitive knowledge, which germinates the entire process of Thought (Understanding). Hence, Wisdom is regarded as masculine and Understanding as feminine. Harmony is related to Wisdom as a son. It is grounded in Wisdom, and, like it, is not the product of analysis. The aesthetics of morality, as well as of art, belong to the dimension of unmediated experience. The final phase of this configuration is the feminine quality of Sovereignty which is the vast sea into which flow all the forces which make possible the emergence and maintenance of the lower realms of Being. The total structure of the world of Emanation (*Azilut*) thus consists of a configuration taking the form of a family of father, mother, son, and daughter,[104] and is known as the Supernal Man. It is in the image of Supernal Man that earthly man is created. The human family, consisting of father, mother, son, and daughter (according to the normative view of the House of Hillel), is thus the earthly embodiment of Supernal Man. The family together makes up a person. Where the family is incomplete, personality remains fragmented, and the Divine potencies, which are to find their expression in the life of man through human activity, remain unfulfilled. Man's failures thus turn into cosmic tragedies.

The original source of the concept of the family as related to heavenly roots is found in the Zohar:[105]

> When is man called complete after the supernal pattern? When he is joined with his mate in unity, in joy, and in affection, and there issue from their union a son and a daughter, then is man complete below like the Holy Name above, and the Holy Name is attached to him. But if a man is not willing to complete the Holy Name below, it were better for him that he had not been born, for he has no portion at all in the Holy Name, and when his soul leaves him, it never joins him again, because he diminished the likeness of his Master, until it has been wholly rectified.

This view of the family as the true fulfillment of man is based on the Talmudic statement:

> Any man who has no wife is no proper man; for it is said, Male and female created He them and called their name Adam (Man).[106]

From the Talmudic views on the significance of marriage and procreation, the mystics have drawn the profoundest implications. He who refrains from fulfilling the commandment pertaining to fruitfulness has denied the essential purpose for which man was created, namely, to serve as a witness for the Creator.[107] Man testifies to the Power and Love of God, being built in the form of the Heavenly Man, the Supernal Chariot, or Celestial Tabernacle,[108] and, in this sense, every man is a Microcosm.[109] The diminution of the race deprives God, so to speak, of witnesses to His glory.

Moreover, when the commandment of fruitfulness is neglected, the Divine Presence departs from Israel. The fulfillment of man's destiny upon the earth will be achieved in the Messianic era, when new souls will be created (at the present time very few newly created souls come into being), after all the souls in their treasure-house have come into the world. He who does not carry out his obligation of fruitfulness is delaying the return to the earth of the Divine Presence in its full splendor and glory. In addition, he is also guilty of bloodshed. The Divine energy which is ready to create new life is deflected from its course into unproductive, or even destructive, channels. Thus, there results a diminution of the Image of God, of Torah, whereby His indwelling among men becomes possible, and of Israel.

In the writings of the *Ḥabad* mystics, the question is raised as to the reason for the descent of the soul from the spheres of celestial delight to the earthly regions, where pleasures are ephemeral and joys are totally dissimilar to those on high. The answer is typical for this school of thought. All existence, *Ḥabad* teaches, is permeated with a Divine vitality. Hence, God is to be regarded as dwelling within this world. But God not only fills all worlds, He also envelops them. He is immanent as well as infinitely transcendent. Because He is transcendent, His Presence is wholly hidden from the eyes of man, and the light of the Infinite *(Ein-Sof)* remains unrevealed within mundane existence. By entering into the material world, the soul enables its bodily counterpart to achieve a lofty spiritual character through the study of Torah and the fulfillment of the Divine commandments. The Divine light that envelops all existence thus manifests its presence within the realm of physical reality, and the soul, through the performance of the commandments, enables the revelation of the Infinite in His transcendent glory to take place within the sphere of His immanence. The commandment of propagation makes it possible for souls to achieve this ineffable delight of knowing the *Sovev* (Transcendent) within the *Memalei* (Immanent)—thereby accelerating the advent of the Messianic era and the Resurrection, when this knowledge will become the heritage of all flesh.[112]

The sexual character of man's life is also discussed in *Ḥabad* writings. Man's existence is sexual because the spiritual grounds of his being are sexual. Man's life in all it phases and ramifications is a composite of contradictory, paradoxical, and complementary qualities. It contains the active and passive, the creative and receptive, the positive and negative, compassion and cruelty, mercy and judgment, tenderness and sternness, knowledge and ignorance, breadth and narrowness, in contradistinction to the angels, who are not complex beings but rather essences of a single spiritual component. Because the roots of his character and spiritual make-up are highly intricate and involved, it is through the union of the sexes that the soul is brought down to earth to be joined with the body, in order ultimately to achieve a bliss it never knew before.[113]

NOTES

1. Gen. 1:22.
2. *Ibid.,* 1:28.
3. *Ibid.,* 1:12.
4. *Ibid.,* 3:17; 5:29.
5. *Ibid.,* 26:15.
6. Deut. 28:4.
7. Ex. 23:25.
8. See Naḥmanides to Gen. 1:22; Baḥya, *ibid.*
9. *Midrash Aggadah* (ed. Buber) to Gen., *ibid.,* Naḥmanides, Baḥya, Ḥizkuni, *ibid.*
10. Cf. Ex. 23:29. [I later found this reason given in *Adderet Eliyahu* by the *Gaon* of Vilna, *ad locum.*]
11. Gen. 9:1–17.
12. *Ibid.,* 17:15.
13. *Ibid.* 17:20.
14. *Ibid.,* 26:16.
15. *Ibid.,* 28:14; 32:13.
16. *Ibid.,* 35:11.
17. *Ibid.,* 12:2.
18. *Ibid.,* 46:3.
19. *Ibid.,* 24:60.
20. *Ibid.,* 28:3.
21. *Ibid.,* 48:16.
22. *Ibid.,* 48:25.
23. Ex. 1:7; Cf. Deut. 26:5.
24. Ex. 32:10, 13.
25. Nu. 23:10.
26. Deut. 1:10–11.
27. Ex. 23:29.
28. Deut. 7:13–14; 28:4; Cf. Lev. 26:9.
29. Deut. 28:62; Cf. Lev. 26:22.
30. Cf. Naḥmanides, Gen. 1:29; Baḥya, *ibid.;* Cf. also Naḥmanides to Lev. 26:4.
31. Ps. 104:31.
32. *Ḥullin* 60a.
33. Gen. 1:31.
34. *Ibid.,* 1:26–28.
35. See *Gen. Rabbah* 39, 2 on Gen. 12:2; *Da'at Zekenim,* Abravanel, and R. Samson Raphael Hirsch to Gen., *ibid.,* Cf. Nu. 6:22–27. Other commentators to Genesis, however, differ.
36. Gen. 1:28.
37. *Ibid.,* 1:22.
38. See commentaries of Samuel David Luzzatto, R. Samson Raphael Hirsch, R. Naphtali Zevi Judah Berlin, and R. David Hoffmann to Gen. 1:28. See also R. Nissim quoted by Abravanel.
39. Gen. 9:1.
40. Cf. Naḥmanides, *ibid.,* and references in note by C. B. Chavel in his edition of Naḥmanides' Commentary (likewise in edition by Rabbi M. Z. Eisenstadt).
41. Commandment 212.

42. *Sefer ha-Ḥinnukh,* Commandment 1.

43. *Berakhot* 13a; *et passim; Melo ha-Ro'im* by Rabbi Jacob Ẓevi Yolles, p. 138 ff.

44. *Melo ha-Ro'im,* p. 138, sec. 8.

45. *Ibid.,* See, also, Maim., *De'ot,* III 2 and *Shemonah Perakim,* chap. 5. Perhaps Maimonides' statement in *Sefer ha-Mitzvot* should be understood in the light of his views enunciated in *De'ot* and *Shemonah Perakim.*

46. See below, section VII.

47. *Yevamot* 55b.

48. Gen. 1:27–28.

49. Cf. Rabbi Levi ben Gershom (Gersonides) in his commentary to Genesis (ed. Venice, photographed edition, New York), folio 13a.

50. *Kiddushin* 2b. Text in Deut. 22:13. The institution of *shadkhanut* developed in Jewish life testifies to the extent of modesty achieved by our people, that even young men were not possessed of the aggressiveness required to seek out a mate. The right of the father to betroth his minor daughter (*Ketubbot* 45b) may have similar grounds.

51. *Yevamot* 65b; *Tosafot, ibid.;* cf. also R. Samuel Edels' commentary to *Sanhedrin* 59b. See also *Ha'amek Davar* to Gen. 35:11 and notes of R. Jacob Emden to *Yevamot, ibid.*

52. *Meshekh Ḥokhmah* to Genesis 9:7.

53. 45:18.

54. *Gittin* 41b.

55. Cf. Maim., *Sefer ha-Mitzvot,* Root 1.

56. *Tosafot, Gittin, ibid.* The Tosafists cite the passage in *Megillah* 27a to confirm their opinion. In that passage the right to sell a scroll of the Torah to facilitate marriage is based on the Isaianic text.

57. *Issurei Biah,* XXI, 26.

58. *Ishut,* XV, 16.

59. *Yevamot* 65b; also *Shabbat* 111a. The laws of sterilization are a supplement to the laws pertaining to the prohibition of injury and apply even to animals.

60. *Ketubbot* 86a.

61. Cf. Maim., *Avel,* XIV, 1: Ritva to *Rosh ha-Shanah* 12a; *Or Same'aḥ, Keriat Shema,* beginning. Cf. *Ḥagigah* 18a; *et passim.*

62. *Meshekh Hokhmah, ibid.*

63. See *Ketubbot* 75a.

64. The reference here is, or course, to Biblical, not rabbinic, law.

65. *Ketubbot* 64b.

66. *Kiddushin* 41a.

67. Commentary to Alfasi, *Kiddushin,* beginning of chap. 2; *Responsa* of R. Nissim, No. 27.

68. *Beit ha-Beḥirah* to *Kiddushin* 41a. Cf. *Korban Netanel* to *Asheri, Kiddushin,* chap. 2, no. 1.

69. *Ishut,* III, 19.

70. See *Korban Netanel, ibid.* Cf. also R. Jacob Ettlinger, *Responsa Binyan Ẓiyyon,* No. 123.

71. Jer. 29:6.

72. See *Ketubbot* 52b. See, however, Ritva, quoted in *Shittah Mekubeẓet, ibid.*

73. Section 21; see *Kiddushin* 30b.

74. *Ishut,* XX, 1; cf. *Ketubbot* 68a.
75. *Yevamot* 62b.
76. *Issurei Bi'ah,* XXI, 25.
77. Lev. 19:29.
78. *Yevamot,* end of Chap. 6.
79. *Noah,* 12; however, in the Buber edition (*Noah,* 18) it appears that this is the view of Rabbi Yoḥanan ben Beroka.
80. Gen. 9:1.
81. *Midstream,* August 1959 in article by Edward Wakin "Veiled Revolution," p. 81. Cf. Genesis 30:23.
82. *Quaestiones et Solutiones in Genesin,* Bk. 1, No. 29.
83. *She'eltot,* no. 165. Cf. the disputation between Rabbi Yoḥanan and Resh Lakish in *Yevamot* 62a and *Tosafot, ibid.*
84. *Sanhedrin* 59a.
85. Cf. *Bava Kamma* 38a. Except insofar as it manifests itself in various religious traditions, both ancient and more recent.
86. Maim., *Melakhim,* VIII, 11, according to the correct reading.
87. See formal argument in *Sanhedrin* 58a.
88. *Ibid.,* 59b; cf. *Tosafot, ibid.*
89. See Gen. 6:1.
90. Cf. *Meshekh Ḥokhmah* quoted above.
91. Deut. 7:7.
92. *Yevamot* 61b. *Bet Shammai*-School of Shammai; *Bet Hillel*-School of Hillel.
93. *Ibid.*
94. *Ibid.,* 62a.
95. See *Sanhedrin* 6b and cf. with *Shabbat* 30b–31a, *Eruvin* 13b, and *Avot* I, 12. The generally more rigorous views of the Shammaites also reflect their preference for the quality of justice. The statement that the Shammaites maintained that the commandment of procreation is fulfilled through sons because of their more militant outlook does not contradict our statement above that the Divine blessing of fruitfulness was not intended to increase hands for defense. The historical situation of the Jewish people determined the character of the commandments imposed upon it, as well as their application.
96. Maim., *Ishut,* XV, 16; *Shulḥan Arukh, Even ha-Ezer* I, 8.
97. *Yevamot* 63b–64a.
98. *Tanḥuma, Naso,* 16.
99. *Yevamot* 63b.
100. The tree is a symbol of the realm of the *Sefirot.*
101. *Zohar,* I, 12b.
102. *Shenei Luḥot ha-Berit,* (ed. Amsterdam), 270b.
103. Cf. Maim., *Guide,* I, 17; see also *Bava Batra* 75b.
104. The notion of the heavenly family (of angels) corresponding to the earthly family (of nations) is already found in the Talmud (*Berakhot* 17a). Needless to say, these are terms which do not apply to the Godhead, but to the manifestations of Divine activity as they first appear in the paradigmatic world of the Supernal or Primordial Man *(Adam Kadmon),* which is the primeval pattern of all creation and particularly of Man.
105. III, 7a.
106. *Yevamot* 63a.
107. *Sifre* to Deut. 33:5.
108. Cf. Malbim to Ex. 25ff.

109. Cf. Maim., *Guide,* I, 72.
110. *Shenei Luḥot ha-Berit, ibid.*
111. *Ibid.*
112. *Derekh Mitzvotekha* by Rabbi Menahem Mendel of Lubavich *(Ẓemaḥ Ẓedek),* pp. 1–8.
113. *Ibid.,* 45–8. The sexual character of animals is also undoubtedly related, according to this view, to their composite character, although in a different sense from that of man.

4

Test-Tube Babies

J. DAVID BLEICH

With the birth of Louise Brown in the obscure mill town of Oldham in northwest England, science fiction of yesteryear became the reality of today. The legend of Faust and Homunculus, the little man-like creature created in a vial, has now become reality through successful development of in vitro fertilization.

Under normal circumstances pregnancy occurs when an ovum, an egg-cell which has been released by the ovary during ovulation, is fertilized by the sperm of the male as it passes through the Fallopian tube. Conception takes place when the ovum is penetrated by a single sperm from among the literally millions of sperm contained in the ejaculate deposited in the vagina. This occurs only when the sperm, after having successfully traversed the uterus, finds its way into the Fallopian tube and succeeds in making contact with the ovum. Thereupon, the fertilized egg undergoes a number of cell divisions and subsequently descends into the uterus where it becomes implanted in the uterine wall.

A significant percentage of infertility problems are the result of a disorder of the Fallopian tubes. When the Fallopian tubes are blocked or missing, it is impossible for the sperm and ovum to make contact. The newly-developed technique enables conception to occur outside the Fallopian tubes. The procedure involves surgically removing the mature ovum from the ovary, placing it in a petri dish in an appropriate culture medium, and adding the male sperm to the solution. The fertilized ovum is allowed to incubate in order to undergo the cell divisions which in normal pregnancy occur in the Fallopian tube and is then introduced into the uterus through the cervical os by means of a pipette. The fetus continues to develop in the uterus in an apparently normal manner. The identical technique may also be utilized to overcome moderate male infertility due to a low sperm count. A single ejaculate of a fertile male contains as many as 100 or 150 million sperm. Even though conception results from the meeting of the ovum and a

Reprinted from *Tradition* (Summer, 1978). Copyright © 1978 by the Rabbinical Council of America.

single sperm, vast numbers of sperm are destroyed or rendered impotent in the process of traversing the female genital tract. Hence, males whose ejaculate contains a significantly diminished number of sperm experience difficulty in fathering children. In vitro fertilization would overcome this difficulty. Since the sperm are placed directly in a petri dish together with the ovum, fertilization is likely to occur even in the presence of only a small number of sperm.

As might have been anticipated, perfection of in vitro fertilization has given rise to a host of moral, theological and halakhic questions. Addressing the 1978 annual *Torah she-be' al Peh* convocation in Israel, the Sephardic Chief Rabbi, Rabbi Ovadiah Yosef, gave his qualified approval to this procedure.[1] The Ashkenazic Chief Rabbi, Rabbi Shlomoh Goren, is reported to view conception by such means as morally repugnant, although halakhically unobjectionable.[2] We shall endeavor to delineate the specific questions involved and to show how those questions may be resolved in light of earlier precedents in Jewish law.[3]

In vitro fertilization has been condemned by some Catholic theologians on the grounds that such interference is not morally acceptable because it is a violation of natural law. This is precisely the same consideration which forms the basis of the Church's opposition to contraception and artificial insemination. This argument is, however, alien to Judaism. Since Judaism does not posit a doctrine of natural law as such, these practices must be examined solely in light of possible infraction of Biblical and rabbinic proscriptions. In the absence of a specific prohibition, man is free to utilize scientific knowledge in order to overcome impediments to procreation.

The first question which must be examined is the moral legitimacy of research involving fetal experimentation. The birth of a test-tube baby could not, at present, have taken place in the United States. All such research was abruptly terminated in 1975 when the Department of Health, Education and Welfare was barred from funding in vitro fertilization experiments in the absence of prior approval of a national ethics advisory board. Such a board was not constituted until January 1978 and has, as yet, not approved experimentation of this nature. The crucial issue is that of increased risk of chromosomal abnormalities leading to physical and mental defects when the ovum is fertilized outside of the body. It is entirely possible that some aspect of the experimental technique may cause genetic damage. Moreover, it is estimated that as many as a half of all pregnancies are spontaneously terminated by the time of implantation. The mechanism responsible for this phenomenon is not fully known, but there is reason to believe that in many instances this is nature's method of providentially preventing the development of a deformed fetus. Artificial maintenance of the zygote outside the body during this early stage of gestation may prevent the natural elimination of a deformed fetus.

The ethical implications of experimentation which may result in the birth of a defective fetus have been analyzed by a leading bioethicist, Professor Paul Ramsey of Princeton University.[4] Professor Ramsey argues that in vitro fertilization followed by implantation is an immoral experiment upon a possible future life since no researcher can exclude the possibility that he will do irreparable damage to the child-to-be: "We ought not to choose for another the hazards he must bear, while choosing at the same time to give him life in which to bear them and to suffer our chosen experimentations."[5]

This argument, insofar as it applies to artificial conception, is entirely consistent with the norms of Torah ethics. Jewish law does not sanction abortion motivated solely by a desire to eliminate a defective fetus, nor does it sanction sterile marriage as a means of preventing transmission of hereditary disorders.[6] However, it does discourage marriages which would lead to the conception of such children. The Gemara, *Yevamot* 64b, declares that a man should not marry into an epileptic or leprous family, i.e. a family in which three members have suffered from these diseases. This ruling is obviously a eugenic measure designed to prevent the birth of defective children.[7] While the rabbinic decree is presumably limited to the specifically delineated circumstances insofar as establishment of a binding prohibition is concerned, the ethical concerns reflected in this legislation are equally applicable with regard to contemplated marriages which would result in issue afflicted with other genetic defects. Furthermore, the Gemara discusses only situations in which defective children would be born as the result of natural procreation. While natural misfortunes may not be avoidable, man does not have the right to act in a manner which will result in harm to others. It follows, *a fortiori*, that overt intervention in natural processes which might cause defects in the fetus would be viewed by Judaism with opprobrium.

Despite the happy initial success in the case of the Brown infant, it will require the birth and maturation through adolescence and into adulthood of a significant number of healthy and normal test-tube babies before the technique may be viewed as morally acceptable. When, and if, it has in fact been demonstrated that the procedure poses no risk to the fetus, there can be no objection to the utilization of this technique on the basis of the fact that the original experimentation was morally unconscionable. As observed by Dr. Daniel Callahan, "The history of medicine is full of instances where things were done unethically but led to benefits for people."[8] An obvious example, from the perspective of Jewish law, is that of post-mortem examinations which were halakhically unwarranted at the time of their performance but which have led to acquisition of potentially life-saving information. Jewish ethics knows of no "Miranda" principle which would bar the use after the fact of information obtained by illicit means.

It should also be stressed that, even in the absence of moral or halakhic objections, no woman is required to submit to in vitro fertilization. The obligations of women, whether by reason of the scriptural exhortation to populate the universe, "He created it not a waste, He formed it to be inhabited" (Isaiah 45:18), or by virtue of marital contract, are limited to bearing children by means of natural intercourse. In a different context, *Iggerot Moshe, Even ha-Ezer,* III, no. 12, expresses the view that a woman, while bound to assume the pain usually associated with normal childbirth, is under no obligation to conceive when faced with the likelihood of unusual and extraordinary pain. Furthermore, it appears to this writer that the comments of *Tosafot, Yevamot* 70a and *Pesaḥim* 28b, establish the principle that one need not assume the pain and risk of a surgical procedure for purposes of fulfilling even an obligatory *mitzvah.*[9] The husband's obligations with regard to procreation under such circumstances are discussed by the *Shulḥan Arukh, Even ha-Ezer* 154: 10-11, and commentaries thereon.

The means employed in procuring sperm for purposes of in vitro fertilization do, however, pose a halakhic problem. Jewish law forbids ejaculation other than within the context of intercourse as *hoẓa'at zera le-vatalah* — destruction of the seed. The question is whether or not semen procurement designed to promote procreation is deemed to be *le-vatalah.* The identical question has been raised in the past, both with regard to semen testing in cases of suspected male infertility and in connection with artificial insemination utilizing the semen of the husband. This question is analyzed in detail by many halakhic authorities.[10]

Removal of semen from the vaginal tract following normal coitus for in vitro fertilization would appear to be regarded by most authorities as the optimal method. Although some authorities forbid emission of semen for subsequent insemination other than in the course of coitus, others sanction this practice but disagree with regard to the means of procurement. Some authorities advise that semen be obtained by means of coitus interruptus. Others sanction the use of a condom as well. The permissibility of masturbation for this purpose is a matter of dispute. Such procedures can, of course, be sanctioned only if the sperm of the husband is used exclusively. Under no circumstances should the sperm of any person other than the husband be utilized. Proper safeguards must be established in order to assure that this should not occur even unwittingly.

There are of course a host of other questions which present themselves: Does the husband fulfill his obligation with regard to procreation by means of in vitro fertilization? Does a filial relationship exist between the father and a child born in this manner? Does the child enjoy the status of the father as a Kohen or Levite? Is the child considered to be an heir to his father's estate? These questions have been analyzed with regard to children born of artificial insemination, and such discussions appear to be equally germane to the case of children born as a result of in vitro fertilization. In any event, the resolution of these questions has no bearing upon the permissibility of in vitro fertilization.

It should be noted that one aspect of the in vitro procedure—as reportedly performed—does present particular cause for concern. The human female is endowed at birth with as many as a million or more ova. These egg-cells mature, ripen and are normally released between puberty and menopause at the rate of approximately one a month. It is reported that, in order to enhance the chances of success of in vitro fertilization without resorting to repeated surgical removal of mature ova, hormones are administered in order to hasten maturation of the egg-cells, so that multiple ova may be removed at one time. All ova removed in this manner are exposed to the male sperm. This permits the fertilization of more than a single ovum. The fertilized ova are then examined and carefully monitored for any sign of chromosomal abnormality. Finally, a single blastocyst is selected for implantation and the remainder are destroyed.

The procedure, when carried out in this manner, poses the question of the permissibility of destroying a developing embryo. Many halakhic authorities have ruled that the prohibition against feticide is operative immediately following conception, while others maintain that no prohibition exists within the first forty days of gestation. In the case of in vitro fertilization the entire question may, of course, readily be side-stepped by limiting the procedure to the fertilization of a single ovum.

Development and perfection of in vitro techniques may, in time, make it possible to select not only the sex but also other genetic characteristics, such as the color of the baby's eyes, I.Q., adult height, etc. Indeed, given the almost infinite number of ova and sperm available and the rapid advances now being made in the field of genetics, it is not at all inconceivable that genetic characteristics may be ordered to conform with virtually any parental preference or whim. The moral, genetic and societal implications of such practices are truly awesome. Nevertheless, the distinction between capricious genetic manipulation and in vitro fertilization which simulates natural procreation and is designed solely to alleviate infertility due to abnormality of the Fallopian tubes should be readily apparent.

In vitro fertilization may, in time, prove to be a highly beneficial development if properly safeguarded. Certainly, indiscriminate tampering with nature is dangerous and immoral. Utmost vigilance must be maintained lest we fashion a Huxley-type world in which eugenic selection becomes the norm. Yet, if properly controlled and not permitted to become a substitute for normal human procreation, this revolutionary technique can be a welcome means of bestowing the happiness and fulfillment of parenthood upon otherwise childless couples.

NOTES

1. *J.T.A. Daily News Bulletin,* Aut. 16, 1978.
2. *J.T.A. Daily News Bulletin,* July 28, 1978; *Be-Olam ha-Rabbanut,* Av 5738, p. 1.
3. See also J. David Bleich, *Or ha-Mizraḥ,* Tishri 5739; R. Judah Gershuni, *ibid.;* and R. Meir Amsel, *Ha-Ma'or,* Tammuz, 5738.
4. "Shall We 'Reproduce'?" *Journal of the American Medical Association,* vol. 220, no. 10 (June 5, 1972), pp. 1346-1350 and vol. 220, no. 11 (June 12, 1972), pp. 1480-1485 and *The Ethics of Fetal Research* (Yale University Press, 1975).
5. *Journal of the American Medical Association,* p. 1350.
6. See *Levushei Mordekhai,* II, no. 68; *Teshuvot Afarkasta de-Anya,* no. 169; R. Isaac Weiss, *Minḥat Yiẓhak,* III, no. 26; R. Moshe Feinstein, *Iggerot Moshe, Even ha-Ezer,* I, no. 62.
7. See *Pri ha-Areẓ,* cited by *Levushei Mordekhai,* II, no. 68; and *Minḥat Yiẓhak,* III, no. 26. CF., however, *Teshuvot Ḥatan Sofer,* no. 136, who offers the unlikely explanation that the concern reflected in this declaration is that the prospective *groom* may contract epilepsy or leprosy.
8. *The New York Times,* July 27, 1978, p. A16, col. 3.
9. Cf., however, Rashba and Me'iri, *Yevamot* 71b.
10. The most significant of these discussions are those of Rabbi Shalom Mordecai Schwadron, *Teshuvot Maharsham,* III, no. 268; Rabbi Aaron Walkin, *Teshuvot Zekan Aharon,* II, no. 97; Rabbi Malkiel Zvi Tanenbaum, *Teshuvot Divrei Malki'el,* IV, nos. 107-108; Rabbi Ben Zion Uziel, *Mishpetei Uzi'el, Even ha-Ezer,* I, no. 19; Rabbi Yehoshua Baumel, *Teshuvot Emek Halakhah,* no. 68; Rabbi Ovadiah Hadaya, *No'am* I, (5718), pp. 130-137; Rabbi Ya'akov Breisch, *Teshuvot Ḥelkat Ya'akov,* I, no. 24; Rabbi Yitzchak Weisz, *Teshuvot Minḥat Yiẓhak,* IV, no. 5; Rabbi Eliezer Waldenberg, *Ẓiẓ Eli'ezer,* IX, no. 51, secs, 4-6; Rabbi Shlomoh Zalman Auerbach, *No'am,* I, (5718), pp. 145-166; Rabbi Ovadiah Yosef, *Teshuvot Yabbi'a Omer,* II, no. 1 and Rabbi Moshe Feinstein, *Iggerot Moshe, Even ha-Ezer,* I, nos. 70 and 71, II, nos. 16 and 18, and III, no. 13.

5

Contraception in Jewish Law

FRED ROSNER

Introduction

Controversy surrounding the problems associated with contraception is by no means on the decline. On the contrary, a veritable recent flood of books and articles in the medical and lay press, as well as innumerable programs on the mass communication media devoted to family planning, contraceptive practice and birth control, attest to the widespread and increasing interest in this subject. Introduction of the pill in the early 1960's revolutionized many people's thinking toward birth control and has had a major impact on the overall picture of world population limitation.

It is beyond the scope of this essay to provide the reader with a comprehensive discussion of the various contraceptive methods, their effectiveness or lack thereof, the physiological mechanisms involved and the possible side effects that may be encountered. For such information the reader is referred to the standard texbooks of obstetrics and gynecology. Suffice it simply to enumerate the major methods employed: the condom, coitus interruptus, the diaphragm and cervical caps, chemical contraceptives, the safe period or rhythm method, oral contraceptives and the intrauterine devices. Sterilization and abortion should also be mentioned, as well as a variety of minor methods, such as douching, sponges and tampons, scrotal hyperthermia and coitus reservatus and saxonicus.

Moral Aspects of Contraception

The morality (or immorality) of contraception boils down to a two-sided

Reprinted from *Tradition* (Fall, 1971). Copyright © 1971 by the Rabbinical Council of America.

argument. On the one hand, many people claim that there is no moral difference between preventing the natural process of conception by contraception and preventing the natural process of obesity by diet or pills. On the other hand, traditional Judaic-Christian teaching maintains that by the mind and will of God there is an objective standard of right and wrong in the universe, and that men are possessed with the rational faculty to choose one or the other. Thus, if the Torah considers any interference with the act of procreation as morally wrong, then such interference is legally prohibited in Jewish law. The commandment of *be fruitful and multiply* (Genesis I:28) interdicts the indiscriminate use of contraceptives.

The argument that contraceptive chemicals may kill a fertilized ovum (i.e., a potential person) is more germane to a treatise on abortion and will not be discussed here. Furthermore, such an argument is not applicable to most modern methods of contraception including the pill. The problem of eugenics and population control is as much a moral dilemma as it is a matter of social ethics.

The economic argument for contraception emphasizes that parents should only have the number of children they can support in an adequate fashion. This argument possesses its greatest strength and appeal when it is applied to large families with below-average income. That some good may be derived from contraception employed for economical reasons does not, however, make such a practice morally right. In order that all children in a family be provided with adequate food, clothing, shelter and education, contraception may be no more morally justified than robbery by the parents to provide for the needs of the children. Robbery and contraception are both immoral, although both might achieve a desirable outcome. The solution to the economic argument for contraception is a better organization of society, with sufficient work and distribution of wealth for all.

Medical indications for the use of contraceptive devices and methods are many and include diseases wherein pregnancy would result in a marked deterioration of the mother's health or even threaten her life. Such conditions are rheumatic heart disease, tuberculosis, certain kidney diseases, severe diabetes and others. However, to masquerade behind a medical indication, particularly psychiatric illness, where none exists, or where the risks are minimal, is certainly immoral.

It is sometimes asserted that the stability, or even the preservation, of a marriage depends upon the practice of contraception. Reasons may include the desire of a wife to continue working after marriage, the lure of a professional career, unwillingness to give up an active social life and reluctance to financially drain the marriage by having children. Such reasons, purely of convenience, for the use of contraceptives, are certainly immoral.

Catholic Attitude Toward Contraception

The most thorough, scholarly, objective analysis of Catholic doctrine on birth control throughout history is the recently published work of John T. Noonan, Jr.[1] This book traces the development of the Church's position on contraception, and analyzes the historical situations that influenced various church decisions over the centuries from the year 50 C.E. until 1965.

The traditional Catholic viewpoint is to prohibit all forms of contraception, except the rhythm method. This position is based upon the doctrine that the primary purpose of marriage is procreation, not companionship. Any method of birth control which violates the "natural law" is thus prohibited. Birth control by natural means, that is using the rhythm method or abstinence, is not considered a violation of the "natural law."

Recent pronouncements by several Popes have reaffirmed the traditional Catholic teaching on this matter. In his famous 1930 Encyclical *Casti Connubii* (On Christian Marriage), Pope Pius XI solemnly restated the condemnation of contraception, but gave his approval to the rhythm method. This approval was repeated by Pope Pius XII in 1951 when he said:

> We affirm the legitimacy and, at the same time, the limits — in truth very wide — of a regulation of offspring which, unlike so-called "birth control," is compatible with the law of God. One may even hope that science will succeed in providing this licit (rhythm) method with a sufficiently secure basis.[2]

In a second address in 1951 the Pope elaborated on the conditions under which Catholics may use the rhythm method and be exempt from the duty of procreation and parenthood. Examples are "serious reasons, such as those often provided in the so-called indications of the medical, eugenical, economic and social order."[3] In an address to hematologists in 1958, Pope Pius XII approved the use of oral contraceptives for the treatment of disease, but condemned their use for birth control.

In 1966, a papal commission, appointed two years earlier to re-examine the church's position on marriage and the family, submitted its report to Pope Paul VI. There were both minority and majority reports. The former recommended continued adherence to the traditional beliefs, whereas the latter urged changes in past teachings to allow chemical and mechanical contraceptives. In July 1968, in his Encyclical *Humane Vitae,* the Pope rejected the majority report and condemned the use of techniques other than abstinence or the rhythm method. Dissent within the Catholic hierarchy was considerable with progressive views being voiced by Catholic theologians and laymen alike.

Protestant Views on Contraception

Protestant churches are virtually unanimous in their endorsement of birth control as enunciated in the 1961 statement of the National Council of Churches, the federation of 32 major Protestant denominations. Such an endorsement stems from the view that the basic purposes of marriage include not only procreation but also the "nourishment of the mutual love and companionship of husband and wife and their service to society."[4]

Jewish Attitude Toward Contraception

The most extensive study of the principles of Judaism concerning contraception, based on a wealth of primary sources, is that of David Feldman.[5] In his book, Feldman examines the relevant precepts of the Talmud, codes, commentaries and rabbinic responsa.

A brief discussion of the Biblical commandment *be fruitful and multiply* as decreed first to Adam and Eve (Gen. 1:28) and later to Noah and his sons (Gen. 9:1 and 7) and to Jacob (Gen. 35:11) seems appropriate. The importance of this commandment is stated in the Babylonian Talmud (*Yevamot* 63b):

> Rabbi Eliezer stated: He who does not engage in propagation of the race is as though he sheds blood; for it is said, "Who so sheddeth man's blood by man shall his blood be shed" (Gen. 9:6); and this is immediately followed by the text "And you, be ye fruitful and multiply" (Gen. 9:7). Rabbi Jacob said: As though he has diminished the Divine Image; since it is said, "For in the image of God made He man" (Gen. 9:6), and this is immediately followed by "And you, be ye fruitful and multiply" (Gen. 9:7). Ben Azzai said: As though he sheds blood *and* diminishes the Divine Image . . .

The explanation of the commandment is provided by the Mishnah (*Yevamot* 6:6) where it states:

> A man shall not abstain from the performance of the duty of the propagation of the race unless he already has children. (As to the number), Bet Shammai ruled: two males, and Bet Hillel ruled: A male and a female, as it is written (Gen 1:27 and 5:2); *"male and female* created He them."

It is beyond the scope of the present essay to delve in depth into the rabbinic ramifications of the commandment of procreation. Suffice it to say that "the moral obligation, if not the commandment of propagating the race, still rests upon the husband when he already has two children." The role of the woman in procreation is described by Feldman and summarized in a quote from the fourteenth century Talmudic commentary of Rabbi Nissim (*Hiddushei ha-Ran* to *Kiddushin* 41a):

> . . . even though she is not personally commanded concerning procreation, she performs a *mitzvah* (meritorious act) in getting married because she thereby assists her husband in the fulfillment of his *mitzvah* (religious duty) of *be fruitful and multiply.*

In a Jewish marriage, over and above the question of procreation, there exist the conjugal rights of the wife, technically termed *onah*. Thus, non-procreative intercourse such as occurs if the wife is too young to bear children, or is barren, or is pregnant, or post menopausal, or following a hysterectomy, is not only allowed but required. Improper emission of seed (*hashhatat zera*) is not involved, or is cancelled out so long as the intercourse is in the manner of procreation. Not only are such sexual activities permitted, but they are in fact required by Biblical law based on Exodus 21:10. "Marriage and marital relations are both independent of procreation, achieving the many desiderata spoken of in Talmudic, responsa and mystic literatures."[6] Such goals include fulfilling the wife's desire, physical release of the husband's sexual pressures, and the maintenance of marital harmony and domestic peace.

A lengthy chapter in Feldman's book is devoted to a discussion of the legitimacy of sexual pleasure in Judaism. He quotes Nahmanides who said that

> Sexual intercourse is holy and pure when carried on properly, in the proper time and with the proper intentions. No one should claim that it is ugly or unseemly. God forbid! . . .

In a similar vein, Rabbi Jacob Emden is cited as having said:

> . . . to us the sexual act is worthy, good and beneficial even to the soul. No other human activity compares with it; when performed with pure and clean intention it is certainly holy. There is nothing impure or defective about it, rather much exaltation . . .

Thus, whereas Christian teaching promulgates that procreation is the sole purpose of marriage and sexual intercourse, Judaism requires that not only need procreation result from sex, but mutual pleasure is sufficient reason for the sex act.

There are at least six methods of contraception mentioned in the Bible and Talmud. The first of these is "coitus interruptus" which is unequivocally prohibited as stated by Maimonides (*Mishneh Torah, Hilkhot Issurei Bi'ah* 21:18):

> It is forbidden to expend semen to no purpose. Consequently, a man should not thresh within and ejaculate without . . . As for masturbators, not only do they commit a strictly forbidden act, but they are also excommunicated. Concerning them it is written, "Your hands are full of blood" (Isaiah 1:15), and it is regarded as equivalent to killing a human being.

A similar prohibition is found in Asheri (*Teshuvot ha-Rosh* 33:3), and in Caro's *Shulḥan Arukh* (*Even ha-Ezer* 23:5) as well as in other codes of Jewish law.

The scriptural source upon which is based the prohibition of improper emission of seed is not clear, although many consider the act of Er and Onan (Gen. 38:7–10) to be the classic case of coitus interruptus. The Talmud, however (*Yevamot* 34b), views the act of Er and Onan as unnatural intercourse. Er wanted to preserve his wife's beauty by preventing her from becoming pregnant, and Onan sought to frustrate the Levirate law.

Other possible Biblical sources outlawing emission of seed for naught have been suggested. The Decalogue's commandment against adultery is said to have wider application, perhaps to immorality in general. The generation destroyed by the great flood is thought to have been liquidated because of the sin of improper emission of seed. Others say that this cardinal sin is implied in the commandment to *be fruitful and multiply*. Finally, states Feldman, the injunction (in Leviticus 18:6) against incest, literally, "immorality with one's own flesh" *(ish ish el kol she'er besaro)* includes improper emission of seed.

Whether this offense is considered homicide or only immoral as self-defilement is also a matter of argumentation. The *Zohar* apparently espouses both reasons. Bringing forth semen in vain would also be prohibited if a man were to use a condom during intercourse, even if the sex act were performed in the natural way. Procurement of sperm for medical reasons (i.e., not in vain) is permitted under certain circumstances, such as sterility testing.

Since the commandment of procreation in Judaism rests primarily on the man, any contraceptive method employed by him such as coitus interruptus or the condom would be strictly prohibited because of the Onanite nature of these methods. Even in situations where contraception is permitted by Jewish law, such as for situations in which pregnancy might endanger the life of the mother, these methods are not allowable.

The Talmud discusses four methods and techniques employed by the woman to prevent conception: The safe period, twisting movements following cohabitation, an oral contraceptive, and the use of an absorbent material during intercourse.

The period of fertility of a woman is mentioned in the Talmud (*Niddah* 31b) as follows:

> Rabbi Isaac . . . stated: A woman conceives only immediately before her menstrual period, for it is said "Behold, I was brought forth in iniquity" (Psalms 51:7). But Rabbi Yohanan stated: A woman conceives only immediately after her ritual immersion for it is said "And in cleansing did my mother conceive me" (Psalms 51:7).

Feldman cites rabbinic responsa that call attention to cycles of fertility and sterility as a possible method of contraception. He concludes that there is no impropriety in the use of this method when birth control is required, such as in situations of hazard to the mother. However, by its use, the commandment of procreation and the wife's conjugal rights (*Onah*) are both frustrated. Furthermore, the unreliability of this method makes it unacceptable in cases of danger to life.

An ancient method of contraception is when the woman makes violent and twisting movements following cohabitation in order to spill her husband's seed. This method is described in the Talmud (*Ketubbot* 37a) by Rabbi Yose, who is of the opinion that "a woman who plays harlot turns over in order to prevent conception." The Talmud (*ibid.* 72a) further entitles a woman to receive her marriage settlement *(Ketubbah)* if the husband imposes a vow on her to produce violent movements immediately after intercourse to avoid conception.

Throughout the centuries, numerous recipes have been recommended for oral contraception, from Pliny the Elder's parsley and mint, to Dioscorides' willow leaves in water; from Soranes' opapanix, with cyrenaiac sap, to the marjoram, parsley and thyme of medieval Germany. In the Talmud, there are at least two discussions of a "cup of roots" or sterility potion. In *Yevamot* 65b we find the following:

> . . . Judith, the wife of Rabbi Hiyya, having suffered agonizing pains of childbirth, changed her clothes [on recovery] and appeared [in her disguise] before Rabbi Hiyya. She asked, "Is a woman commanded to propagate the race?" He replied, "no." And relying on this decision [literally: she went], she drank a sterilizing potion.

Elsewhere the Talmud states (*Shabbat* 109b-110b) that a potion of roots may be imbibed on the Sabbath because it is a cure for jaundice and gonorrhea. However, the imbiber may become impotent thereby. Thus, a woman may drink a sterilizing (i.e., contraceptive) potion as a cure for jaundice. A smaller dose recommended to treat gonorrhea does not produce permanent sterility. The ingredients of this "cup of roots" are enumerated by Rabbi Yoḥanan (*ibid.* 110a) and include Alexandrian gum, liquid alum, and garden crocus, powdered and mixed with beer (for jaundice) or wine (for gonorrhea). The Tosefta in tractate *Yevamot* 8:2 specifically states that a man is not allowed to drink any potion in order not to be fertile, because he is commanded to propagate the race, whereas a woman is permitted to drink the potion in order not to conceive.

The latter ruling is codified by both Maimonides (*Hilkhot Issurei Bi'ah* 12:12) and Caro (*Shulḥan Arukh, Even ha-Ezer* 5:12) unconditionally. Later rabbis, however, stipulate that there must be some medical indication as in the case of Rabbi Ḥiyya's wife (*vide supra*) to allow the use of the potion of roots. Furthermore, as pointed out by Feldman, "the bulk of the legal discussion surrounding the cup of roots is based on the crucial assumption that the sterilizing effect of this potion is permanent," thus raising the problem of castration, an act prohibited by Jewish law.[7]

The oral contraceptive pill of today seems to embody within itself the Talmudic "cup of roots." It allows intercourse to proceed in a natural and unimpeded manner, thus allowing fulfillment of the wife's conjugal rights. Furthermore, whereas the effect of the "cup of roots" is permanent, the effect of the pill is temporary, thereby setting aside the question of castration. No improper emission of seed is involved in the use of the pill.[8] However, without medical indication it appears as if the oral contraceptives should not be employed prior to the fulfillment of the commandment of procreation (i.e., at least two children). Furthermore, the question of the safety of the pill is both of medical and Jewish legal concern. Certainly, women in whom medical contraindications make the use of oral contraceptives dangerous, would be prohibited by Jewish law from taking them. Other deleterious side effects must also be taken into consideration. However, at the moment, the pill seems to be the least objectionable method of birth control in Jewish law.

Virtually all rabbinic rulings on the subject of contraception are based upon a key Talmudic statement which has been called the *"Baraita* of the Three Women" (*Yevamot* 12b).

> Rabbi Bebai recited before Rabbi Naḥman: Three [categories of] women may [or must] use an absorbent [Hebrew: *mokh*] in their marital intercourse [to prevent conception]: a minor, a pregnant woman and a nursing woman. The minor, because [otherwise] she might become pregnant and as a result might die. A pregnant woman because [otherwise] she might cause her fetus to become a *sandal* [a flat fish-shaped abortion due to superfetation]. A nursing woman, because [otherwise] she might have to wean her child prematurely [owing to her second conception], and he would die. And what is a minor? From the age of eleven years and one

day until the age of twelve years and one day. One who is under or over this age [when conception is not possible or where pregnancy involves no fatal outcome, respectively] carries on her marital intercourse in the usual manner. This is the opinion of Rabbi Meir. But the Sages say: The one as well as the other carries on her marital intercourse in the usual manner, and mercy be vouchsafed from Heaven [to save her from danger], for Scripture says "The Lord preserveth the simple" (Psalms 116:6).

The nature and the status of the absorbent (or *mokh*) in Talmudic law is explored in an entire chapter of Feldman's book. Subsequent chapters are devoted to an in-depth consideration of the three categories of women in the *baraita,* the many levels of debate concerning the meaning of the *baraita.*

Does the *baraita* allow or require the three women to use the absorbent? Rashi states that Rabbi Meir means "may use" and the Sages mean "may not," whereas Rabbenu Tam reports that Rabbi Meir means "must" and the Sages mean "must not but may." A second level of debate is concerned with whether the absorbent is to be used before (i.e., during) or after coitus? The outcome of the argumentation in the interpretation of the *baraita* is summarized by Rabbi Immanuel Jakobovits, as follows:

> . . . several authorities assume that this dispute applies only to these particular cases (i.e., three women) where the danger of a conception is in any event rather remote: hence, they infer that, in cases of a more definite threat to the mother's life arising from a pregnancy, there would be no objection at all to the use of contraceptives. Others hold that the three women are mentioned to illustrate the attitude to cases of resultant danger to life in general; while yet others regard the entire sanction as limited to these three women only.[8a]

Rabbis Jakobovits, Feldman and others express surprise at the omission of reference to the pivotal *baraita* by the major codes of Jewish law, Maimonides and Caro. Even the codes which mention the *baraita (Asheri* and *Alfasi)* only relay it verbatim without deriving any legal ruling therefrom. To perhaps compensate for this silence, there is available an enormous rabbinic responsa literature dealing with contraception. The most lenient or permissive view is that of 16th century Rabbi Solomon Luria[9] who allows the wife to apply a tampon before intercourse, if a conception and pregnancy would prove dangerous. Many subsequent writers including Rabbis Solomon Zalman of Posen,[10] Simḥah Bunem Sofer,[11] Mordecai Horowitz,[12] Ḥayyim Ozer Grodzinsky,[13] Shalom Mordecai Schwadron,[14] David Hoffmann[15] and others agree with Luria. On the other hand, there is a school of non-permissivists who do not allow any impediment to natural intercourse. The chief proponents of this school are Rabbis Akiva Eger,[16] Jacob Ettlinger,[17] and Moses Schreiber.[18]

For situations of pregnancy hazard, the pessary or diaphragm is allowed by numerous authorities including Rabbis Joshua Baumol,[19] Shalom Mordecai Schwadron,[20] Ḥayyim Sofcr,[21] and Moses Feinstein.[22] The reason is that the normal coital act is not interfered with. This is not the case with the condom, which constitutes an improper interference and is strictly prohibited. Chemical spermicides and douches are other contraceptive methods which leave the sex act alone and are thus permitted by many responsa writers but only in a case of danger to the mother from pregnancy. Whether spermicides are preferable to the use of a diaphragm or vice versa is a matter of debate. On the one hand, the occlusive diaphragm does in fact constitute a mechanical barrier. On the other hand, "spermicides destroy the seed immediately upon its entry into the canal."[23]

As to the intrauterine contraceptive devices, recent medical evidence seems to indicate that these produce contraception by inhibiting proper implantation of the fertilized ovum in the wall of the uterus. If this is so, then their abortifacient action would prohibit their use, as it is akin to abortion.

Conclusion

The Jewish attitude toward contraception by any method is a non-permissive one if no medical or psychiatric threat to the mother or child exists. The duty of procreation, which is primarily a commandment on man, coupled with the wife's conjugal rights in Jewish law, mitigates against the use of the condom, coitus interruptus or abstinence under any circumstances. Where pregnancy hazard exists, and where rabbinic sanction for the use of birth control is obtained, a hierarchy of acceptability emerges from the Talmudic and rabbinic sources. Most acceptable are contraceptive means that least interfere with the natural sex act and least interfere with the full mobility of the sperm and its natural course. "Oral contraception by pill enjoys preferred status as the least objectionable method of birth control."[24] Since many different factors must be brought to bear on the final decision, it is suggested that competent rabbinic opinion be sought to adjudicate any given case, such opinion to be based upon expert medical testimony.

NOTES

1. Noonan, J. T., Jr., *Contraception—A History of Its Treatment by the Catholic Theologians and Canonists,* 1966, Cambridge, Mass., Harvard Univ. Press, 1966, pp. 561.

2. Guttmacher, A., *Birth Control and Love,* London, McMillan Co., 1969, 2nd edit., pp. 141–168.

3. *Ibid.*

4. *Ibid.*

5. Feldman, D., *Birth Control in Jewish Law,* 1968, New York Univ. Press, 322 pp.

6. *Ibid.*

7. *Ibid.*

8. Feinstein, M., *Iggerot Moshe, Even ha-Ezer,* no. 65 and Waldenberg, *Ziz Eli'ezer,* vol. 9, no. 51. Talmud, tractate *Shabbat* 110b–11a and based upon the Biblical phrase *that which has its stones bruised or crushed or broken or cut, ye shall not offer unto the Lord; neither shall ye do thus in your land* (Levit. 22:24).

8a. Jakobovits, I., *Jewish Medical Ethics,* New York, Block Publishers, 1959, pp. 389.

9. *Yam shel Shelomo, Yevamot* 1:8.

10. *Hemdat Shelomo, Even ha-Ezer, no. 46.*

11. *Shevet Sofer, Even ha-Ezer, no. 2.*

12. *Mattei Levi,* vol. 2, no. 31.

13. *Ahie'zer, Even ha-Ezer, no. 23.*

14. *Maharsham,* vol. 1, no. 58.

15. *Melammed Leho'il, Even ha-Ezer, no. 18.*

16. *Akiva Eger,* no. 71.

17. *Binyan Ziyyon,* no. 137.

18. *Hatam Sofer, Yoreh De'ah,* no. 172.

19. *Emek Halakhah,* no. 66.

20. *Maharsham,* vol. 1, no. 58.

21. *Mahaneh Hayyim, Even ha-Ezer, no. 53.*

22. *Iggerot Moshe, Even ha-Ezer, no. 63.*

23. Rabbi Eliezer Waldenberg, *Ziz Elie'zer,* vol. 9, no. 51, 2, 3.

24. Feldman, p. 248.

6

Population Control
–the Jewish View
MOSES D. TENDLER

The world's increasing population is viewed by many as one of the basic problems of our time. The "demographic problem" or, as referred to in the lay press, the "population explosion," has received the attention of the best minds of the fields of medicine, economics, law, and religion. Reports of authoritative decisions reflecting the Catholic, Protestant and Jewish viewpoints appear with annoying repetition. This paper is offered firstly to summarize and clarify the Torah view of the demographic problem, and secondly as a cry of protest against those who took unto themselves the mantle of spokesman for the Jewish people on this complex and delicate issue.

The penalty for the failure of the Orthodox community to speak out on the great issues of the day is twofold. The truths of our Torah are unavailable as guidelines for our people, and many who should be silent represent themselves as prophets of Judaism. The validation of a prophecy occurs when there is absolute concurrence between the prophetic message and the prophecy of Moses — our Torah teachings. Based on this criterion, we must conclude that the topic of population control has attracted a disproportionate number of false prophets whose teachings weaken rather than strengthen the hearts of our people.

For almost a decade, I have had the unique opportunity of conducting a seminar series in *Hilkhot Niddah* for the senior students at Yeshiva University. The laws relevant to the principle and practices of birth-control techniques comprise a significant part of these seminars. Despite the lucidity and accuracy that is the teacher's reward from the student-teacher countercurrent,[1] I approach my task with trepidation. What right do I have to don the mantle of spokesman? Indeed I claim none. Let no one read into my words the language of *Pesak Din* — a language reserved for

Reprinted from *Tradition* (Fall, 1966). Copyright © 1966 by the Rabbinical Council of America.

the ears or eyes of the individual questioner on this complex, intimately personal problem. I present for considered judgment a point of view based on the primary sources of our faith — the words of the Talmud and its commentaries. It is my hope that it will serve to counterbalance the views already expressed by others.

Definition of the problem: Recent advances in disease control have given new impetus to the recurring Malthusian nightmare of world population outstripping world food supply. Unless vigorous action is taken to correct the imbalance of a declining death rate coupled to a burgeoning birth rate, mankind is irrevocably committed to a catastrophic famine.

The Torah attitude consists of the composite answer to the following questions:

(a) Are the facts presented accurate?

In the many publications presented to the lay public, the basic mathematics of the Malthusian nightmare goes unchallenged. Historically speaking, the projections of Malthus were totally inaccurate. He failed to allow for the scientific and technological advances that have kept food production increases ahead of population growth. Indeed, at the World Conference on Populations, organized under the auspices of the United Nations in September 1965, many expressed the opinion that [2] "there was no problem of excessive rates of growth in under-developed areas and therefore no public or private action was needed."

At a recent symposium the view that the world faces a choice between birth control and famine was not at all unanimous. Many maintained that "despite the stresses imposed upon our food supply by the unprecedented population explosion, we could feed everyone well."[3]

(b) What are the philosophical or ethical implications of projected programs to reduce the birth rate?

The conflict of science and religion was once limited to the question of the authenticity of the Torah. In the 19th century the challenge to the Torah came from the evolutionists. In our time the spotlight is focused on the methodology of natural science. The challenge to Torah values stems from the claim that the methods of natural science constitute man's only reliable access to the knowledge of reality.

Those familiar with the personal letters of Charles Darwin know that he first lost faith in God as a Judge and Ruler and then rejected Him as a Creator. Evident from the writings of many of the leaders in the study of the demographic problem is the conviction that the Darwinian refutation of God, the Creator, compels us to discount Him as an active force in the affairs of mankind. In the halakhic sense, if the God of Shabbat does not exist then the God of the Exodus is equally non-existent.

Such is not the Torah view! The management of the world's population is relegated unto God.[4] The insistence that God erred in not realizing the mathematical certainty of a geometrically increasing population outstripping arithmetical increases in food supply is but another manifestation of the theology of blasphemy which is in vogue today. Inherent in our concept of a Personal God is the philosophy of the verse in Psalm 145 in which God is praised for providing sustenance for all His creatures. Food supply and world population are areas of divine concern.

However, man has been granted a junior partnership in the management of this world. Imbued with the spark of Divine Intelligence, man is permitted, even required, to use his partnership rights to regulate his own affairs, on condition that he does not violate the by-laws of this God-man relationship that are formulated in the Torah. What if the present projections prove to be more accurate than those made by Malthus? We are told that at the present rate of increase in world population, 300 million tons of *additional* grain annually will be needed by 1980. This is more grain than is now produced by all of North America! What guidelines have been set down for our instruction in this yet hypothetical situation?

The Jew as a world citizen is personally concerned with famine in India and China.[5] However the Noachidic laws which serve as Torah (instruction) for all humanity demand a proper sequence of actions. Before a Jew can support birth-control clinics in overpopulated areas of the world, he must insist that there be heroic efforts made to utilize fully the agricultural potential of the world. This implies the extension of modern farming technology to all parts of the world, as well as a more effective and more morally responsible distribution of food surpluses. It is ludicrous to maintain that an Indian will allow himself to be surgically sterilized, his wife aborted or implanted with a plastic loop, bow, or spiral, yet he will obstinately refuse to use a better grain seed, add chemical fertilizers to his land, or adjust his plowing pattern so as to minimize water loss.

It is equally untenable to insist that the logistics of world-wide food distribution present insurmountable obstacles. A nation that can transport the men and material needed to wage modern war in Korea and Vietnam can, with efficiency and dispatch, overcome all obstacles in the way of food distribution. Surely we have adequate motivation. Is it more immoral to allow a family to lose its political freedom than to sit idly while it loses its personal freedom to bear children? At the symposium previously referred to[3], a leading professor of political science bravely presented a prognosis that clearly spells the doom of the concept of the integrity and worth of the individual upon which all democratic principles depend. He predicted, "Inescapably there will be changes in our most intimate habits and patterns of living. It is not enough to have a pill. People must be willing to take it — in many cases not merely to prevent the birth of unwanted children, but even to prevent the birth of deeply wanted, even longed-for children. The time may not be far off when some societies, at least, may find themselves pressed by unyielding circumstances into an extraordinary invasion of human privacy — the limitation of births by legal ordinance, with severe penalties for infraction." The threat of communism pales in comparison with this summary of the fantasy of "1984" materializing because man lacks the humility to admit that there are areas that are immune to his encroachments. Can any moral individual concern himself with abortion clinics before he has suggested, nay demanded, that our resources be committed to increase meat and poultry production, tap the wealth of the oceans, and then develop new sources of high quality proteins from the algal and microbial cultures studied experimentally these last few years? The idea that an illiterate African, Asian, or South American would rather starve than accept a diet "strange" to him, has been fully disproved by the Incaparina Program in South America. Under this program, teams of nutritionists educated the protein-starved masses to accept a flour composed of corn, sesame or soy oil, peas, and vitamin A. New recipes were accepted by the "illiterate masses" with the resultant upgrading of the national diet of millions of people. There must be unanimity in the conviction that we dare not dump potatoes, burn excess wheat, cut back on production quotas, and then make impassioned pleas for free distribution of contraceptive devices as a humanitarian effort to prevent world-wide famine.

Let us assume, once again, the hypothetical situation of world-wide food shortages uncompensated by our best utilization of the latest technological advances in food production. The question to be answered is: (c) *Are there religiously acceptable means of artifically limiting family size?*

All people, Jew and non-Jew, are enjoined to procreate. The philosophy of the Halakhah is clearly opposed to any limitation of family size.[4] Abstinence is hardly more in compliance with the spirit of the Halakhah than are other more artificial means of contraception. Only when proper motivation for family planning can be ascertained does specific methodology become the critical issue. Any halakhic principle that requires the prior determination of unexpressed motivations proves to be most difficult to legislate. Thought processes are so variable among different people, that whenever possible overt acts are substituted by our Sages for the equally authoritative intellectual commitments.[6]

Poverty that threatens a family's physical and spiritual welfare may indeed be adequate motivation for the use of acceptable contraceptive methods or for delaying marriage until there is an improvement in the financial situation.[7] However, poverty has many interpretations. The psychological poverty of the $15,000 income family surrounded by families with $50,000 yearly incomes must be clearly differentiated from the physiological poverty of the protein-starved Peruvian or Indian. The demarcation line between necessity and luxury has been obliterated so often during the maturation of the economies of the western nations, that objective criteria for a universal standard of living must be established before the need for population control can be evaluated.[8]

Many of the population-control techniques being proposed for mass use are categorically unacceptable to Judaism. Surgical intervention, in the form of vasectomies (male), oophorectomies and tubal ligations (female), or abortions, is forbidden to both Jew and non-Jew unless necessitated by life-threatening medical emergencies. Abortion is included in the Noachidic prohibition of murder. Surgical induction of male infertility *(sirus)* may likewise be proscribed in the universally applicable Noachide laws. The use of the intrauterine contraceptive devices (I.U.C.D.) such as the Grafenberg rings of the 1920's or their modern counterparts designed by Margulies and others, present unique problems to halakhic authorities. Medical scientists have yet to fully elucidate the mechanism of contraceptive action of the I.U.C.D. If the evidence we now have proves accurate, contraception is accomplished by increasing uterine or tubal contractions. The resulting expulsion of the fertilized ovum is actually an early abortion. Abortions prior to 40 days of conception are halakhically differentiated from true abortion that is equated with murder. However it is clearly prohibited unless there be adequate justification based on medical or other equally valid grounds. The recently proposed post-coital contraceptive pills must be equated with the I.U.C.D. since their effectiveness is the result of abortifacient action.[9]

If all ancillary criteria for their use are met, the anovulatory pills, or the use of a mechanical barrier with or without chemical spermicides (condom and diaphragm method) may be acceptable for use by the non-Jewish populace that is obligated to the observance of the Noachide laws. Three experimental techniques, unavailable as yet for mass use, may also prove to be acceptable. I refer to the use of various drugs by the husband to inhibit sperm formation; the injection of a silicone plug into the sperm duct to prevent the passage of sperm, but with the important feature of easy removal to restore fertility; and the infertility that can be induced by immunological means.

There are different guidelines for the Jew on this question of population control. If reduction in the birth rate of the famine-threatened population of the world is indeed the proper response, then the Jew as a world citizen should join in the world-wide effort of providing contraceptive materials to those desirous of limiting family size. The Jew as a Jew must at this time reject the suggestion that he, too, limit the size of his family. We have unique problems created for us by world citizenry. Six and one half million Jews destroyed at the hands of world citizenry in one generation represents a staggering loss. When calculated on the Malthusian geometric tables it represents an astronomical loss of our life blood. Only a total lack of moral and historic responsibility can explain the present-day statistics which show our brethren leading the list of ethnic groups with the lowest birth rates in America. Their motivation is that of an egotistic hedonist, rather than of a world citizen sleepless from nights of Malthusian nightmares. Reduction of family size must be justified only on a personal, familial basis, not as part of the demographic problem.

For the observant Jew, the use of any contraceptive device introduces new halakhic considerations. The basic prohibitions are well known. Onanism, and the *condom method* which is tantamount to onanism, are clearly Biblical prohibitions. Many halakhic authorities classify the *diaphragm method* as "casting the seed on wood and stones" and prohibit its use even if life-threatening medical consideration demands contraception.[10] The use of non-mechanical barriers to conception such as chemical spermicidals or hormonal repression of ovulation present us with the least objectionable methodology for contraception. However the hormonal contraceptives pose a new problem. Many women find that the "pill" induces intermenstrual bleeding. The earlier dosage forms caused such major or minor spotting in 65% of the women, especially during the first 3 months of use. Such spotting induces the state of *niddah* (menstrual bleeding) which necessitates abstinence and *mikvah* with all the Halakhot of menstrual bleeding. The use of I.U.C.D. likewise is often accompanied by intermenstrual spotting. If this spotting be due to physiological modification rather than mechanical damage to the uterine wall, then this too is true *niddah*. The newer low-dosage "pills", and new designs of the I.U.C.D., may minimize the problem of *niddah*. However, no observant Jew can consider their use except under the constant supervision of a competent halakhic authority.

The use of hormonal or chemical inhibitors of spermatogenesis, or of the temporary interference with sperm passage, is prohibited to the Jew. The use of chemical spermicides or the yet experimental induction of immunological infertility, or the use of injected high dosage progesterones which appear to inhibit ovulation without the problem of intermenstrual spotting, offer the best possibilities for halakhically acceptable contraception for the family that must use artificial contraceptive techniques.

The concept of proper motivation as a prerequisite for any halakhic evaluation of the contraceptive technique to be used, requires further elaboration. *Emunah* (Faith) and *Bittaḥon* (Trust) are not psychological crutches. They are the natural laws of our existence. The big sacrifice, the *Akedat Yizḥak* (the sacrifice of Isaac) is rarely demanded of us. However the small daily acts of sacrifice that are the basis of our survival as a Holy Nation, should be woven into the personality fabric of every Jew. It may be "inconvenient" to measure every thought and act against the yardstick of Torah right and wrong. Indeed to live the life of a human being clearly differentiated by his every act from those infrahuman species that are his co-tenants on this planet, is a major inconvenience. The Torah concerns itself with every aspect of our personal and interpersonal life.[11] When probing one's own motivation for family planning there must be a differentiation between proper motives and those that reflect the flaws in the

Torah personality. When a yeshiva trained young man presents to the halakhic authority motives such as: We want time to get to know each other better; we would like to travel first; if my wife can work we can raise our standard of living, he simultaneously reveals that the years of Torah training had little impact on his personality. Even if the absence of a second income necessitates continued parental support, there is little validity to the claim of financial hardship. It is a misdirected sense of dignity that dictates that money may be borrowed from parents for the purchase of a car, a home, even for travel tickets, but not to permit fuller compliance with our Torah regulations.

Competent halakhic authority may under specific circumstances permit the use of some contraceptive techniques. Any permission granted is based on major and minor details of the particular situation. Such permission is "non-transferable" and "non-extendable" in time. It is a *Pesak Halakhah* in its finest, purest, and most legalistic form. In general the following factors would first be carefully evaluated:

(a) What are the true motivations of husband and wife that induced them to seek halakhic permission?
(b) Has there been minimum compliance with the commandment, "to be fruitful"?
(c) What specific contraceptive technique is being considered?
(d) What is the medical status of husband and wife? Psychological as well as physiological factors are most significant.
(e) What is the financial status of the family?

The Torah attitude toward family planning is the consequence of its teachings about the function and purpose of the marital act. A full treatment of these teachings is beyond the scope of this paper. We are taught that the purpose of the sexual union is far more encompassing than merely the biological generative function. The laws of *niddah,* the commandment "to be fruitful", the details of *mitzvat onah* that recognizes the sexual rights of the wife, the laws of *mikvah* and the laws that determine our position on contraception, all join to formulate a philosophy of family life for the Jew. It is a program of refinement in thought and act so that the individual can fulfill his duties and obligations inherent in this intimate association of a man, his wife, his people and his God.

NOTES

1. *Ta'anit* 7a.
2. *Science,* vol. 151, Jan. 14, 1966.

3. "Time for Decisions: The Biological Crossroads," University of Colorado School of Medicine, June 1966.

4. *Rosh Ha-Shanah* 1:5; *Yevamot* 62b–63; cf. Rashi *ad locum*.

5. *Ta'anit* 11a. Cf. *Derishah* on *Oraḥ Ḥayyim* 574:5.

6. Cf. *Yevamot* 39b. Rabbenu Nissim, *Pesaḥim* 1, comment on need for *bedikah* and *bitul*.

7. *Shulḥan Arukh, Even ha-Ezer* 1, 3 and 8; Maimonides, *Hilkhot De'ot* 5:11.

8. *Ta'anit* 11; *Oraḥ Ḥayyim* 574:5. This reference has little relevance despite its erroneous application to our discussion by previous authors. Firstly the prohibition is one of abstaining from pleasurable activity when the populace is in distress and applies with equal force to calamitous childhood epidemics or wide-spread infertility. Secondly, the exemption of the *tevilah* night from this prohibition minimizes its impact on the birth rate since this is usually the period of peak fertility for the wife.

9. Recent findings raise the question of a possible abortifacient action by the anovulatory pills. At the *Third Teratology Workshop* in April 1966, experimental evidence was presented of direct damage to pre-implanted embryos by these drugs. Likewise the observation that contraception occurred even in subjects in whom ovulation was not surpressed, suggests an abortifacient role.

10. Rabbi Akiva Eger, *Responsa,* 71.

11. The health safety aspect of contraceptive pills or mechanical devices is also of halakhic concern. Man is required by Torah Law to avoid all acts that may prove injurious. In May 1966, the "pills" were reported on by a 12-member Scientific group of the World Health Organization. In general they found risks to be "minimal" with the warning that doctors keep alert to individual idiosyncracies, and that the possibility of long-term harmful effects cannot be excluded.

7
Artificial Insemination in Jewish Law
FRED ROSNER

Definition and Introduction

Artificial insemination is the instrumental deposition of semen into the female genital tract without sexual intercourse. There are two types of insemination, and they are frequently referred to by their abbreviations which are, respectively, A.I.H. (artificial insemination, husband) and A.I.D. (artificial insemination, donor). One can also use a mixture of semen obtained from husband and donor. Results of artificial insemination employing the husband's semen are good if the indication for the procedure is an anatomical defect, but fair to poor if there is moderate infertility in the male. Women can conceive two or more times from donor insemination.[1]

Artificial insemination has been practiced in animals for many years, primarily to increase the usefulness of the best male animals. For example, a single prize bull can provide enough semen to inseminate and impregnate 500 cows. In the human, John Hunter is known to have artificially inseminated a woman in London in 1790, although earlier accounts are described, while in the United States, J. Marion Sims is credited with the first insemination in 1866. Today, there are an estimated 250,000 people in this country who are the offspring of such inseminations, thousands of which are performed annually.

These days, there is much writing — books, articles, reviews and monographs — in the medical and lay press, concerning this subject from the moral, legal, religious, medical, psychological, sociological, genetic and

Reprinted from *Judaism* (Fall, 1970). Copyright © 1970 by the American Jewish Congress.

other standpoints. The present paper deals primarily with the Jewish religious viewpoint.

Since many moral, legal and religious problems may arise from artificial insemination, one might well ask why a barren couple should not simplify matters and adopt a baby? The psychological stress on women who consider themselves adulteresses following A.I.D. would be bypassed if adoption were resorted to, and, similarly, the emotional strains on some husbands, perhaps due to feelings of inadequate masculinity, might vanish if an adopted child, rather than one conceived from A.I.D., became part of the family.

There are, however, numerous reasons why a woman prefers to carry and give birth to her own child. First, her emotional craving to be pregnant is fulfilled; she has proven her femininity. Second, both the husband and the wife are part of the conception, the antenatal care, the whole pregnancy and the delivery, whereas an adopted child is usually not granted until after it is born. Third, the child physically resembles the siblings and the father, if A.I.H. is resorted to; with an adopted child this resemblance is impossible. Fourth, the adopted child's new parents always fear the appearance of the real mother, a fear which does not exist with a child born following artificial insemination. Finally, since two-thirds of the adopted infants are born to unwed mothers and the other third are unwanted babies, the genetic background of these children may be poor and less desirable to the couple wishing to acquire a child, whereas semen from donors is frequently obtained from college and graduate students.

Around the major parties who may be involved in artificial insemination, namely the husband, the wife, the child, the physician, the donor and the donor's wife, any number of legal questions may arise. Can the husband sue for divorce on the grounds of adultery following A.I.D. if he can prove that he is sterile? Can the physician and/or donor also be implicated as having participated in the adultery? Would the question of adultery vanish if the husband made the injection? Is the doctor responsible if a defective child is born? Is the doctor guilty of perjury when he signs the birth certificate, since he knows that the true father is not the one named on the birth certificate? Is the child considered legitimate? What are his rights concerning inheritance, support and custody? Can he sue for the donor's estate? Can the mother sue the donor for support of the child? Can the donor sue for custody of the child? Should the husband legally adopt the child when his wife gives birth? How do adoption laws apply here, if at all? If insemination is performed without the woman's consent, is it considered rape? If so, by whom — the physician, the donor or the husband?

Surprisingly, with only one exception, artificial insemination does not exist in the law books of any state in the union. Only Oklahoma, in 1967, passed a statute which resolves the legitimacy, support, custody and inheritance rights of a child born of A.I.D.

Jewish Viewpoint

ANCIENT SOURCES — Before entering into Jewish legal discussions in the rabbinic responsa literature dealing with artificial insemination, it might be useful to cite three major ancient sources in the Talmud and the codes of Jewish law upon which these discussions are based. They are a passage of the Babylonian Talmud, a pronouncement in the 13th century by Rabbi Perez ben Elijah of Corbeil, and the Midrashic legend of Ben Sira.

In the Talmud we find: ". . . Ben Zoma was asked: May a high priest marry a maiden who has become pregnant (yet who claims she is still a virgin)? Do we take into consideration Samuel's statement, for Samuel said: I can have repeated sexual connections without (causing) bleeding (i.e., without the woman losing her virginity) or is the case of Samuel rare? He replied: The case of Samuel is rare, but we do consider (the possibility) that she may have conceived in a bath (into which a male has discharged semen). . ."[2]

From this 5th century Talmudic passage we see that generation *sine concubito* was recognized as possible by the Sages of old. Though Rabbi Judah Rozanes of Constantinople, the renowned commentator on Maimonides' *Mishneh Torah,* expresses doubt that impregnation through bathing in water into which a man had previously discharged semen can occur,[3] many authorities, including Rabbi Hayyim Joseph David Azulai,[4] Rabbi Jonathan Eybeschuetz[5] and Rabbi Jacob Ettlinger[6] differ with him and interpret the Talmudic passage literally. Others,[7] however, agree with Rabbi Rozanes.

The second major ancient source indicating the possibility of pregnancy without sexual intercourse is by Rabbi Perez ben Elijah of Corbeil in his work *Haggahot Semak,* who states: ". . . a woman may lie on her husband's sheets but should be careful not to lie on sheets upon which another man slept lest she become impregnated from his sperm. Why are we not afraid that she become pregnant from her husband's sperm and the child will be conceived of a *niddah* (menstruating female)? The answer is that since there is no forbidden intercourse, the child is completely legitimate (literally: kosher) even from the sperm of another just as Ben Sira was legitimate. However, we are concerned about the sperm of another man because the child may eventually marry his sister. . . ."[8]

Several things emerge from this statement. First, generation *sine concubito* was recognized. Second, the offspring is considered legitimate. Third, no prohibition is mentioned concerning cohabitation of the woman with her husband afterwards, even if she has become pregnant from another. The only reason for her to avoid contact with the linen upon which another has lain is to prevent incest at a later date, i.e., the child marrying its own sibling. Finally, only forbidden intercourse would make her forbidden to her husband, whether or not she has lost her virginity, and irrespective of whether or not her male partner has emitted sperm into her genital tract during the forbidden sexual act.

The third ancient source for artificial insemination is the legend of Ben Sira, first mentioned by Rabbi Jacob Moellin Segal (1365–1427) in his work entitled *Likutei Maharil*. This Midrashic legend relates that Ben Sira was conceived without sexual intercourse by the prophet Jeremiah's daughter, in a bath, the father having been Jeremiah himself who, coerced by a group of wicked men, emitted semen into the water.[9] The legend has since been quoted many times in medical literature[10] as well as in nearly all of the rabbinic responsa dealing with artificial insemination.

Some authorities, notably Rabbi David Gans,[11] deny the legend of Ben Sira's birth having followed a conception *sine concubito*. Rabbi Gans claims that he could not find the legend of Ben Sira in either the Talmud or the Midrash, and quotes Rabbi Solomon ibn Verga, who says that Ben Sira was the son of the daughter of Joshua ben Jehozadak the High Priest mentioned in the book of Ezra.[12]

RECENT RULINGS — Since there is a vast rabbinic literature which addresses itself to the question of artificial insemination, and since the problem is so complex from the Jewish legal viewpoint, it seems desirable to subdivide the discussion into the major questions involved. Some of these are: Is the woman prohibited to her husband following an artificial insemination? Is it considered an act of adultery? What is the status of the child? Is the child a *mamzer* (illegitimate)? Is artificial insemination permitted at all? Is it permissible to use the sperm of the husband, or a donor, or a gentile? Does the donor fulfill the commandment of procreation? Is the offspring considered the child of the donor? Is the woman considered to be the pregnant or nursing wife of another and prohibited to marry again for a certain interval if her husband should die or divorce her? Is the husband permitted to provide his sperm for analysis and subsequent insemination if it is found suitable? How should one obtain the sperm from husband or donor? If artificial insemination is permitted, may it be performed during the woman's unclean period (menstruation and the ritual cleansing period thereafter)?

Is the Woman Prohibited to her Husband Following A.I.D.? — The question obviously does not apply to A.I.H. since the problem of possible adultery arises only with the semen of a man other than the husband. The case in the Talmud of the High Priest marrying a pregnant maiden who claims to be a virgin, as cited above, concludes that Samuel's capacity to impregnate a woman without producing bleeding or loss of virginity is extremely rare. Thus, the maiden is permitted to marry the High Priest as she is deemed trustworthy when she claims to be a virgin despite having been impregnated in a bath into which a man had previously discharged semen. It would seem from this Talmudic passage that only the act of sexual intercourse makes a maiden ineligible to marry a High Priest.

The analogy between these situations can, however, be invalidated. The case of a High Priest requires only that the girl's virginity be preserved to comply with the Biblical commandment (Levit. 21:14) ". . . but a virgin *(betulah)* of his own people shall he take to wife." Thus, if she becomes pregnant *sine concubito* or if she cohabits with a man without her virginity being lost, as in the case of Samuel, she is still permitted to a High Priest. However, to prohibit a woman to her husband requires only a sexual union between the woman and another *(be'ulat ba'al)* as enunciated in Deut. 22:22. Therefore, even without the loss of virginity, she is considered an adulteress.

The question remains: Does A.I.D. constitute an adulterous act or not? Rabbi Judah Rozanes states that even without loss of virginity the sexual act makes a maiden prohibited to marry a High Priest. [13]

Rabbi Hananel ben Hushi'el (11th century), in his commentary on the Talmud, interprets the discussion of the maiden and the High Priest entirely differently. He states that the whole question revolves around the requirement of the pregnant maiden to bring a sacrifice to purify herself from the ritual impurity of birth. Does the Biblical phrase "if a woman conceive seed and bear a man child, then she shall be unclean for seven days" (Levit. 12:2) apply only to a woman who has become pregnant as a result of sexual intercourse, or is it also applicable for conception *sine concubito?* This, says Rabbi Hananel, is the major question discussed in the Talmud and the problem of the maiden's permissibility to a High Priest is only coincidental.

Thus, whether or not we subscribe to Rabbi Hananel's interpretation of the Talmudic passage, it seems impossible, from this source, to resolve the question as to whether A.I.D. constitutes an act of adultery which would prohibit the woman to her husband.

We then turn to another ancient source, namely the pronouncement of Rabbi Perez ben Elijah of Corbeil, who doubts the feasibility of conception *sine concubito* and specifically states that a married woman who becomes impregnated in a bathouse is not forbidden to her husband because there has been no prohibited intercourse involved.

In our times, Rabbi Ben-Zion Uziel also states that no adultery or incest can occur unless there is a physical union of man and woman. [14] Rabbi Moses Feinstein agrees that, without an act of sexual intercourse, the woman is not prohibited to her husband even if she has been inseminated with the semen of another without the husband's consent. The law of an adulteress, says Rabbi Feinstein, applies only for the sexual act and is involved even if there is no emission of sperm or even if the act is performed in an unnatural manner, i.e. sodomy. [15] Other authorities, such as Rabbi Shalom Mordecai Schwadron, [16] Rabbi Joshua Baumol [17] and Rabbi Aaron Wolkin [18] also permit the woman to her husband if no sexual contact has occurred between her and the donor of the semen.

Others disagree vehemently. Rabbi Judah Leib Zirelson looks upon
A.I.D. as adultery, plain and simple.[19] The same view is held by Rabbi
Abraham Lurie of South Africa[20] and Rabbi Ovadiah Hadaya.[21] Rabbi
Eliezer Judah Waldenberg of Jerusalem is of the opinion that A.I.D. is akin
to adultery, and cites numerous rabbinic responsa to support his
viewpoint.[22] He dismisses the Talmudic passage and the pronouncement of
Rabbi Perez ben Elijah, stating that in both instances impregnation of the
woman occurred passively and as an accident. On the other hand, A.I.D.
entails the active participation of woman, physician and donor and thus
constitutes a prohibited act. The husband, continues Rabbi Waldenberg, is
entitled to divorce his wife on these grounds and she forfeits the monetary
settlement written into the marriage contract (ketubbah).

What is the status of the child? Is it illegitimate (mamzer)?—Here there is
marked difference of opinion in the rabbinic literature. Rabbis Zirelson,
Lurie, Hadaya, Mordecai Jacob Breisch[23] and others consider the child to
be a *mamzer,* while Rabbi Waldenberg and others consider the child a
questionable or possible *mamzer* (literally: *safek mamzer*). On the other
hand, Rabbis Uziel, Weinberg, Feinstein, Baumol, Wolkin, Joseph Saul
Nathanson,[24] Menahem Kirshbaum,[25] Raphael Pladi,[26] Abraham Y.
Neemrok[27] and Shlomoh Zalman Auerbach,[28] as well as others, are of the
opinion that the child is perfectly legitimate and not a *mamzer.*

Is Artificial Insemination from a Donor Permissible? — The previous
questions dealt with the result of A.I.D., but the question as to whether
A.I.D. is permitted at all has not yet been definitively answered. Rabbi
Waldenberg categorically prohibits it as an utter abomination, and cites
Rashi's comment on a Talmudic passage. Rashi interprets the Biblical
phrase ". . . to be a God unto thee and to thy seed after thee" (Genesis
17:7) to mean that God favors only those whose genealogy (i.e., paternity)
is known.[29] The phrase in the Talmud itself reads "to distinguish between
the seed of the first (husband) and the seed of the second." Thus, Rabbi
Waldenberg prohibits A.I.D. because the genealogy of the child is
unknown. Another reason given by Rabbi Waldenberg and in many other
responsa is "lest he marry his sister" as mentioned in the Talmud.
Therefore, avoidance of possible incest would interdict A.I.D. A third
reason for prohibiting it is that after the "proxy" father's death, his other
children may "steal" the portion of inheritance belonging to the child
produced by A.I.D. Alternatively, the child may wrongly receive
inheritance from his mother's husband upon the latter's death. Therefore,
the question of stealing an inheritance makes A.I.D. forbidden.

Even if the donor's identity is known, continues Rabbi Waldenberg,
A.I.D. is still prohibited, one reason being that the scriptural phrase "And
thou shalt not lie carnally with thy neighbor's wife to defile thyself with
her" (Levit. 18:20) includes the prohibition of having one's semen enter
another's wife even without the sexual act. There is, generally, strong

rabbinic opinion, including that of Jakobovits, that A.I.D. should be condemned as "an act of hideousness" or "an abomination" or "human stud farming." Although, technically, A.I.D. does not produce an illegitimate offspring, according to most viewpoints, it should be outlawed lest it pave the way to increased promiscuity. Only under situations of extreme need does rabbinic opinion, as stated by Schwadron and Baumol, permit A.I.D.

Does the Donor Fulfill the Commandment of Procreation? Is the Child Considered the Child of the Donor? — Again, there are differing viewpoints on this problem. The specific question is asked by Rabbi Moses of Brisk in his commentary on Caro's code as follows:

". . . one may raise the question, in the case of a woman who became pregnant in a bathhouse, whether the father has fulfilled (the precept) of 'be fruitful and multiply' (Gen. 1:28; 9:1 and 9:7) and if the child is considered his son in all respects. And in the *Likutei Maharil* we find that Ben Sira was the son of Jeremiah who washed in the bathhouse because Sira numerically equals Jeremiah . . ." i.e., the arithmetical sum of the Hebrew letters of the name Sira is identical with that of Jeremiah.[30]

Another commentary on Caro's code, that of Rabbi Samuel ben Uri, answers that the child is considered the man's son in all respects.[31] He bases his answer on the pronouncement of Rabbi Perez ben Elijah *(Haggahot Semak)* quoted above. Rabbi Rozanes quotes both Rabbi Moses of Brisk and Rabbi Samuel ben Uri and states that he agrees with them. Others, such as Rabbis Jacob ben Samuel,[32] Israel Ze'ev Mintzberg,[33] Simeon ben Zemah Duran[34] and Jacob Ettlinger[35] also subscribe to this viewpoint. Some, such as Rabbis Jacob Emden[36] and Moses Schick disagree, and claim that although the child is considered the son of the donor, the donor has not fulfilled the precept of procreation because there has been no sexual act involved. Yet others, such as Rabbis Hadaya and Moses Ayreh Leib Shapiro state that the child is neither his nor has he fulfilled the commandment of procreation.[37]

One might argue that if the case of impregnation in the bathhouse, where there was no intent on the part of the true father to impregnate the woman, results in a child considered to be his son in all respects and he has fulfilled the commandment of procreation (according to most authorities), then certainly *a fortiori* the same results should pertain to A.I.D. where at least the doctor and the woman intentionally seek a pregnancy. This argument can be countered by the fact that anonymous donors provide their sperm to semen banks without intention as to their use for a specific woman, but on the other hand, there is the intent on the part of the donor that his sperm be utilized for the purpose of artificial insemination. Thus, the argument of intent seems to have little if any validity or applicability to the problem under discussion.

Is the Woman Following A.I.D. Considered to be the Pregnant or

Nursing Wife of Another? — Should the woman's husband die or divorce her following A.I.D., is she allowed to remarry while she is still pregnant or, following delivery, while she is still nursing? A Talmudic pronouncement states that a man should not marry the pregnant wife of another or the nursing wife of another, even though she has been divorced or widowed, until after the child is born or until she stops nursing, respectively.[38] Three reasons are given. First, we are concerned lest the woman conceive again while she is pregnant, thus making it impossible to identify which part of the child is the offspring of the first husband and which is the offspring of the second. Whether a woman can conceive by two different men and produce one child has been stated as fact by some[39] and denied by others.[40] Second, there may be danger to the fetus from abdominal pressure from sexual relations with the new husband, who might not be as careful to avoid harming the unborn fetus as would the true father. Third, if the woman conceives during the nursing period, her milk would become turbid and the nursing baby might die of starvation.

This rule has been codified by Maimonides who states: "And the Sages also ordained that a man not marry the pregnant wife of another or the nursing wife of another even though (in the former case), the owner of the seed which made her pregnant is known— lest the fetus be harmed during intercourse because he is not careful with the child of another. And (in the case of) a nursing woman lest her milk become turbid and he does not pay attention to heal the milk with things which improve turbid milk."[41]

Rabbi Jacob ben Asher and Rabbi Joseph Caro in their codes also state that "the Sages decreed that a person should not marry nor betroth the pregnant wife of another or the nursing wife of another . . .". [42]

With this discussion as background, Rabbi Waldenberg ponders whether the decree against a man marrying the pregnant or nursing wife of another is applicable to the husband whose wife has undergone A.I.D. He concludes in the affirmative and the new husband must, as a result, abstain from cohabitation with his wife until after she stops nursing. Some rabbis, such as Malchiel Zevi ha-Levi Tanenbaum,[43] Zirelson and Uziel agree with Waldenberg, whereas others, such as Hayyim Joseph David Azulai,[44] are in doubt whether the decree applies to A.I.D.

Artificial Insemination Using the Husband's Semen — Using the husband's sperm to inseminate the woman would eliminate many of the objections raised regarding A.I.D., such as possible adultery, the offspring possibly marrying a sibling, "stealing" of an inheritance and licentiousness, among others. Is then A.I.H. permissible? Difference of opinion exists on this question in the responsa literature. Rabbis Feinstein, Schwadron, Wolkin, Zevi Pesah Frank and others state that A.I.H. is permissible.[45] Others, such as Rabbis Tanenbaum and Waldenberg frown upon it, stating it is permissible only in extreme situations. The rabbis who normally forbid

A.I.H. claim that Rabbi Elijah ben Perez' pronouncement allowing a woman to lie on sheets upon which her husband has lain (and possibly emitted sperm) is because impregnation in that situation is extremely rare. However, A.I.H. commonly leads to pregnancy. Furthermore, in the case described by Rabbi Elijah, pregnancy occurred passively and by accident, whereas in A.I.H. the physician, the donor and the woman are active participants. Furthermore, claim the rabbis who object to A.I.H., if A.I.H. were permitted, the physician might be tempted to add foreign semen to that of the husband in order to facilitate conception, thus performing A.I.D., which is certainly prohibited. Even the rabbis who permit A.I.H. would prohibit the use of a mixture of the husband's and another man's sperm. Thus, Rabbi Feinstein states that such an admixture of semens is a trick to overcome the weakness of the husband's sperm and is, therefore, considered like A.I.D. and is not A.I.H. Rabbis Waldenberg, Henkin and others agree. One must be sure that only the husband's sperm is employed and only trustworthy physicians must be sought.

Insemination While the Woman is Ritually Unclean (Niddah)—If we follow the permissive ruling regarding A.I.H., then the question arises as to whether it is allowed to perform artificial insemination on a woman during the period of her ritual uncleanliness.

It is related about Rabbi Abraham Isaiah Karelitz, known as *Ḥazon Ish* (*Ha-Ish ve-Ḥazono,* p. 33), that he was asked about a woman who had very short menstrual cycles so that her fertile periods always occurred during her counting of the "seven clean days." Physicians recommended that A.I.H. be performed during this period prior to the woman's *tevilah* (ritual immersion for purification). Rabbi Karelitz, who was opposed to artificial insemination, answered that she should abbreviate her unclean period to four days but that she should not be inseminated while ritually unclean prior to *tevilah*.

Rabbis Schwadron, Waldenberg, Hadaya, Tanenbaum and others permit A.I.H. but not while the woman is ritually unclean, whereas Rabbis Feinstein, Wolkin, Auerbach and others permit A.I.H. even during this period if no other way proves successful.

An additional requirement before A.I.H. can be performed is an interval of time after the wedding during which pregnancy has been attempted in the usual manner of cohabitation, but without results. This interval must be ten years, according to Rabbi Isaac Jacob Weiss,[46] five years in the opinion of Rabbi Feinstein,[47] two years according to Rabbi Karelitz and long enough to establish the medical necessity for A.I.H., in the opinion of Rabbi Waldenberg.

Procurement of Semen for Artificial Insemination — Since most rabbinic opinion sanctions A.I.H. under circumstances where pregnancy can be achieved in no other way, the question arises as to how to obtain the semen for the insemination without transgressing the prohibition of improper emission of seed or emission of semen for naught. This was the sin of Er and Onan (Genesis 38:7-10). This subject alone is of such broad dimensions as to require a separate essay and the interested reader is referred to extensive discussions elsewhere. [48]

In brief, most rabbis (Frank, Feinstein, Waldenberg, Schwadron, Wolkin, Shapiro, Auerbach, Mintzberg, Baumol) state that procurement of semen by acceptable means from the husband for insemination into his wife is permissible and does not constitute emission of seed for naught, since the semen will be used to fulfill the commandment of procreation. Some, like Rabbis Tanenbaum, Uziel, Hadaya and Breisch disagree, but they are in the minority. Two methods of obtaining the sperm are mentioned in the Talmud where we find a discussion concerning a Priest who is wounded in his testicles *(pezu'a dakkah)* or whose membrum is cut off *(kerut shafkhah)*:

". . . Rabbi Judah stated in the name of Samuel: If it (the membrum) had a small perforation which was closed up, the man is deemed to be unfit if the wound re-opens when semen is emitted, but if it does not reopen the man is regarded as fit. . . . Raba, the son of Rabbah, sent to Rabbi Joseph: Will our Master instruct us how to proceed (to test whether the semen will re-open the closed perforation). The other replied: Warm barley bread is procured and placed upon the man's anus. Thereby the flow of semen sets in, and the effect can be observed . . . said Abaye, colored (women's) garments are dangled before him (exciting his passions thus causing semen emission). . . ." [49]

Both of these two methods, as well as others, are perfectly acceptable, according to Rabbi Feinstein. [50] In addition, it is permissible to think of a woman in order to excite the emotions and to cause semen emission for the purpose of artificial insemination into one's wife. The least objectionable method is the procurement of sperm from coitus interruptus, or, if this is unsatisfactory for any reason, a condom may be applied on the male membrum prior to coitus. These latter two procedures involve the natural sex act and are, therefore, most acceptable to Jewish law. Masturbation to obtain sperm is strongly condemned by Rabbi Feinstein, based upon the following Talmudic passage: ". . . Rabbi Eleazar stated: Who are referred to in the scriptural text "Your hands are full of blood" (Isaiah 1:15)? Those that commit masturbation with their hands. It was taught at the school of Rabbi Ishmael "Thou shalt not commit adultery" (Exod. 20:13) implies that thou shalt not practice masturbation either with hand or with foot. . .". [51]

To have sexual intercourse in the physician's office and for the physician to retrieve the sperm from the vagina of the woman to combine several ejaculates for subsequent insemination is considered licentious and improper, according to Rabbi Feinstein, although Rabbi Waldenberg allows this practice.[52] Rabbi Waldenberg also permits masturbation to obtain semen if all the other methods cannot be employed. He states that, if possible, the physician should perform the masturbation but, if that is not feasible, the husband can do it. Rabbi Waldenberg further states that one is permitted to extract semen directly from the testicle.

Conclusions

Artificial insemination using the semen of a donor other than the husband is considered by most rabbinic opinion to be an abomination and strictly prohibited for a variety of reasons, including the possibility of incest, lack of genealogy and the problems of inheritance. Some authorities regard A.I.D. as adultery, requiring the husband to divorce his wife and her forfeiture of the *ketubbah,* and even the physician and the donor are guilty when involved in this act akin to adultery. Most rabbinic opinion, however, states that without a sexual act involved, the woman is not guilty of adultery and is not prohibited to cohabit with her husband.

Regarding the status of the child, rabbinic opinion is divided. Most consider the offspring to be legitimate as was Ben Sira, the product of conception *sine concubito,* a small minority of rabbis consider the child illegitimate, and at least two authorities take a middle view and label the child a *safek mamzer.* Considerable rabbinic opinion regards the child (legitimate or illegitimate) to be the son of the donor in all respects (i.e., inheritance, support, custody, incest, Levirate marriage, and the like). Some regard the child to be the donor's son only in some respects but not others. Some rabbis state that although the child is considered the donor's son in all respects, the donor has not fulfilled the commandment of procreation. A minority of rabbinic authority asserts that the child is not considered the donor's son at all.

The woman, following A.I.D. or A.I.H., is considered to be the nursing or pregnant wife of another and, if her husband dies or divorces her, she cannot remarry another until after she has finished nursing the child. Several rabbis also invoke this rule to prohibit a man to cohabit with his pregnant or nursing wife following A.I.D.

There is near unanimity of opinion that the use of semen from the husband is permissible if no other method is possible for the wife to become pregnant. However, certain qualifications exist. There must have been a reasonable period of waiting since marriage (2, 5, or 10 years or until medical proof of the absolute necessity for A.I.H.), and, according to many authorities, the insemination may not be performed during the wife's period of ritual impurity.

It is permitted by most rabbis to obtain sperm from the husband both for analysis and for insemination, but difference of opinion exists as to the method to be used in the procurement of it. Masturbation should be avoided if at all possible and *coitus interruptus,* retrieval of sperm from the vagina, or the use of a condom seem to be the preferred methods.

Since many important legal and moral considerations which cannot be enunciated in the presentation of general principles may weigh heavily upon the verdict in any given situation it seems advisable to submit each individual case to rabbinic judgment which, in turn, will be based upon expert medical advice and other prevailing circumstances.

NOTES

1. D. P. Murphy and E. F. Torrano, "The Day of Conception: A Study of 48 Women Having 2 or More Conceptions by Donor Insemination," *Fertility and Sterility,* 14:410–415, 1963.

2. Babylonian Talmud *Hagigah* 14b.

3. J. Rozanes, *Hilkhot Ishut,* commentary *Mishneh Le-Melekh* on Maimonides' code, 15:4.

4. Quoted by I. Jakobovits in "Artificial Insemination, Birth Control and Abortion," *Ha-Rofe ha-Ivri* 2:169–183 (Eng.) and 114–129 (Heb.), 1953.

5. J. Eybeschuetz, *"Hilkhot Ishut,"* commentary *Benei Ahuvah* on Maimonides' code, 15:6.

6. J. Ettlinger, Commentary *Arukh la-Ner* on *Yevamot* 12b.

7. Moses Schick (Maharam Schick), *Taryag Mitzvot,* chapter 1; Solomon Schick, *"Even ha-Ezer," Responsa Rashbam,* chapter 8.

8. Quoted by Rabbi Joel Sirkes *(Bah* or *Bayit Hadash),* in his commentary on Rabbi Jacob ben Asher's *Tur Shulhan Arukh, Yoreh De'ah,* 195. Also quoted by Rabbi David ben Samuel ha-Lev *(Taz* or *Turei Zahav),* in his commentary on *Shulhan Arukh, Yoreh De'ah,* 195:7.

9. I. D. Eisenstein, *"Alfa Beta de-Ben Sira,"* in *Ozar Midrashim* (New York, 1928), p. 43.

10. J. Preuss, *Biblical and Talmudic Medicine,* tr. by Fred Rosner (New York, Sanhedrin Press, 1978), pp. 463-464; H. Friedenwald, *The Jews and Medicine* (Baltimore, Johns Hopkins Press, 1944), vol. I, p. 386; I. Jakobovits, *Jewish Medical Ethics* (New York, Bloch Publishers, 1959), Appendix on "Artificial Insemination," pp. 244–250.

11. D. Gans, *Zemah David* (Offenbach, 1968), 1:1:441, p. 14b.

12. S. Verga, *Shevet Yehudah* (Lemberg, 1846).

13. J. Rozanes, *Hilkhot Issurei Bi'ah* (Laws of Forbidden Sexual Connections), op. cit., 17:13.

14. B. Uziel, *"Even ha-Ezer," Mishpetei Uzi'el* (Tel Aviv, 1935), no. 19.

15. M. Feinstein, *"Even ha-Ezer," Iggerot Moshe* (New York, 1961), no. 10.

16. S. M. Schwadron, *Maharsham* (Brezany, 1910), vol. 3, no. 268.

17. Y. Baumol, *Emek Halakhah* (New York, 1934), no. 68.

18. A. Wolkin, *"Even ha-Ezer," Zekan Aharon* (New York, 1951), part 2, no. 97.

19. J. L. Zirelson, *Ma'arekhei Lev* (Kishinev, 1932), no. 73.
20. A. Lurie, *Haposek* (Tel Aviv, [Heshvan-Kislev 5710] 1949).
21. O. Hadaya, *Hazra'a Melakhutit* (Artificial Insemination), *No'am* vol. 1, 1958 (5718), pp. 130-137.
22. E. Y. Waldenberg, *Ziz Eli'ezer* (Jerusalem, 1967). vol. 9, no. 51, section 4.
23. M. J. Breisch, *Helkat Ya'akov* (Jerusalem, 1951), no. 24.
24. J. S. Nathanson, *Sho'el u-Meshiv* (Lemberg, 1868), part 3. vol. 3, no. 132.
25. M. Kirshbaum, *Menahem u-Meshiv,* quoted by D. B. Kranzer in *Hazra'a Melakhutit* (Artificial Insemination). *No'am,* vol. 1, 1958 (5718), pp. 111–123.
26. R. Pladi, *Yad Rama* quoted by D. B. Kranzer, *loc. cit.*
27. A. Y. Neemrok, *Kashrut ha-Yilad* (The Legitimacy of the Offspring), *No'am,* vol. 1, 1958 (5718), pp. 143–144.
28. S. Z. Auerbach, *Hazra'a Melakhutit* (Artificial Insemination), *No'am* vol. 1, 1958 (5718), pp. 145–166.
29. Commentary of Rashi in *Yevamot* 42a.
30. *Helkat Mehokek* on *Even ha-Ezer, Shulhan Arukh,* 1:6.
31. *Beit Shemu'el* on *Even ha-Ezer, Shulhan Arukh,* 1:6.
32. Jacob Ben Samuel, *Beit Ya'akov* (Dyrenfurth, 1696), no. 122.
33. I. Z. Mintzberg, *No'am,* vol. 1, 1958 (5718), p. 129.
34. S. Duran, *Tashbez* (Amsterdam, 1739), part 3, no. 263.
35. J. Ettlinger, *Arukh le-Ner on Yevamot* (Pietrkow, 1914), p. 10.
36. J. Emden, *She'elat Yavez* (Altona, 1739), part 2, no. 96.
37. M. A. L. Shapiro, *Hazra'a Melakhutit* (Artificial Insemination), *No'am,* vol. 1, 1958 (5718), pp. 138–142.
38. *Yevamot* 36b and 42a.
39. *Tosafot* on *Sotah,* 42b s.v., *Me'ah Pappi;* Jerusalem Talmud, *Yevamot* 4:2.
40. Rashi on *Sotah,* 42b s.v. *Bar Me'ah Pappi.*
41. Maimonides, *Hilkhot Gerushin* (Laws Pertaining to Divorce) *Mishneh Torah,* 11:25.
42. Jacob ben Asher, *Even ha-Ezer, Tur Shulhan Arukh,* 13:11; J. Caro, *Even ha-Ezer, Shulhan Arukh,* 13:11.
43. M. Z. Tanenbaum, *Divrei Malki'el* (Vilna, 1901), part 4, nos. 107 and 108.
44. H. J. D. Azulai, *Birkei Yosef* quoted by Waldenberg, see note 19.
45. M. Feinstein, *Even ha-Ezer, Iggerot Moshe,* part 2, no. 18 (New York, 1963), supplement to *Hoshen Mishpat;* A. Wolkin, *Even ha-Ezer, Zekan Aharon,* part 2, no. 97; Zevi Pesah Frank, as quoted by Waldenberg; *Yabbi'a Omer,* part 2, no. 1, as quoted by Feinstein.
46. I. J. Weiss, *Minhat Yizhak* (London, 1955).
47. M. Feinstein, *Even ha-Ezer, Iggerot Moshe* (New York, 1963), part 2, no. 16. Supplement to *Hoshen Mishpat.*
48. L. M. Epstein, "Wasting Nature," *Sex Laws and Customs in Judaism* (New York, Ktav, 1967), pp. 144–147; S. J. Zevin, *Hashhatat Zera, Talmudic Encyclopedia* (Jerusalem, 1965), vol. 11, pp. 129–141.
49. *Yevamot* 76a.
50. M. Feinstein, *Even ha-Ezer, Iggerot Moshe* (New York, 1961), no. 70.
51. *Niddah* 13b.
52. E. J. Waldenberg, Op. cit., section 1, chapter 2.

8

Jewish Views on Abortion

IMMANUEL JAKOBOVITS

With the staggering rise in the rate of abortions — the overwhelming majority of them illegal according to most states' laws — and with the motives for such operations now including the fear of abnormal births as well as birth control considerations, abortion has lately become the most widely debated medico-moral subject.* What was previously either a therapeutic measure for the safety of the mother or a plainly criminal act is now being widely advocated as a means to prevent the birth of possibly defective children, to curb the sordid indignities and hazards imposed on women resorting to clandestine operators, and simply to contain the population explosion. Under the mounting pressure of these new factors, combined with the widespread violation of the existing laws even by reputable practitioners, there is increasing agitation for a liberalization of these laws, particularly among physicians.[1] Many physicians, individually and as organized groups, are pressing for legislative modifications which would give them far more discretionary power than they presently enjoy. They claim that, within some broad general guidelines, the decision whether or not legally to terminate a pregnancy should be left to their judgment. In part, this claim is already being asserted on a wide scale through the establishment at numerous hospitals of "abortion boards," composed solely of physicians, charged with the responsibility of sanctioning all such operations.

In the Jewish view, this line of argument cannot be upheld. The judgment that is here required, while it may be based on medical evidence, is clearly of a moral nature. The decision on whether, and under what circumstances, it is right to destroy a germinating human life depends on the assessment and weighing of values, on determining the title to life in any given case. Such

*This paper was written prior to the U.S. Supreme Court decision on abortion.

Reprinted from D. T. Smith (ed.), *Abortion and the Law.* Copyright © 1965, 1967 by Western Reserve University Press.

value judgments are entirely outside the province of medical science. No amount of training or experience in medicine can help in ascertaining the criteria necessary for reaching such capital verdicts, for making such life-and-death decisions. Such judgments pose essentially a moral, not a medical, problem. Hence they call for the judgment of moral, not medical, specialists.

Physicians, by demanding that as the practitioners in this field they should have the right to determine or adjudicate the laws governing their practice, are making an altogether unprecedented claim not advanced by any other profession. Lawyers do not argue that, because law is their speciality, the decision on what is legal should be left to their conscience. And teachers do not claim that, as the profession competent in education, the laws governing their work, such as on prayers at public schools, should be administered or defined at their discretion. Such claims are patently absurd, for they would demand jurisdiction on matters completely beyond their professional competence.

There is no more justice or logic in advancing similar claims for the medical profession. A physician, in performing an abortion or any other procedure involving moral considerations, such as artificial insemination or euthanasia, is merely a technical expert; but he is no more qualified than any other layman to pronounce on the rights or legality of such acts, let alone to determine what these rights should be, relying merely on the whims or dictates of his conscience. The decision on whether a human life, once conceived, is to be or not to be, therefore, belongs to moral experts, or to legislatures guided by such experts.

Jewish Law

A. The Claims of Judaism   Every monotheistic religion embodies within its philosophy and legislation a system of ethics — a definition of moral values. None does so with greater precision and comprehensiveness than Judaism. It emphatically insists that the norms of moral conduct can be governed neither by the accepted notions of public opinion nor by the individual conscience. In the Jewish view, the human conscience is meant to enforce laws, not to make them. Right and wrong, good and evil, are absolute values which transcend the capricious variations of time, place, and environment, just as they defy definition by relation to human intuition or expediency. These values, Judaism teaches, derive their validity from the Divine revelation at Mount Sinai, as expounded and developed by sages faithful to, and authorized by, its writ.

B. The Sources of Jewish Law   For a definition of these values, one must look to the vast and complex corpus of Jewish law, the authentic expression of all Jewish religious and moral thought. The literary depositories of Jewish law extend over nearly four thousand years, from the Bible and the Talmud, serving as the immutable basis of the main principles, to the great medieval codes and the voluminous rabbinical responsa writings recording practical verdicts founded on these principles, right up to the present day.

These sources, to be detailed below, spell out a very distinct attitude on all aspects of the abortion problem. They clearly indicate that Judaism, while it does not share the rigid stand of the Roman Catholic Church which unconditionally proscribes any direct destruction of the fetus from the moment of conception, refuses to endorse the far more permissive views of many Protestant denominations. The traditional Jewish position is somewhere between these two extremes, corresponding roughly to the law as currently in force in all but five American states, namely, recognizing only a grave hazard to the mother as a legitimate indication for therapeutic abortion. [2]

1.   *Abortion in the Bible.* — The legislation of the Bible makes only one reference to our subject, and this is by implication:

> And if men strive together, and hurt a woman with child, so that her fruit depart, and yet no harm follow, he shall be surely fined, according as the woman's husband shall lay upon him; and he shall pay as the judges determine. But if any harm follow, then shalt thou give life for life. . . .[3]

a.   *The Jewish Interpretation.* — This crucial passage, by one of the most curious twists of literary fortunes, marks the parting of the ways between the Jewish and Christian rulings on abortion. According to the Jewish interpretation, if "no harm follow" the "hurt" to the woman resulting in the loss of her fruit refers to the survival of the woman following her miscarriage; in that case there is no capital guilt involved, and the attacker is merely liable to pay compensation for the loss of her fruit. "But if any harm follow," *i.e.,* if the woman is fatally injured, then the man responsible for her death has to "give life for life"; in that event the capital charge of murder exempts him from any monetary liability for the aborted fruit.[4]

This interpretation is also borne out by the rabbinical exegesis of the verse defining the law of murder: "He that smiteth *a man,* so that he dieth, shall surely be put to death . . ."[5] which the rabbis construed to mean "a man, but not a fetus."[6]

These passages clearly indicate that the killing of an unborn child is not considered as murder punishable by death in Jewish law.

b.   *The Christian Interpretation.* — The Christian tradition disputing this view goes back to a mistranslation in the Septuagint. There, the Hebrew for "no harm follow" was replaced by the Greek for "[her child be born] imperfectly formed."[7] This interpretation, distinguishing between an unformed and a formed fetus and branding the killing of the latter as murder, was accepted by Tertullian, who was ignorant of Hebrew, and by later church fathers. The distinction was subsequently embodied in canon law as well as in Justinian Law.[8] This position was further reinforced by the belief that the "animation" (entry of the soul) of a fetus occurred on the fortieth or eightieth day after conception for males and females respectively, an idea first expressed by Aristotle,[9] and by the doctrine, firmly enunciated by Saint Augustine and other early Christian authorities, that the unborn child was included among those condemned to eternal perdition if he died unbaptized.[10] Some even regarded the death or murder of an unborn child as a greater calamity than that of a baptized person.[11] Eventually the distinction between animate and inanimate fetuses was lost; and since 1588, the Catholic Church has considered as murder the killing of any human fruit from the moment of conception.[12]

This position is maintained to the present day.[13] It assumes that potential life, even in the earliest stages of gestation, enjoys the same value as any existing adult life. Hence, the Catholic Church never tolerates any direct abortion, even when, by allowing the pregnancy to continue, both mother and child will perish;[14] for "better two deaths than one murder."[15]

2. *Abortion in the Talmud.* — Jewish law assumes that the full title to life arises only at birth. Accordingly, the Talmud rules:

> If a woman is in hard travail [and her life cannot otherwise be saved,] one cuts up the child within her womb and extracts it member by member, because her life comes before that of [the child]. But if the greater part [or the head] was delivered, one may not touch it, for one may not set aside one person's life for the sake of another.[16]

This ruling, sanctioning embryotomy to save the mother in her mortal conflict with her unborn child, is also the sole reference to abortion in the principal codes of Jewish law.[17] They add only the further argument that such a child, being in "pursuit" of the mother's life, may be destroyed as an "aggressor" following the general principle of self-defense.[18]

This formulation of the attitude toward abortion in the classic sources of Jewish law implies (1) that the only indication considered for abortion is a hazard to the mother's life, and (2) that, otherwise, the destruction of an unborn child is a grave offense, although not murder.

3. *Abortion in Rabbinical Writings.* — Some of these conclusions, and their ramifications, are more fully discussed in later rabbinical writings, notably the prolific responsa literature. Before some of these writings are detailed, it should be pointed out that criminal abortion, as distinct from therapeutic abortion, is scarcely mentioned in Jewish sources at all. This omission seems all the more glaring in view of the extraordinary attention given to the subject in Christian literature and other legislation in ancient, medieval, and modern times. Criminal abortion was, with few exceptions,

simply nonexistent in Jewish society. Consequently, the legal and moral problems involved were rarely submitted to rabbinical judgment, and their consideration thus did not enter into the responsa, at least not until comparatively recent times. [19]

Elaborating on the law as defined in the Talmud and the codes, the responsa add several significant rulings. While the status of a child conceived by rape is not discussed, several opinions are expressed on the legality of aborting a product of incest or adultery, both capital offenses in Biblical law. One eighteenth-century authority considered the case of an adulteress different insofar as her capital guilt would also forfeit the life of the fruit she carried. [20] But others maintained that there could be no distinction between a bastard and a legitimate fetus in this respect, and that any sanction to destroy such a product would open the floodgates to immorality and debauchery. [21] A later responsum also prohibited such an operation. [22]

Since the Talmud permits the sacrifice of the child to save the mother only prior to the emergence of its head or the greater part of its body from the birth canal, [23] a widely discussed question concerns the right to dismember the fetus even during the final stage of parturition if it is feared that otherwise both mother and child may die. As the danger to the mother usually is likely to occur before that stage is reached, this is mainly a hypothetical question, but it may be of some practical significance in the case of a breech-birth if the child's head cannot be extracted following the delivery of the rest of the body. Notwithstanding the rule that the child in principle assumes full and equal human rights once the major part is born, and that consequently one may not thereafter save one life (the mother's) at the cost of another (the child's), this particular case may be an exception because (1) the child is liable to die in any event, whether the operation is carried out or not, while the mother can be rescued at the expense of the child, and (2) in the Jewish view the viability of a child is not fully established until it has passed the thirtieth day of its life, so that of the two lives here at stake the one is certain and established, while the other is still in some doubt. This slight inequality in value is too insignificant to warrant the deliberate sacrifice of the child for the sake of the mother if, without such sacrifice, the child would survive; but it is a sufficient factor to tip the scales in favor of the mother if the alternative is the eventual loss of both lives. Hence, with one exception, [24] rabbinical verdicts are inclined to countenance the intervention, provided the physician is confident of the success of the operation. [25]

4. *Deformed Children in Rabbinical Writings.* — More recently the tragic problem of abortions indicated by suspected fetal defects has occupied considerable space in rabbinical writings. The recognition of this problem only dates from 1941, when an Australian medical journal first drew attention to the incidence of abnormalities resulting from rubella [26] in the mother during her early pregnancy. Since then, the legal, moral, and

religious issues involved have been widely but still inconclusively debated in medical as well as non-medical circles. They aroused much public controversy when it was established that the birth of thousands of deformed babies could be traced to drugs, notably thalidomide, taken by pregnant mothers and when many such mothers sought to have their pregnancies terminated for fear that they would deliver malformed children.

All the authorities of Jewish law are agreed that physical or mental abnormalities do not in themselves compromise the title to life, whether before or after birth. Cripples and idiots, however incapacitated, enjoy the same human rights (though not necessarily legal competence) as normal persons.[27] Human life being infinite in value, its sanctity is bound to be entirely unaffected by the absence of any or all mental faculties or by any bodily defects: any fraction of infinity still remains infinite.

5. *Monster-Births in Rabbinical Writings.*—The absolute inviolability of any human being, however deformed, was affirmed in the first responsum on the status of monster-births. Early in the nineteenth century, a famous rabbinical scholar advised a questioner that it was forbidden to destroy a grotesquely misshapen child; he ruled that to kill, or even starve to death, any being born of a human mother was unlawful as homicide.[28] Indeed, in a somewhat less legal context, a twelfth-century moralistic work referred to a ruling against terminating the life of a child born with teeth and a tail like an animal, counseling instead the removal of these features.[29]

C. Arguments against the Destruction of Defectives   Based on these principles and precedents, present-day rabbis are unanimous in condemning abortion, feticide, or infanticide to eliminate a crippled being, before or after birth, as an unconscionable attack on the sanctity of life. Further considerations leading to this conclusion include the arguments that, conversely, the saving of an unborn child's life justifies the violation of the Sabbath (permitted only when human life is at stake);[30] that such a child is not in "pursuit" of the mother, thus excluding an important condition for the right to perform a therapeutic abortion;[31] that the interruption of a pregnancy is not without hazards to the mother, particularly the danger of rendering her sterile and the increase in maternal mortality resulting from abortions, as attested by physicians;[32] and that the killing of an embryo, while technically not murder due to a "scriptural decree," yet constitutes "an appurtenance of murder" because "in matters affecting human life we also consider that which is going to be [a human being] without any further action, following the laws of nature."[33]

These considerations would be valid even if it were known for certain that the expected child would be born deformed. The almost invariable doubts about such a contingency only strengthen the objections to abortion in these circumstances, especially in view of the Talmudic maxim that in matters of life and death the usual majority rule does not operate; any chance, however slim, that a life may be saved must always be given the benefit of the doubt.[34]

A similar attitude was adopted in a recent rabbinical article on the celebrated trial in Liege (Belgium) in which a mother and others were acquitted of guilt for the confessed killing of a thalidomide baby.[35] The author denounces abortion for such a purpose as well as the Liege verdict. "The sole legitimate grounds for killing a fetus are the urgent needs of the mother and her healing, whereas in these circumstances the mother's efforts to have the child aborted are based on self-love and plain egotism, wrapped in a cloak of compassion for this unfortunate creature, and this cannot be called a necessity for the mother at all."[36]

D. Psychological Considerations   On the other hand, Jewish law would consider a grave psychological hazard to the mother as no less weighty a reason for an abortion than a physical threat. On these grounds a seventeenth-century responsum permitted an abortion in a case where it was feared the mother would otherwise suffer an attack of hysteria imperiling her life.[37] If it is genuinely feared that a continued pregnancy and eventual birth under these conditions might have such debilitating effects on the mother as to present a danger to her own life or the life of another by suicidal or violent tendencies, however remote this danger may be, a therapeutic abortion may be indicated with the same justification as for other medical reasons. But this fear would have to be very real, attested to by the most competent psychiatric opinion, and based on previous experiences of mental imbalance.[38]

Moral and Social Considerations

The legalistic structure of these conclusions must be viewed in the context of Judaism's moral philosophy and against the background of contemporary social conditions.

A. The "Cruelty" of the Abortion Laws   At the outset, it is essential, in order to arrive at an objective judgment, to disabuse one's mind of the often one-sided, if not grossly partisan, arguments in the popular (and sometimes medical) presentations of the issues involved. A hue and cry is raised about the "cruelty" of the present abortion laws.[39] Harrowing scenes are depicted, in the most lurid colors, of girls and married women selling their honor and their fortunes, exposing themselves to mayhem and death at the hands of some greedy and ill-qualified abortionist in a dark, unhygienic back-alley, and facing the prospect of being hunted and haunted like criminals for the rest of their lives — all because safe, honorable, and reasonably priced methods to achieve the same ends are barred from hospitals and licensed physicians' offices by our "barbaric" statutes. Equally distressing are the accounts and pictures of pitifully deformed children born because our "antiquated" abortion laws did not permit us to forestall their and their parents' misfortune. And then there are, of course, always heart-strings or sympathy to be pulled by the sight of "unwanted" children taxing the patience and resources of parents already "burdened" with too large a brood.

There is, inevitably, some element of cruelty in most laws. For a person who has spent his last cent before the tax bill arrives, the income tax laws are unquestionably "cruel"; and to a man passionately in love with a married woman the adultery laws must appear "barbaric." Even more universally "harsh" are the military draft regulations which expose young men to acute danger and their families to great anguish and hardship.

B. Moral Standards in Society   All these resultant "cruelties" are surely no valid reason for changing those laws. No civilized society could survive without laws which occasionally spell some suffering for individuals. Nor can any public moral standards be maintained without strictly enforced regulations calling for extreme restraints and sacrifices in some cases. If the criterion for the legitimacy of laws were to be the complete absence of "cruel" effects, we should abolish or drastically liberalize not only our abortion laws, but our statutes on marriage, narcotics, homosexuality, suicide, euthanasia, and numerous other laws which inevitably result in personal anguish from time to time.

So far our reasoning, which could be supported by any number of references to Jewish tradition, has merely sought to demolish the "cruelty" factor as a valid argument per se by which to judge the justice or injustice of any law. It still has to be demonstrated that the restrictions on abortion are morally sound enough and sufficiently important to the public welfare to outweigh the consequential hardships in individual cases.

C. The Hidden Side of the Problem   What the fuming editorials and harrowing documentaries on the abortion problem do not show are pictures of radiant mothers fondling perfectly healthly children who would never have been alive if their parents had been permitted to resort to abortion in moments of despair. There are no statistics on the contributions to society of outstanding men and women who would never have been born had the abortion laws been more liberal. Nor is it known how many "unwanted" children eventually turn out to be the sunshine of their families.

A Jewish moralistic work of the twelfth century relates the following deeply significant story:

> A person constantly said that, having already a son and a daughter, he was anxious lest his wife become pregnant again. For he was not rich and

asked how would he find sufficient sustenance. Said a sage to him: "When a child is born, the Holy One, blessed be He, provides the milk beforehand in the mother's breast; therefore, do not worry." But he did not accept the wise man's words, and he continued to fret. Then a son was born to him. After a while, the child became ill, and the father turned to the sage: "Pray for my son that he shall live." Exclaimed the sage: "To you applies the Biblical verse: 'Suffer not thy mouth to bring thy flesh into guilt.' "[40]

Some children may be born unwanted, but there are no unwanted children aged five or ten years.

D. Abortion Statistics   There are, then — even from the purely utilitarian viewpoint of "cruelty" *versus* "happiness" or "usefulness" — two sides to this problem, and not just one as pretended by those agitating for reform. There are the admittedly tragic cases of maternal indignities and deaths as well as of congenital deformities resulting from our restrictive abortion laws. But, on the other hand, there are the countless happy children and useful citizens whose births equally result from these laws. What is the ratio between these two categories?

If one considers that even with the existing, rigid laws there are well over one million abortions performed annually in the United States (most of them by reputable physicians), it stands to reason that a relaxation of these laws would raise the abortion rate by many millions. In Hungary, for instance, where abortions were legalized in 1956, state physicians have terminated about two million pregnancies since then (in a population of ten million), amounting to three abortions for every live birth.[41] Even allowing for the more widespread recourse to birth control and for some stricter controls in the proposed abortion laws in this country, there can be little doubt that the American abortion rate would soar to at least two or three times the present number (probably a gross underestimate) if the proposed changes were adopted.

Out of the three million pregnancies that would probably be terminated every year, no more than thirty thousand[42] would have resulted in deformed births, while the remaining 99 per cent would have been healthy children, had their mothers been allowed or forced to carry them to term. Subtract from this latter figure the number of mothers whose hazards would be minimized if they did not feel compelled to resort to clandestine operations, and one would still have only a relatively minute proportion of abortions that would be fully justified for the reasons advanced by the advocates of liberalization. Well over 95 per cent, if not 98 per cent, of all abortions would eliminate normal children of healthy mothers. In fact, as for the mothers, the increased recourse to abortion (even if performed by qualified physicians), far from reducing hazards, would increase them, since such operations leave at least 5 per cent of the women sterile,[43] not to mention the rise in the resultant mortality rate. One can certainly ask if the extremely limited reduction in the number of malformed children and maternal mortality risks really justify the annual wholesale destruction of three million germinating, healthy lives, most of them potentially happy and useful citizens, especially in a country as underpopulated as America (compared to Europe, for instance, which commands far fewer natural resources).

E. The Individual's Claim to Life These numerical facts alone make nonsense of the argument for more and easier abortions. But moral norms cannot be determined by numbers. In the Jewish view, "he who saves one life is as if he saved an entire world";[44] one human life is as precious as a million lives, for each is infinite in value. Hence, even if the ratio were reversed, and there was only a 1 per cent chance that the child to be aborted would be normal — in fact the chances invariably exceed 50 per cent in any given case[45] — the consideration for that one child in favor of life would outweigh any counterindication for the other 99 per cent.

But, in truth, such a counterindication, too, is founded on fallacious premises. Assuming one were 100 per cent certain (perhaps by radiological evidence) that a child would be born deformed, could this affect its claim to life? Any line to be drawn between normal and abnormal beings determining their right to live would have to be altogether arbitrary. Would grave defect in one limb or in two limbs, or an anticipated sub-normal intelligence quotient of seventy-five or fifty make the capital difference between one who is entitled to live and one who is not? And if the absence of two limbs deprives a person of his claim to life, what about one who loses two limbs in an accident? By what moral reasoning can such a defect be a lesser cause for denying the right to live than a similar congenital abnormality? Surely life-and-death verdicts cannot be based on such tenuous distinctions.

F. The Obligations of Society The birth of a physically or mentally maldeveloped child may be an immense tragedy in a family, just as a crippling accident or a lingering illness striking a family member later in life may be. But one cannot purchase the relief from such misfortunes at the cost of life itself. So long as the sanctity of life is recognized as inviolable, the cure to suffering cannot be abortion before birth, any more than murder (whether in the form of euthanasia or of suicide) after birth. The only legitimate relief in such cases is for society to assume the burdens which the individual family can no longer bear. Since society is the main beneficiary of restrictive public laws on abortion (or homicide), it must in turn also pay the price sometimes exacted by these laws in the isolated cases demanding such a price.

Just as the state holds itself responsible for the support of families bereaved by the death of soldiers fallen in the defense of their country, it ought to provide for incapacitated people born and kept alive in the defense of public moral standards. The community is morally bound to relieve affected families of any financial or emotional stress they cannot reasonably bear, either by accepting the complete care of defective children in public institutions, or by supplying medical and educational subsidies to ensure that such families do not suffer any unfair economic disadvantages from their misfortune.

G. Illegitimate Children Similar considerations apply to children conceived by rape. The circumstances of such a conception cannot have any bearing on the child's title to life, and in the absence of any well-grounded challenge to this title there cannot be any moral justification for an abortion. Once again, the burden rests with society to relieve an innocent mother (if she so desires) from the consequences of an unprovoked assault upon her virtue if the assailant cannot be found and forced to discharge this responsibility to his child.

In the case of pregnancies resulting from incestuous, adulterous, or otherwise illegitimate relations (which the mother did not resist), there are additional considerations militating against any sanction of abortion. Jewish law not only puts an extreme penalty on incest and adultery, but also imposes fearful disabilities on the products of such unions. It brands these relations as capital crimes,[46] and it debars children born under these conditions from marriage with anyone except their like.[47]

1. *The Deterrent Effect.* — Why exact such a price from innocent children for the sins of their parents? The answer is simple: to serve as a powerful deterrent to such hideous crimes. The would-be partners to any such illicit sexual relations are to be taught that their momentary pleasure would be fraught with the most disastrous consequences for any children they might conceive. Through this knowledge they are to recoil from the very thought of incest or adultery with the same horror as they would from contemplating murder as a means to enjoyment or personal benefit. Murder is comparatively rare in civilized society for the very reason that the dreadful consequences have evoked this horror of the crime in the public conscience. Incest and adultery, in the Jewish view, are no lesser crimes,[48] and they require the same horror as an effective deterrent.

2. *Parental Responsibility.* — Why create this deterrent by visiting the sins of the parents on their innocent children? First, because there is no other way to expose an offense committed in private and usually beyond the chance of detection. But, above all, this responsibility of parents for the fate of their children is an inexorable necessity in the generation of human life; it is dictated by the law of nature no less than by the moral law. If a

careless mother drops her baby and thereby causes a permanent brain injury to the child, or if a syphilitic father irresponsibly transmits his disease to his offspring before birth, or if parents are negligent in the education of their children, all these children may innocently suffer and for the rest of their lives expiate the sins of their parents. This is what must be if parental responsibility is to be taken seriously. The fear that such catastrophic consequences would ensue from a surrender to temptation or from carelessness will help prevent the conception of grossly disadvantaged children or their physical or mental mutilation after birth.

H. Public Standards v. Individual Aberration   In line with this reasoning, Jewish law never condones the relaxation of public moral standards for the sake of saving recalcitrant individuals from even mortal offenses. A celebrated Jewish sage and philosopher of the fifteenth century, in connection with a question submitted to his judgment, averred that it was always wrong for a community to acquiesce in the slightest evil, however much it was hoped thereby to prevent far worse excesses by individuals. The problem he faced arose out of a suggestion that brothels for single people be tolerated as long as such publicly controlled institutions would reduce or eliminate the capital crime of marital faithlessness then rampant. His unequivocal answer was: It is surely far better that individuals should commit the worst offenses and expose themselves to the gravest penalties than publicly to promote the slightest compromise with the moral law.[49]

Rigid abortion laws, ruling out the *post facto* "correction" of rash acts, compel people to think twice *before* they recklessly embark on illicit or irresponsible adventures liable to inflict lifelong suffering or infamy on their progeny. To eliminate the scourge of illegitimate children more self-discipline to prevent their conception is required, not more freedom to destroy them in the womb. For each illegitimate child born because the abortion laws are strict, there may be ten or more such children *not* conceived because these laws are strict.

The exercise of man's procreative faculties, making him (in the phrase of the Talmud) "a partner with God in creation," is man's greatest privilege and gravest responsibility. The rights and obligations implicit in the generation of human life must be evenly balanced if man is not to degenerate into an addict of lust and a moral parasite infesting the moral organism of society. Liberal abortion laws would upset that balance by facilitating sexual indulgences without insisting on corresponding responsibilities.

I. Therapeutic Abortions   This leaves only the concern for the mother's safety as a valid argument in favor of abortions. In the view of Judaism, all human rights, and their priorities, derive solely from their conferment upon man by his Creator. By this criterion, as defined in the Bible, the rights of the mother and her unborn child are distinctly unequal, since the capital guilt of murder takes effect only if the victim was a born and viable person. This recognition does not imply that the destruction of a fetus is not a very grave offense against the sanctity of human life, but only that it is not technically murder. Jewish law makes a similar distinction in regard to the killing of inviable adults. While the killing of a person who already suffered from a fatal injury (from other than natural causes) is not actionable as murder,[50] the killer is morally guilty of a mortal offense.[51]

This inequality, then, is weighty enough only to warrant the sacrifice of the unborn child if the pregnancy otherwise poses a threat to the mother's life. Indeed, the Jewish concern for the mother is so great that a gravid woman sentenced to death[52] must not be subjected to the ordeal of suspense to await the delivery of her child.[53] (Jewish sources brand any delay in the execution, once it is finally decreed, as "the perversion of justice" *par excellence*,[54] since the criminal is sentenced to die, not to suffer.)

Such a threat to the mother need not be either immediate or absolutely certain. Even a remote risk of life invokes all the life-saving concessions of Jewish law,[55] provided the fear of such a risk is genuine and confirmed by the most competent medical opinions. Hence, Jewish law would regard it as an indefensible desecration of human life to allow a mother to perish in order to save her unborn child.

Conclusion

This review may be fittingly concluded with a reference to the very first Jewish statement on deliberate abortion. Commenting on the Septuagint version of the above-quoted Exodus passage,[56] the Alexandrian-Jewish philosopher, Philo, at the beginning of the Current Era declared that the attacker must die if the fruit he caused to be lost was already "shaped and all the limbs had their proper qualities, for that which answers to this description is a human being . . . like a statue lying in a studio requiring nothing more than to be conveyed outside."[57] The legal conclusion of this statement, reflecting Hellenistic rather than Jewish influence, may vary from the letter of Jewish law; but its reasoning certainly echoes the spirit of Jewish law. The analogy may be more meaningful than Philo could have intended or foreseen. A classic statue by a supreme master is no less priceless for being made defective, even with an arm or a leg missing. The destruction of such a treasure can be warranted only by the superior worth of preserving a living human being.

NOTES

1. The New York Academy of Medicine, in a report by its Committee on Public Health, has pleaded that "permissive medical practices based on *sound medical judgment* should be recognized, not forbidden by law . . ." and it recommended an amendment to the State Penal Law "to legalize therapeutic abortion when there is substantial risk that the continuance of the pregnancy would gravely impair the physical or mental health of the mother, or that the child would be born with grave physical or mental defects." The report argued that the present law "places the physician who performs the therapeutic abortion and the hospital where it is done in the position of *breaking the law,* even when they are adhering to what they believe to be *sound medical practice."* N.Y. Times, Dec. 14, 1964, p. 48, col. 5. (Emphasis added.) A subsequent report indicated that 87.6 per cent of New York obstetricians answering a questionnaire favored the change in the law, and that the President of the Association for Humane Abortion, who called the existing law "inhumane and unrealistic," had admitted that "reputable physicians often perform therapeutic abortions, in respectable New York hospitals, which are not strictly legal." N.Y. Times, Jan. 31, 1965, p. 73, col. 5.

2. The only states in which health risks, too, are recognized as a legal ground for abortion are Alabama, Colorado, Maryland, New Mexico, and Oregon. See ALA. CODE tit. 14 § 9 (1958); COLO. REV. STAT. ANN. § 40-2-23 (1963); MD. ANN. CODE art. 27, § 3 (1957); N.M. STAT. ANN. § 40A-5-3 (1953); ORE. REV. STAT. § 163.060 (1957).

3. Exodus 21:22-23.

4. *Mekhilta* and Rashi. For a translation of these sources, see 3 Lauterbach, *Mekhilta* 66-67 (1935); Rosenbaum & Silbermann, *Pentateuch with Rashi's Commentary,* 112-13 (1930).

5. Exodus 21:12. (Emphasis added.)

6. *Mekhilta* and Rashi. For a translation of these sources, see 3 Lauterbach, *op. cit. supra* note 4, at 32-33; Rosenbaum & Silbermann, *op. cit. supra* note 4, at 110-10a.

7. The mistranslation, also followed in the Samaritan and Karaite versions, is evidently based on reading *zurah* or *surah* (meaning "form") for *ason* (meaning "harm" or "accident"). See Kaufmann, *Gedenkschrift* 186 (1900).

8. See Westermarck, *Christianity and Morals* 243 (1939).

9. Aristotle, *De Anim. Hist.,* vii. 3; see 1 *Catholic Encyclopedia* 46-48 (1907).

10. See 1 Ploss & Bartels, *Woman* 483 (1935); 2 *Catholic Encyclopedia* 266-67 (1907).

11. See 2 Lecky, *History of European Morals* 23-24 (3d ed. 1891).

12. See 1 Ploss & Bartels, *op. cit. supra* note 10, at 484; Bonnar, *The Catholic Doctor* 78 (1948).

13. See, *e.g.,* Catholic Hospital Association of the United States and Canada, *Ethical and Religious Directives for Catholic Hospitals* 4 (1949).

14. See Bonnar, *op. cit. supra* note 12, at 84.

15. Tiberghien, "Principles et Conscience Morale," *Cahiers Laennac,* Oct. 1946, p. 13.

16. *Tohorot II Oholot* 7:6.

17. Maimonides, *Hil. Roze'ah,* 1:9; *Shulhan Arukh, Hoshen Mishpat* 425:2.

18. This is based on a discussion of the Mishnah, *Sanhedrin* 72b. See generally Jakobovits, *Jewish Medical Ethics,* 184-91 (1962).

19. See Jakobovits, *op. cit. supra* note 18, at 181.

20. Emden, *She'elat Yavez,* pt. 1, no. 43. *Cf.* note 53 *infra.*

21. Bacharach, *Havvot Ya'ir* no. 31.

22. Halevi, *Lehem ha-Panim, Kunteres Aharon* no. 19.

23. See text accompanying notes 16–18 *supra*.

24. Sofer, *Mahaneh Hayyim Hoshen Mishpat,* pt. 2, no. 50. Some authorities left the question unresolved, see Eger, *Oholot* 7:6; Meir of Eisenstadt, *Panim Me'irot,* pt. 2, no. 8.

25. Schick, *Maharam Shick, Yoreh De'ah* no. 155; Hoffmann, *Melamed le-Ho'il, Yoreh De'ah* no. 69.

26. German measles. See Gregg, *Congenital Cataract Following German Measles in Mother,* 3 Transactions of the Ophthalmological Society of Australia 35–46 (1941); see also Swan, Tostevin, Mayo & Black, *Congenital Defects in Infants Following Infectious Diseases During Pregnancy,* 2 *Medical Journal of Australia* 201–10 (1943).

27. See *Mishnah Berurah, Bi'ur Halakhah,* on *Orah Hayyim* 329:4. An idiot can even sue for injuries inflicted on him. *Bava Kamma* 8:4. Again, the killing of even a dying person is culpable as murder. Maimonides, *Hil. Roze'ah* 2:7.

28. Eleazar Fleckeles, *Teshuvah me-Ahavah,* pt. 1, no. 53. See Zimmels, *Magicians, Theologians and Doctors* 72 (1952).

29. *Sefer Hasidim,* no. 186 (Zhitomir ed., 1879).

30. See Bacharach, *op. cit. supra* note 21. But there is some rabbinical dispute on this opinion. See Jakobovits, *op. cit. supra* note 18, at 279 n.38.

31. See text accompanying notes 16–18 *supra*.

32. Unterman, 6 *No'am* 1 (1963). Unterman, Chief Rabbi of Israel, refers to medical evidence given him by Professor Asherman, Director of the Maternity Department of the Municipal Hadassah Hospital in Tel Aviv. See also note 43 *infra*.

33. *Ibid*.

34. *Yoma* 84; *Shulhan Arukh, Orah Hayyim,* 329:2. See also note 45 *infra*.

35. Zweig, 7 *No'am* 36 (1964).

36. *Ibid*.

37. Mizrahi, *Peri ha-Arez, Yoreh De'ah* no. 21.

38. Unterman, *Ha-Torah ve-ha-Medinah* 25, 29 (4th ser. 1952); Friedman, *Nezer Mata'ai* pt. 1, no. 8; Feinstein, *Iggerot Moshe Orah Hayyim* pt. 4, no 88. These authorities permit the violation of the Sabbath for the sake of psychiatric patients.

39. See editorial in N.Y. Times, April 7, 1965, p. 42, col. 2, commenting on CBS TV program of April 5, 1965; see also editorial in N.Y. Times, Feb. 13, 1965, p. 20, col. 2.

40. *Sefer Hasidim, op. cit. supra* note 29, no. 520.

41. See N.Y. Times, Oct. 28, 1965, p. 14, col. 3.

42. This is the number of defective births resulting from German measles anticipated for 1965 in the United States. To this number may have to be added anticipated abnormalities for other reasons, but from it would have to be subtracted the considerably larger number of cases in which affected mothers would not resort to abortion, either because of their opposition to abortion or because the condition is undetected during pregnancy. The total of abortions fully justified by actual (not suspected) fetal defects due to factors that could be recognized during pregnancy could thus scarcely exceed thirty thousand.

43. See N.Y. Times report, note 41 *supra*.

44. *Sanhedrin* 4:5. For this reason, Jewish law forbids the surrender of a single life even if any number of other lives may thereby be saved. Maimonides, *Hil. Yesodei ha-Torah* 5:5.

45. Estimates of the rate of abnormalities from German measles have varied widely, but none approaches 50 per cent. The rate among live-born babies was

recently found to be under 10 per cent, and "one can conclude [from various studies] that the incidences of congenital malformations reported by early workers are fantastically high and incorrect. The recommendation of therapeutic abortion based on those rates is not medically justified." Greenberg, Pellitteri & Barton, *Frequency of Defects in Infants Whose Mothers Had Rubella During Pregnancy,* 165 *A.M.A.J.* 675, 678 (1957). *Cf.* note 26 *supra.*

46. See Leviticus 20:10-20.

47. See Deuteronomy 23:3, and Jewish commentaries.

48. Compare the juxtaposition of murder and adultery in the Ten Commandments. Exodus 20:13.

49. Arama, *Akedat Yizhak* ch. 20, at 41(b) (ed. Frankfurt a/o, 1785).

50. *Sanhedrin* 78a.

51. Maimonides acquits such a murderer only before "a human court." *Hil. Roze'ah* 2:7-8. *Cf.* note 4 *supra.*

52. In practice Jewish law virtually abolished capital punishment thousands of years ago, as it insisted on numerous conditions whose fulfillment was almost impossible (such as the presence of, and prior warning by, two eyewitnesses).

53. *Arakhin* 1:4; *Tosafot, Arakhin* 7a.

54. *Ethics of the Fathers* 5:8.

55. *Shulhan Arukh, Orah Hayyim* 329:2-4.

56. See text accompanying note 3 *supra.*

57. *De Spec. Legibus* 3:108-10, 117-18; *De Virtut.* 138. But in the latter two passages, Philo himself qualified his statement by calling only a person who killed a child already born "indubitably a murderer."

9

Abortion in Halakhic Literature

J. DAVID BLEICH

There are three [persons] who drive away the Shekhinah *from the world, making it impossible for the Holy One, blessed be He, to fix His abode in the universe and causing prayer to be unanswered. . . . [The third is] he who causes the fetus to be destroyed in the womb, for he destroys the artifice of the Holy One, blessed be He, and His workmanship. . . . For these abominations the Spirit of Holiness weeps . . .*

ZOHAR, SHEMOT 3b

Throughout the history of civilization, abortions have been performed on a surprisingly wide scale among even the most primitive of peoples; feticide is singled out as one of the "abominations of Egypt" which the Torah sought to suppress. Despite the clause in the Hippocratic oath in which the physician declares, "nor will I give to a woman a pessary to procure abortion," artificial interruption of pregnancy, both legal and illegal, remains a widespread practice. While Judaism has always sanctioned therapeutic abortion in at least limited circumstances, the pertinent halakhic discussions are permeated with a spirit of humility reflecting an attitude of awe and reverence before the profound mystery of existence and a deeply rooted reluctance to condone interference with the sanctity of individual human life.

In recent years many attempts were made in the legislative bodies of

Reprinted from *Tradition* (Winter, 1968). Copyright © 1968 by the Rabbinical Council of America.

various states to implement changes in the laws governing the performance of induced abortions. Such proposals were designed to liberalize existing statutes both by enlarging the criteria under which legal sanction would be granted for the interruption of pregnancy and by treating abortion, at least in the early stages of pregnancy, as a private matter between a woman and her physician. These efforts culminated in the now historic Supreme Court decision in *Roe* v. *Wade*, issued in January 1973, which had the effect of rendering most existing abortion statutes unconstitutional. The ensuing discussion led to numerous requests for clarification of religious teachings with regard to these pressing problems. The inevitable demands made upon individual rabbis and communal spokesmen for an explication of the position of normative Judaism regarding this question has made it imperative that we examine this issue and acquaint ourselves with the teachings of our tradition regarding this area of serious concern.

There can be no doubt that a pregnancy contraindicated by considerations of social desiderata and personal welfare poses grave and tragic problems. We are, indeed, keenly aware of the anguishing emotional ramifications of such problems and are acutely sensitive to their moral implications. Yet when we are confronted by these and similar dilemmas, our response cannot simply echo humanistic principles and values, but must emerge from the wellspring of Halakhah. An authentically Jewish response must, by definition, be found in and predicated upon halakhic prescriptions. To us, in the words of one of the foremost rabbinic authorities of the last generation, Rabbi Abraham Isaiah Karelitz, popularly known as the *Hazon Ish*, "Ethical imperatives are . . . at one with the directives of Halakhah; it is Halakhah which determines that which is permitted and that which is forbidden in the realm of ethics."[1]

Judaism regards all forms of human life as sacred, from the formation of germ plasm in the cell of the sperm until the decomposition of the body after death. While applicable Halakhot vary in an appropriate manner from stage to stage along this continuum, fetal life is regarded as precious and may not be destroyed wantonly. This analysis of the halakhic literature concerning abortion has been undertaken as an attempt to refer the reader to the basic sources and relevant responsa and to direct attention to the halakhic intricacies upon which the issues revolve.

Basis of the Prohibition

The basic halakhic principle governing abortion practices is recorded in the Mishnah, *Oholot* 7:6, in the declaration that when "hard travail" of labor endangers the life of the mother an embryotomy may be performed and the embryo extracted member by member. This ruling is cited as definitive by Rambam, *Hilkhot Roze'ah* 1:9, and *Shulḥan Arukh, Hoshen Mishpat* 425:2. The halakhic reasoning underlying this provision is incorporated in the text of the Mishnah and succinctly couched in the explanatory phrase "for her [the mother's] life has priority over its [the fetus'] life." In the concluding clause of the Mishnah, a distinction is sharply drawn between the status of the fetus and that of a newly born infant. The Mishnah stipulates that from the moment at which birth, as halakhically definied,[2] is considered to have occurred, no interference with natural processes is permitted, since "one life is not to be set aside for the sake of another life."

It may readily be inferred from this statement that destruction of the fetus is prohibited in situations not involving a threat to the life of the pregnant mother. Incorporation of the justificatory statement "for her life takes precedence over its life" within the text of the Mishnah indicates that in the absence of this consideration abortion is not sanctioned.[3] *Tosafot (Sanhedrin* 59a; *Hullin* 33a) states explicitly that feticide, although entailing no statutory punishment, is nevertheless forbidden.[4] Elsewhere we find that according to rabbinic exegesis (*Mekhilta,* Exod. 21:12; *Sanhedrin* 84a) the killing of an unborn child is not considered to be a capital crime — an implication derived from the verse "He that smiteth a *man* so that he dieth, shall surely be put to death" (Exod. 21:12). *Tosafot,* on the basis of the Mishnah, apparently reasons that although feticide does not occasion capital punishment, the fetus is nevertheless sufficiently human to render its destruction a moral offense.

An offense not entailing statutory punishment is certainly not an anomaly. Many such prohibitions are known to be Biblical in nature. Others are recognized as having been promulgated by the Sages in order to create a "fence" around the Torah or in order formally to prohibit conduct which could not be countenanced on ethical grounds. Under which category is the prohibition against feticide to be subsumed? Is this offense Biblical or rabbinic in nature? At least three diverse lines of reasoning have been employed in establishing the Biblical nature of the offense. Rabbi Hayyim Ozer Grodzinski demonstrates that the remarks of *Tosafot,* taken in context, clearly indicate a Biblical proscription rather than a rabbinic edict.[5] Feticide, as *Tosafot* notes, is expressly forbidden under the statutes of the Noachide Code. The Noachide prohibition is derived by R. Ishmael (*Sanhedrin* 57b) from the wording of Genesis 9:6. Rendering this verse as "Whoso sheddeth the blood of man, *within man* shall his blood be shed," rather than "Whoso sheddeth the blood of man, *by man* [i.e., through a human court] shall his blood be shed," R. Ishmael queries, "Who is a man *within* a man? . . . A fetus within the womb of the mother." *Tosafot* deduces that this practice is prohibited to Jews as well by virtue of the Talmudic principle, "Is there anything which is forbidden to a Noachide yet permitted to a Jew?'' Application of this principle clearly establishes a Biblical prohibition.

R. Meir Simḥah of Dvinsk, in his Biblical novellae, *Meshekh Ḥokhmah,* Exod. 35:2, offers an interesting scriptural foundation for this prohibition, demonstrating that, while not a penal crime, the killing of a fetus is punishable by ''death at the hands of heaven.''[6] He observes that Scripture invariably refers to capital punishment by employing the formula *"mot yumat* — he shall surely be put to death.'' The use of the single expression *"yumat*—he shall be put to death'' as, for example, in Exodus 21:29, is understood in rabbinic exegesis as having reference to death at the hands of heaven. Thus, R. Meir Simḥah argues, the verse ''and he that smiteth a man shall be put to death — *yumat"* (Lev. 24:21) is not simply a reiteration of the penalty for homicide but refers to such destruction of life which is punishable only at the hands of heaven, i.e., the killing of a fetus. Reference to the fetus as ''a man'' poses no difficulty since the fetus is indeed described as ''a man'' in the above cited verse (Gen. 9:6) prescribing death for feticide under the Noachide Code.

Most interesting is the sharply contested view advanced by R. Elijah Mizraḥi, in his commentary on Exodus 21:12, that in principle feticide and murder are indistinguishable. The Biblical ban on murder extends equally to all human life, including, he claims, any fetal life which, unmolested, would develop into a viable human being. In theory, continues Mizraḥi, feticide should be punishable by death since the majority of all fetuses will indeed develop into viable human beings.[7] In practice it is technically impossible to impose the death penalty because punishment may be inflicted by the *Bet Din* only if the crime is preceded by a formal admonition. Since some fetuses will never develop fully, a definite admonition cannot be administered because it cannot be established with certainty that any particular fetus would develop in this manner. Noachides, on the other hand, require no such admonition. Therefore, since the major number of fetuses are viable, feticide is to be punished by death under the Noachide dispensation.

Differing from these various views are the opinions of the many scholars who have espoused the diametrically opposite position that the prohibition against feticide is rabbinic in origin. There is evidence that as early an authority as Rabbenu Nissim is to be numbered among the latter group. R. Ḥayyim Ozer cites Rabbenu Nissim's explanation of the reason for the ruling of the Mishnah (*Arakhin* 7a) that the execution of an expectant mother must not be delayed in order to allow the delivery of her child. Rabbenu Nissim (commentary on *Ḥullin* 58a) fails to offer the explanation adopted by other commentators; namely, that the fetus is regarded as but an organic limb of the mother having no inherent claim of its own to inviolability and hence considerations of its welfare cannot interfere with the statutory provision for immediate execution of the condemned in order to avoid subjecting the convicted criminal to agonizing suspense between announcement of the verdict and execution of the sentence. Rabbenu Nissim offers a simple explanation to the effect that the fetus has not yet emerged into the world and therefore we need not reckon with its well-being. Since Rabbenu Nissim's remarks certainly cannot be construed as sanctioning wanton destruction of a fetus, R. Hayyim Ozer infers that it is Rabbenu Nissim's opinion that the prohibition against taking fetal life is of rabbinic origin.[8] If considered as a rabbinic edict, it is understandable that the Sages suspended their ban in order to mitigate the agony of the condemned woman, giving considerations of her welfare priority over the well-being of the unborn child.

This inference is rejected by R. Moshe Feinstein[9] who asserts that Rabbenu Nissim's comment that no cognizance need be taken of the life of the unborn fetus does not reflect a lack of regard for fetal life but is based upon the Biblical injunction, "they shall also both of them die" (Deut. 22:22), which is adduced by the Gemara, *Arakhin* 7a, as mandating the execution of both the mother and her unborn child. Thus destruction of a fetus under other circumstances constitutes a Biblical offence even according to Rabbenu Nissim.

There are a number of latter-day authorities who are explicit in their opinion that feticide is a rabbinic rather than a Biblical offense. Perhaps the most prominent of these is the renowned seventeenth-century scholar, R. Aaron Samuel Koidonover, author of the famed commentary on *Seder Kodashim, Birkat ha-Zevah*. His views regarding this matter are recorded in his collection of responsa, *Emunat Shemu'el* (Frankfort-am-Main, 5443), no. 14. This position is also espoused by R. Hayyim Palaggi, *Teshuvot Hayyim ve-Shalom* (Smyrna, 5632), I, no. 40, and forms the basis for a number of decisions issued by the contemporary halakhic authority, R. Eliezer Judah Waldenberg. The rulings issued by R. Waldenberg, who serves as head of the Jerusalem *Bet Din,* are recorded in his voluminous work, *Ziz Eli'ezer.*[10]

A tentative distinction between the stringency of the prohibition against abortion involving direct physical removal of the fetus and abortion induced by chemical means is found in a responsum bearing the signature of R. Jacob Schor and included in the *Teshuvot Ge'onim Batra'i* (Prague, 5576), a compendium edited by *Sha'agat Aryeh*. While the author of this responsum makes no pertinent halakhic distinction between these two methods, he does draw attention to the fact that Maimonides found it necessary to state definitively that in cases of danger "it is permitted to dismember the fetus in her [the mother's] womb, whether by chemical means or by hand." The implication is that, if not explicitly obviated, a theoretical distinction might have been drawn between physical dismemberment of the fetus and abortion by indirect means *(gerama),*[11] such as imbibing abortifacient drugs in order to induce the expulsion of the fetus. Such a distinction is in fact made by R. Judah Eiyush, *Teshuvot Beit Yehudah* (Livorno, 5518), *Even ha-Ezer,* no. 14, who maintains that abortion induced by chemical potions is of rabbinic proscription, whereas direct removal of the fetus is forbidden on Biblical grounds.[12] On this basis, R. Eiyush grants permission to induce an abortion in a woman who became pregnant while still nursing a previous child in order that the life of the nursing infant not be endangered.[13]

Preservation of human life is commonly seen as the rationale underlying the ban against induced abortion. Each of the diverse authorities heretofore cited considers the essence of the prohibition to be closely akin to that of homicide. There are, however, other authorities who deem the destruction of a fetus to be unrelated to the taking of human life but nevertheless forbidden on extraneous grounds. Chief among these are the opinions of those who maintain that feticide is precluded as constituting a form of destruction of the male seed or that it is forbidden as a form of unlawful flagellation. R. Solomon Drimer (*Teshuvot Beit Shelomoh, Hoshen Mishpat,* no. 132) contends that the destruction of a fetus cannot be a form of homicide since the fetus cannot be viewed as "a life" in its prenatal state.[14] He does not, however, spell out the nature of the crime committed in causing the death of a fetus. The origin of this view can be traced to the *Teshuvot ha-Radbaz,* II, no. 695, in which the author states explicitly that destruction of a fetus is not a form of homicide. R. Ja'ir Hayyim Bacharach (*Havvot Ya'ir,* no. 31), argues that feticide is included in the interdiction against onanism[15] and reasons that destroying the fetus is within the scope of the verse "slaying the children in the valley under the clefts of the rocks" (Isa. 57:5), which is interpreted by the Gemara, *Niddah* 13a, as having reference to the destruction of the male seed.[16] The author of *Zekhuta de-Avraham* offers an identical opinion, adding that feticide and onanism incur the self-same penalty — "death at the hands of heaven."[17] In his responsum *Havvot Ya'ir* accepts the ruling of *Tosafot* (*Yevamot* 12b) that women are also bound by the prohibition against destroying the male seed. He notes that, even according to the view of Rabbenu Tam that women are not included in this specific prohibition,[18] these practices are nevertheless forbidden to them, for women, too (*Tosafot, Gittin* 41b), are bound to bring to fulfillment the divine design of a populated world as stated in the words of Isaiah 45:18, "He created it [the earth] not a waste, He formed it to be inhabited."[19]

A number of objections to *Havvot Ya'ir's* position are raised in later works. R. Meir Dan Plocki[20] expresses the view that with the promulgation of the Sinaitic covenant, Noachides were absolved from the obligation of procreation and also from the prohibition against wanton emission of semen.[21] Granting this point, it follows that according to *Havvot Ya'ir's* reasoning there would be no apparent grounds for denying Noachides the right to commit feticide. Such a conclusion would be contrary to the clear-cut recognition that destruction of a fetus continues to constitute a capital crime under the Noachide code. R. Plocki further states that feticide cannot be punishable by "death at the hands of heaven." Such punishment, he avers, would be incompatible with the exaction of monetary compensation for loss of the fetus, as prescribed by Exodus 21:12, in light of the general rule that a single act cannot result in the infliction of both capital punishment and punitive financial compensation — a principle which R. Neḥunya b. ha-Kanah (*Ketubbot* 30a) extends not only to the forms of capital punishment imposed by the *Bet Din* but to "death at the hands of heaven" as well. R. Plocki arrives at the conclusion that the ban against onanism is operative only with regard to the wasting of one's own seed, since such an act contravenes the obligation "be fruitful and multiply," but is inapplicable with regard to the destruction of fetal progeny other than of one's own parentage.

A somewhat similar objection is voiced by the late Rabbi Jehiel Jacob Weinberg.[22] R. Plocki maintains that women, although not bound by the commandment "be fruitful and multiply," are nevertheless obligated to fulfill the intent expressed in the verse, "He formed it [the earth] to be inhabited." This consideration, R. Plocki maintains, precludes feticide even on the part of women. Rabbi Weinberg rebuts this contention, asserting that the obligation set forth in Isaiah 45:18 is understood by the authorities as paralleling the injunction "be fruitful and multiply" in that such considerations apply only to one's own progeny. Accordingly, argues Rabbi Weinberg, assimilation of the prohibition against feticide to the ban against onanism would lead to the bizarre conclusion that a woman might be permitted to perform an abortion upon any woman other than herself — a conclusion not to be found in any halakhic source.

The early seventeenth-century scholar, R. Joseph Trani of Constantinople, author of *Teshuvot Maharit,* also endeavors to show that the taking of fetal life, while forbidden, nevertheless cannot be considered as constituting a form of homicide.[23] The Mishnah, *Arakhin* 7a, indicates that an expectant mother who has been sentenced to death, as long as she has not already "sat on the birth stool," must be executed without delay in order to spare her the agony of suspense. Whereupon the Gemara in its comments on this Mishnah exclaims *"Peshita!* — Of course!" R. Joseph Trani argues that if destruction of the fetus is tantamount to the taking of human life the amazement registered by the Gemara is out of place. The Gemara provides that the mother be struck on the abdomen against the womb in order to cause the prior death of the fetus. This is done in order to avoid the indignity which would be inflicted upon her body as a result of an attempt on the part of the fetus to emerge after the death of its mother. An act of murder certainly would not be condoned simply in order to spare the condemned undue agony or to prevent dishonor to a corpse.[24] R. Joseph Trani then advances an alternative basis for this stricture. In his opinion, the destruction of an embryo is within the category of unlawful "wounding," which is banned on the basis of Deuteronomy 25:3.[25] This consideration is, of course, irrelevant in the case of one lawfully sentenced to death, and hence the Gemara raises an objection to the need for specific authorization for the execution of a pregnant woman sentenced to death. A more recent authority, Rabbi Joseph Rosen, expresses a similar view.[26]

The dispute concerning the classification of the nature of the stricture against feticide is of more than mere speculative interest. It will be shown that various halakhic determinations regarding the permissibility of therapeutic abortion in certain situations hinge directly upon proper categorization of this prohibition.[27] This issue is also the focal point of an intriguing problem discussed by Rabbi Isser Yehudah Unterman, the former Ashkenazic Chief Rabbi of Israel. Writing in *No'am,* VI, 52, Rabbi Unterman refers to an actual question which arose in the course of the German occupation of Poland and Lithuania during World War I. A German officer became intimate with a Jewish girl and caused her to become pregnant. Becoming aware of her condition, the officer sought to force the young woman in question to submit to an abortion. The German officer ordered a Jewish physician to perform the abortion. Upon the doctor's refusal to do so, the officer drew his revolver and warned the physician that continued refusal would result in the latter's own death. If the prohibition against taking the life of a fetus is not subsumed under the category of murder, thereby constituting one of the *avizraiya,* or "appurtenances," of murder, there arises no question of an obligation on the part of the physician to forfeit his own life; on the contrary, he is halakhically bound to preserve his own life since preservation of life takes precedence over all other considerations. If, however, feticide is considered to be among the *avizraiya* of murder and akin to homicide, which is one of the three grave offenses which dare not be committed even upon threat of death, then the principle "Be killed but do not transgress" is germane.

Rabbi Unterman, however, argues that even if, halakhically, feticide be deemed a lesser form of murder it may be committed in face of a compelling *force majeure.* His reasoning is based upon the ruling of R. Moses Isserles, *Yoreh De'ah* 157:1, that while sacrifice of one's life is required in face of coerced infractions of even *avizraiya,* or "appurtenances," of the three cardinal sins even though the appurtenances themselves do not involve capital culpability, nevertheless, this is demanded only with regard to violation of those *avizraiya* which are themselves explicit negative commandments pertaining to the three cardinal sins. Since feticide is not numbered among the 365 negative precepts recorded in the Bible it does not fall within this category.[28] R. Moshe Feinstein however, disputes Rabbi Unterman's conclusion and asserts that feticide is not an "appurtenance" of murder but murder *per se,* albeit a form of homicide which is not punishable by the death penalty.[29]

Another argument in support of the contention that the admonition "Be killed but do not transgress" does not apply to an act of feticide was advanced at a much earlier date by R. Joseph Babad in his *magnum opus, Minḥat Ḥinnukh.*[30] He reasons that this principle, as enunciated with regard to homicide, is based upon an *a priori* principle propounded in the Gemara's rhetorical question, "How do you know that your blood is sweeter than the blood of your fellow?" The import of this dictum is to emphasize the intrinsic value of every human life and graphically to underscore the fact that no man dare consider his existence to be of higher value than that of his fellow. For in the sight of God all individuals are equally "sweet" and all alike are of inestimable value. Since, however, a fetus is not accounted as being a full-fledged *nefesh,* or "life," and since, as an outgrowth of the unborn child's inferior status, Jewish law exempts its killer from the death penalty, the fetus' "blood" is quite obviously assessed as being "less sweet."[31] Therefore, reasons the author of *Minḥat Ḥinnukh,* when confronted by the impending loss of either one's own life or of the life of the fetus, the killing of the unborn child is to be preferred as constituting the lesser of two evils. This conclusion is inescapable, argues *Minḥat Ḥinnukh,* since the Mishnah specifically authorizes the sacrifice of a fetal life in order to save its mother. The mother's life is of no greater intrinsic value than that of any other individual. If destruction of the fetus is sanctioned in order to preserve the mother, then it must be permitted in order to save the life of any other person.

Abortion within the First Forty Days of Gestation

We find a declaration of Rav Ḥisda (*Yevamot* 69b) to the effect that the daughter of a *kohen* widowed shortly after marriage to an Israelite may partake of *terumah* during the first forty days following consummation of her marriage despite the fact that she has become a widow in the interim. Permission to eat *terumah* is a privilege accorded an unmarried daughter of a *kohen* or a widowed daughter who has no children. The concern in the case presented to Rav Ḥisda is that the widow, unknown to herself, may be pregnant with child, in which case *terumah* would be forbidden to her. Rav Ḥisda argues, if the widow is not pregnant there is no impediment to her partaking of *terumah;* if she is pregnant the embryo is considered to be "mere water" until after the fortieth day of pregnancy. Therefore she may continue to eat *terumah* for a full forty days after her marriage. The ruling of Rav Ḥisda indicates that fetal development within the initial forty days of gestation is insufficient to warrant independent standing in the eyes of Halakhah. Anothcr source for this distinction is the Mishnah (*Niddah* 30a), which declares that a fetus aborted less than forty days following cohabitation does not engender the impurity of childbirth ordained by Leviticus 12:2–5.[32] Similarly, according to *Mishneh le-Melekh, Hilkhot Tumat Met* 2:1, the defilement associated with a dead body is not attendant upon an embryo expelled during the first forty days of gestation. Furthermore, in the opinion of many authorities, a fetus cannot acquire property prior to the fortieth day of development.[33]

The result is that the status of an embryo's claim to life during the first forty days following conception is not entirely clear. Is the prohibition against feticide operative during this early stage of fetal development during which the embryo is depicted as "mere water"? It would appear that according to the grounds advanced by *Ḥavvot Ya'ir* no distinction can be made between the various stages of fetal development since, according to this opinion, feticide is prohibited, not because it is tantamount to the taking of a human life, but because it is a form of "destroying the seed." The fact that no specific reference is made in *Ḥavvot Ya'ir* to the status of the embryo during this period in no way vitiates this conclusion. In the absence of a distinction there is no reason for such reference.[34] Yet the considerations advanced by *Ḥavvot Ya'ir* can explain only the nature of the ban against feticide under the Sinaitic covenant. Feticide, a capital offense in Noachide law, may well be viewed as a form of homicide under that code, leaving the possibility of such a distinction with regard to the conduct of Noachides an open question.

Whether or not there is a halakhic distinction with regard to this prohibition during the first forty days of gestation according to the authorities who advance other considerations as the grounds for the banning of feticide remains to be considered. Rabbi Weinberg states flatly *(op cit.,* p. 349) that R. Joseph Trani's *(Maharit)* thesis, according to which feticide is a case of unlawful wounding, precludes extension of this prohibition to an embryo of less than forty days since it is deemed as "mere water" throughout this period. Rabbi Weinberg interprets *Maharit's* reference to "wounding" as depicting the harm inflicted upon the fetus. Despite the cogency of Rabbi Weinberg's reasoning regarding "wounding" of the fetus, his reasoning is inapplicable in cases of abortion by means of dilation and curretage which certainly involves "wounding" of the mother as well, irrespective of the stage of pregnancy at which this procedure is initiated. Following this line of thought, it should be forbidden other than for therapeutic considerations which constitute licit grounds for "wounding." Moreover, R. Aryeh Lipschuetz, a nineteenth-century scholar, in his

Aryeh de-Bei-Ila'i (*Yoreh De'ah,* no. 14, p. 58a), interprets *Maharit's* view that feticide is forbidden as a form of "wounding" as being predicated upon consideration of the wounding of the mother rather than of the unborn child. R. Lipschuetz contends that it would be somewhat incongruous to prohibit the wounding of a being which one is not specifically forbidden to kill. Approached in this manner, there is no room for differentiating between the various stages of pregnancy.

There is further evidence pointing to a prohibition against destroying the life of a fetus during this early period. Nahmanides notes that according to the opinion of *Ba'al Halakhot Gedolot* the Sabbath may be violated even during this forty-day period in order to preserve the life of a fetus.[35] The author of *Havvot Ya'ir,* citing *Tosafot, Niddah* 44b, shows that the right to violate the Sabbath for the sake of saving a prenatal life is incompatible with permission to kill it deliberately.[36] It follows that, according to *Ba'al Halakhot Gedolot,* induced abortion during this period is forbidden. Responding to a specific inquiry, R. Plocki grants permission for termination of pregnancy within this forty-day period only when the life of the mother is threatened.[37]

Drawing a parallel from the commandment against the kidnapping and subsequent sale of a person into involuntary servitude, Rabbi Unterman[38] cites the opinion of Rashi, *Sanhedrin* 85b, who maintains that this prohibition encompasses the sale of an unborn child as well. Although the fetus may not be considered a fully developed person, his kidnapper is culpable because he has stolen an animate creature whose status is conditioned by its potential development into a viable human being. Rabbi Unterman further notes that the unborn fetus lacks human status. Consequently, it is excluded from the injunction, "And he [man] shall live by them" (Lev. 18:5), which justifies violation of other precepts in order to preserve human life. Numerous authorities nevertheless permit violation of the Sabbath in order to preserve fetal life. Rabbi Unterman views such permission as being predicated upon a similar rationale. Anticipation of potential development and subsequent attainment of human status creates certain privileges and obligations with regard to the undeveloped fetus. Consideration of future potential is clearly evidenced in the Talmudic declaration: "Better to violate a single Sabbath in order to observe many Sabbaths" (*Shabbat* 151b). Rabbi Unterman concludes that reasoning in these terms precludes any distinction which might otherwise be drawn with regard to the various stages of fetal development.

Surprisingly, there is one source which appears to rule that destruction of the fetus by Noachides, at least under some circumstances, does not constitute a moral offense. *Maharit*[39] writes: "I remember having seen in a responsum of the Rashba that he bears witness that Ramban rendered medical aid to a gentile woman in return for compensation in order that she might conceive and aided her in aborting the fruit of her womb.''[40] It is of course inconceivable that an individual of Naḥmanides' piety and erudition would have violated the injunction "Thou shalt not place a stumbling block before a blind person" (Lev. 19:4) or that he would have actively assisted transgressors. Applying the line of reasoning adduced above, Rabbi Unterman draws the conclusion that there is a fundamental distinction between Jewish law and Noachide law with regard to the assessment of potential life. According to many authorities, Noachides are under no obligation to preserve the lives of their fellows, to "be fruitful and multiply" or to refrain from wasting the male seed.[41] They are forbidden to commit homicide and to take the life of "a man within a man" but bear no responsibility for the safeguarding and preservation of seminal life. It would appear, then, that Halakhah holds them accountable only for *actual,* in contradistinction to *potential,* life.[42] Accordingly, there is no objection to Noachides aborting, or to a Jew giving advice and rendering indirect assistance to Noachides in aborting, a fetus within the first forty days of gestation. Since Halakhah considers that during this initial period the embryo has not as yet developed distinctly recognizable organs or an independent circulatory system it cannot be considered "a man within a man" and hence its destruction does not constitute murder under the Noachide dispensation. Naḥmanides, Rabbi Unterman avers, sanctioned the performance of abortions by Noachides only within this forty-day period.[43]

Rabbi Unterman's distinction between Jews and Noachides with regard to termination of pregnancy within the first forty days following conception was anticipated by an earlier authority. Rabbi Plocki, in his *Hemdat Yisra'el* (p. 176), marshals evidence that an embryo may be destroyed with impunity during the first forty days of its development based upon Rabbenu Tam's interpretation of the Talmudic dispute (*Yevamot* 12a) concerning the "three [categories of] women" who may resort to contraceptive devices in order to prevent conception. Rabbenu Tam explains that the dispute concerns the insertion of a tampon *after* cohabitation. The *Tanna,* R. Meir, rules that use of contraceptive devices by these women is mandatory since pregnancy would place their lives in jeopardy; the Sages assert that such action is not incumbent upon these women stating that the verse "The Lord preserves the simple" (Ps. 116:6) permits reliance upon divine providence to avert tragic consequences. However, according to Rabbenu Tam, the Sages *permit* the use of contraceptives after cohabitation reasoning that women are not commanded to refrain from "destroying the seed." R. Plocki points out that fertilization most frequently takes place immediately following cohabitation. Contraception following cohabitation is then, in effect, not destruction of the seed but abortion of a fertilized ovum.[44] If abortion is forbidden even in the earliest stages of gestation, how then can Rabbenu Tam permit the use of contraceptive devices following cohabitation? R.

Plocki concludes that destruction of the embryo during the first forty days following conception does not constitute an act of feticide but rather falls under the category of "destroying the seed." Since we accept the opinion of those authorities who rule that women are also bound by the prohibition against "destroying the seed," R. Plocki's reasoning (as evidenced by his own remarks) finds practical application only with regard to Noachides. According to those authorities who maintain that the ban against destroying the seed does not apply to Noachides, the latter may be permitted to interrupt pregnancy during the first forty days of gestation.

Distinctions pertaining to the early period of gestation are echoed by numerous other authorities. R. Hayyim Ozer (*Teshuvot Ahi'ezer,* III, no. 65, sec. 14) writes, "It appears that a Noachide is not put to death for this and perhaps even with regard to an Israelite there is no Biblical prohibition." *Torat Hesed, Even ha-Ezer,* no. 42, sec. 33, states explicitly that the prohibition against destroying an embryo within the first forty days following conception is rabbinic in nature. R. Joseph Rosen, *Zofnat Pa'aneah,* no. 59, comments, "Before the fortieth day there is not such a stringent prohibition according to many authorities." In an earlier collection of responsa, *Teshuvot Bet Shelomo, Hoshen Mishpat,* no. 162, R. Solomon Drimer of Skole concludes that there is no prohibition against destroying an embryo less than forty days old and notes that in punishment for performing such a deed "even a Noachide is not put to death." An even more permissive view is cited by Rabbi Waldenberg. He quotes a responsum included in *Teshuvot Peri ha-Sadeh* (vol. IV, no. 50) which extends this distinction to the entire first three months of pregnancy.[45] Relying upon this opinion, Rabbi Waldenberg, *Ziz Eli'ezer,* IX, 236, permits the performance of an abortion within the first three months when there are definite grounds to fear that the child will be born deformed or abnormal.[46] Rabbi Waldenberg, however, denies such permission even within this period once fetal movement is perceived. Rabbi Weinberg, in his original responsum (*No'am* IX, 213 f.), also concluded that it is permissible to induce abortion prior to the fortieth day of pregnancy, but later added in a note (*Seridei Esh,* III, 350, note 7) that having seen a contrary opinion expressed by Rabbi Unterman in *No'am* (VI, 8f),[47] he reserves decision pending consultation with other halakhic authorities. The late Rabbi Moses Jonah Zweig of Antwerp, writing in *No'am* (VII, 48), concurs in the view which forbids abortions even during the first forty days of pregnancy other than on medical grounds.[48]

Therapeutic Abortion of Pregnancy Involving Danger to Life

Authority for performance of an embryotomy in order to preserve the life of the mother is derived from the previously cited Mishnah, *Oholot* 7:6. Virtually all authorities agree that the Mishnah does not merely sanction but deems mandatory[49] that the life of the fetus be made subordinate to that of the mother. At the same time the Mishnah expressly forbids interference with natural processes after the moment of birth, which is defined as the emergence from the womb of the forehead or the greater part thereof.[50] In the ensuing Talmudic discussion (*Sanhedrin* 72b), the child is described as being in effect an aggressor "pursuing" the life of its mother. As such, its life is forfeit if necessary to save the innocent victim so pursued.[51] At this point the question is raised, why should an embryotomy not be performed in such circumstances even in the final stages of parturition? It is answered by pointing out that the law of pursuit does not apply when the mother is "pursued by Heaven," i.e., her danger is the result of natural occurrences rather than malevolent human activity. The apparent inference to be drawn from this discussion is that there is no need for resort to the law of pursuit in order to justify destruction of the fetus prior to birth. On the contrary, were there need for such justification, the law of pursuit would be of no avail since it cannot be validly applied in cases where such "pursuit" arises as a result of the processes of nature. Rashi (*ad loc.*) explains that the fetus is sacrificed in order to spare the life of the mother because even though the fetus has a claim to life and is sufficiently human to render its destruction a moral offense, neither this claim nor its status as a human life is equal to that of the mother: "As long as it [the fetus] has not emerged into the light of the world, it is not a human life."

Maimonides codifies the law emerging from this discussion in the following manner: "This also is a negative precept: not to have compassion on the life of a pursuer. Therefore the Sages ruled [regarding] a pregnant woman in hard travail that it is permitted to dismember the fetus in her womb, whether by chemical means or by hand, for it [the fetus] is as one pursuing her in order to kill her; but if it has already put forth its head it may not be touched, for [one] life may not be put aside for the sake of [another] life. This is the natural course of the world" (*Hilkhot Roze'ah* 1:9). This formulation is problematic in that Maimonides invokes the law of pursuit as justification for the performance of an embryotomy in the early stages of labor, whereas the Gemara implies that the deliberate sacrifice of the unborn child is permitted simply because its life is subservient to that of the mother. Furthermore, the explanation offered seems to be contradictory in nature since Maimonides, in his concluding remarks, follows the Gemara in dismissing the applicability of the law of pursuit on the grounds that nature, not the child, pursues the mother. The question of proper interpretation of Maimonides is of the utmost halakhic relevance because in this instance his phraseology is adopted *verbatim* by the *Shulḥan Arukh, Ḥoshen Mishpat* 452:2.

In an attempt to resolve these difficulties, R. Ezekiel Landau[52] points out that the killing of a fetus, while not constituting a capital crime, is nevertheless a form of homicide. Just as there is no justification for the sacrifice of a person suffering from a fatal injury — the killing of whom does not technically constitute murder — for the purpose of preserving the life of a normal person, so also destruction of the embryo in order to safeguard the life of the mother would not be condoned if not for its being, at least in measure, an aggressor. R. Jair Bacharach[53] and Rabbi Ḥayyim Soloveichik[54] employ similar reasoning in explaining Maimonides' position. A somewhat different explanation is offered by R. Isser Zalman Melzer[55] in the name of R. Ḥayyim Soloveichik. Rabbi Unterman, in his work *Shevet me-Yehudah*,[56] attempts a further clarification of Maimonides' position by explaining that the ban against destroying the life of a fetus stems not from an actual prohibition against the act of feticide *per se*, but from an obligation to preserve the life of the fetus.[57] Since the killing of a fetus is antithetical to its preservation, embryotomy is permissible only when the fetus is, in point of fact, an aggressor. Once the child is born, the prohibition against homicide becomes actual and since, technically, it is nature which is the pursuer, the law of pursuit is not operative.

Resolution of the difficulties surrounding Maimonides' ruling and the reasoning upon which it is based is of great significance in terms of practical Halakhah. According to the explanations offered by R. Ezekiel Landau, R. Ḥayyim Soloveichik and others following in the same general mode, therapeutic abortion would be permissible only in instances where the "pursuer" argument may be applied, i.e., where the threat to the life of the mother is the direct result of the condition of pregnancy. R. Ḥayyim Ozer[58] and Rabbi Weinberg[59] both contend that a pregnancy which merely complicates an already present medical condition, thereby endangering the life of the mother, does not provide grounds for termination of pregnancy according to such analyses of Maimonides' position. In these cases the fetus cannot be deemed an aggressor since the mother's life is placed in jeopardy by the disease afflicting her. It is this malady, rather than her pregnant condition, which is the proximate cause of impending tragedy. An identical conclusion was reached much earlier by R. Isaac Schorr (*Ko'aḥ Shor*, no. 20) who points out that the law of pursuit encompasses only cases where the pursuer seeks to perform an overt act of homicide. If the act only leads indirectly to the death of the pursued, e.g., when the pursuer merely seeks to incarcerate the victim so that he die of starvation or seeks to cut off the intended victim's supply of oxygen in order to cause asphyxiation, the law of pursuit is not applicable, for "we have not heard that the pursued may be saved by taking the life of one who is desirous of preventing a benefit necessary for the life of his fellowman." A fetus, which itself is not the cause of danger but whose presence thwarts the efficacy of medical remedies, clearly falls within this category. At least one other authority, R. Isaac Lampronti, the author of *Paḥad Yiẓḥak* (*Erekh Nefalim,* 79b) states unequivocally that danger caused by an extraneous disease does not warrant performance of an abortion in order to save the mother. Rabbi Schorr emphasizes that (according to Maimonides) it must be known with certainty that the pregnancy *per se* constitutes this danger. This rules out abortion in instances where there is doubt as to whether the pregnancy is the actual case of danger or whether the pregnancy merely complicates a previously existing condition.

The aforementioned discussions concern themselves only with cases in which failure to terminate pregnancy will indubitably result in the loss of life to the mother. The question of termination of a pregnancy which, while jeopardizing the life of the pregnant mother, will not *necessarily* result in imminent loss of life again centers around Maimonides' invocation of the law of pursuit. Citing Rashi, *Sanhedrin* 72b and *Pesaḥim* 2b, Rabbi Schorr demonstrates that the law of pursuit cannot be invoked in cases of doubt.[60] Hence abortion may be permitted only when there exists incontravertible medical evidence[61] that the pregnancy *per se* will result in the loss of the life of the pregnant mother. R. Solomon Drimer (*Beit Shelomoh, Ḥoshen Mishpat,* no. 120), however, reaches the opposite conclusion, at least in theory. Following the authorities who maintain that a fetus is "not a life" and hence its destruction does not constitute an "appurtenance" of homicide, Rabbi Drimer concludes that feticide is no different from other transgressions which may be violated even in cases of possible or suspected danger.[62] Nevertheless, in practice, Rabbi Drimer, on the basis of other considerations, withholds permission in cases of merely possible danger to the life of the mother. The Gemara (*Yoma* 82a) specifies that a pregnant woman who becomes agitated at the smell of food on the Day of Atonement may, if necessary, partake of the food which causes this excitement lest she suffer a miscarriage and her fetus be spontaneously aborted. Maimonides, Rabbenu Asher and Rabbenu Nissim interpret this provision as being based, not on a concern for the preservation of the unborn child, but on a concern for the life of the mother. According to their view, expulsion of the fetus *ipso facto* constitutes a threat to the life of the mother. Accordingly, reasons Rabbi Drimer, even if continuation of pregnancy jeopardizes the life of the mother. this consideration is counterbalanced by the fact that termination of pregnancy in itself constitutes a parallel jeopardy. Therefore, a course of "sit and do not act" is preferable. Even if physicians advise that there is no danger involved in the performance of the abortion, their advice is to be disregarded, just as medical opinion is ignored when it fails to recognize cases of "danger" which are delineated by Halakhah as constituting a threat to human life. Halakhah specifies that a woman's life is in jeopardy for a minimum period of three days following childbirth and hence during this time she is permitted to partake of food on the Day of Atonement, the Sabbath is violated on her behalf, etc. Since Halakhah defines childbirth as a "danger," medical opinions to the contrary or protestations of well-being on the part of the patient are disregarded. Rabbi Drimer reasons that the same considerations should apply to the conditions surrounding abortion.

A very different conclusion is reached by R. Mordecai Leib Winkler[63] (*Levushei Mordekhai*), who finds reason to distinguish between miscarriages and abortions performed by medical practitioners. Since there is no explicit reference to the latter, those authorities who state that abortion *per se* constitutes a threat to the life of the mother may not have intended their remarks to encompass therapeutic abortion surrounded by medical safeguards. *Levushei Mordekhai* also introduces the notion of comparative danger and seems to indicate that, while abortion may itself constitute a danger in the opinion of these authorities, this danger may not be acute since dispensation for violation of *Shabbat* and *Yom Kippur* is granted for even the slightest threat to life. Abortion should therefore be sanctioned in order to obviate a more acute danger. Furthermore, the remarks of these authorities fail to demonstrate that miscarriage *per se* jeopardizes the life of the mother. Their pronouncements are consistent with the conclusion that danger will result only if the woman fails to receive proper care pursuant to the expulsion of the fetus. Since such care would involve desecration of *Yom Kippur* in any event, the woman may break her fast in order to prevent the necessity for such later violations. *Levushei Mordekhai* concludes that there is, then, no evidence that a therapeutic abortion performed under proper medical conditions and with provision for proper convalescence constitutes a jeopardy to the life of the mother.

Relevant to this issue is the tragic case of a pregnant woman suffering from a terminal case of cancer which is pondered by R. Waldenberg (*Ẓiẓ Eli'ezer,* IX, 239). Medical authorities predict that continuation of pregnancy to term will foreshorten her life, but the expectant mother is steadfast in her desire to be survived by a child. Normally her desire would be irrelevant to a halakhic determination that preservation of maternal life is sufficient reason to abort the fetus. With regard to this specific question, Rabbi Waldenberg concludes that since *Beit Shelomoh* and other authorities withhold permission to abort the fetus on grounds that the abortion itself also constitutes a danger to the life of the mother, in this case one is justified in acceding to the wishes of the mother and adopting a stance of passive noninterference.

Returning to our central problem, many authorities take a different view with regard to embryotomy in cases where pregnancy endangers the life of the mother by complicating an already present medical condition. Rabbi Weinberg (*No'am* IX, 204; *Seridei Esh,* III, 343 f.) offers a radically different approach to the resolution of the complex difficulties surrounding the previously cited statements of Maimonides, *Hilkhot Roẓ'eaḥ* 1:9, in light of the latter's remarks in *Hilkhot Ḥoveil u-Maẓik* 8:4. Maimonides rules that although property belonging to others may be appropriated in order to preserve one's own life, compensation must nevertheless subsequently be paid to the lawful owner. Rabbi Weinberg notes that the provision is modified in the event that the property itself is the source of danger (*Nizkei Mammon* 8:15). The paradigm case is that of the threat to the lives of the passengers sailing on an overly-laden ship which is in danger of sinking. One who lightens the load by throwing cargo overboard is absolved from payment of property damages since the cargo itself is deemed to be "a pursuer." Rabbi Weinberg opines that Maimonides invokes this provision in his exposition of the law surrounding danger arising from pregnancy. Maimonides does not resort to the law of pursuit, argues Rabbi Weinberg, in order to justify sacrifice of the life of the fetus; this is warranted on the basis of Rashi's explanation that it is not fully "a human life." Rather, continues Rabbi Weinberg, Maimonides invokes the pursuer argument in order to provide a basis for exemption from satisfaction of the husband's claim for monetary damages normally incurred as a result of destruction of a fetus as provided by Exodus 21:22.

R. Ḥayyim Ozer, in another responsum (*Aḥi'ezer,* III, no. 72), points out that Maimonides' phraseology refers specifically to a woman in "hard travail." As previously noted, the Talmud regards a fetus which has "torn itself loose" from the normal uterine position as a separate body. According to R. Ḥayyim Ozer, Maimonides deems it necessary to rely upon the law of pursuit only because he refers to a fetus which, although yet unborn, is already a separate body. The Gemara speaks of earlier stages of pregnancy and hence has no need for recourse to this line of reasoning. According to this interpretation, Maimonides recognizes that prior to the mother's "sitting on the birth stool" the fetus is but an organic limb of her body. It is of course not merely permissible, but mandatory, to amputate a limb in order to save a life. Therefore, concludes R. Ḥayyim Ozer, even according to Maimonides, it is permissible to perform an abortion in cases involving danger to the life of the mother, irrespective of the source of such danger, provided this procedure is performed before the fetus has "torn itself loose."[64] R. Ḥayyim Ozer adds the stipulation that the physicians advising this medical procedure be highly expert and certain in their opinion that the operation itself does not constitute a danger.

Rabbi Weinberg (*No'am,* IX, 205; *Seridei Esh,* III, 344) objects to this line of reasoning because it is predicated upon the consideration that the fetus is to be accounted as "a limb of the mother." His objection is based upon the remarks of *Tosafot* (*Sanhedrin* 80b) that the principle "a fetus is a limb of the mother" applies in all instances save with regard to the laws of *terefah,* of an animal mortally wounded or afflicted with a terminal disease. The prohibition of a *terefah* is based upon the animal's lack of "animation." Since a fetus possesses "independent animation" and may survive even though the mother is doomed, consideration of the fetus as a limb of the mother does not render it a *terefah* simply because the mother has become a *terefah.* Similarly, argues Rabbi Weinberg, since the fetus is possessed of "independent animation," it does not follow that its abortion is comparable to the removal of a limb in order to save the body. Accordingly, Rabbi Weinberg concludes that abortion is not permitted, according to Maimonides, in cases where extraneous illness would lead to the mother's death if pregnancy were allowed to continue.

Therapeutic Abortion of Pregnancy Involving Danger to Maternal Health

A further ramification of these diverse analyses of Maimonides' views relates to the permissibility of therapeutic abortion in situations deleterious to the health of the mother, but not endangering her life. The most permissive ruling with regard to therapeutic abortion, one to which later authorities take strong exception, is that of R. Jacob Emden,[65] who permits performance of an abortion not only when the mother's health is compromised but also in cases of "grave necessity," such as when continuation of the pregnancy would subject the mother to great pain.[66] Such abortions are sanctioned by R. Emden when performed before the onset of labor at which time the fetus has "torn itself loose" from the uterine wall. Citing *Ḥavvot Ya'ir's* explanation that the basis of the law against feticide is the prohibition against destroying the seed, R. Emden maintains that destroying the seed is forbidden only when such emission or destruction is without purpose, but may be permitted when it serves a medical function. It should, however, be noted that *Ḥavvot Ya'ir* himself quotes Rashi's commentary, *Sanhedrin* 72b, "a woman who is in hard labor *and whose life is in danger,"* from which *Ḥavvot Ya'ir* deduces that other than in cases of actual danger to maternal life abortion cannot be sanctioned.

A view similar to that of R. Jacob Emden is voiced by R. Ben-Zion Uziel, the late Sephardic Chief Rabbi of Israel, in his *Mishpetei Uzi'el, Ḥoshen Mishpat,* III, no. 46. The case brought to his attention concerned a woman threatened with approaching deafness if her pregnancy were permitted to run its normal course. Rabbi Uziel, following the line of reasoning advanced by R. Jacob Emden, rules that abortion is permissible when indicated by any consideration of merit, provided it is performed before the onset of labor, at which time the fetus is considered to have "torn itself loose."

This determination leads Rabbi Uziel to the discussion of an interesting question. A pregnant woman is forbidden to contract a levirate marriage since her deceased husband will no longer remain childless if the pregnancy culminates in the birth of a viable infant. If, however, the widow entered into the marriage with her brother-in-law and later discovered that at the time of consummation she was already bearing the child of her previous husband, the marriage is annulled and a sin-offering brought in expiation of this inadvertent transgression. Why, R. Uziel was asked, is she not advised simply to abort the fetus thereby eradicating her transgression *ab initio?* Obviation of sin certainly constitutes a "grave need" and fulfills the criterion established by R. Jacob Emden. Rabbi Uziel answers that since the husband enjoys rights of proprietorship with regard to the fetus and is indeed entitled to monetary compensation for its loss (Exod. 21:22), the woman has no right to destroy her dead husband's property in order to absolve herself retroactively from the prohibition against cohabitation with a brother-in-law.

On a later occasion Rabbi Uziel seems to have reversed his opinion with regard to the salient point of the responsum. In a responsum dated the following month (*op. cit.,* no. 47), Rabbi Uziel specifically cites the opinion of R. Jacob Emden but reserves decision in cases not involving a threat to the very life of the mother.

R. Joseph Trani, in a somewhat more restricted ruling (*Teshuvot Maharit,* I, no. 99), sanctions abortions when performed in the interests of maternal health. This decision follows logically from his thesis that feticide is not a form of homicide but is forbidden because removal of the fetus constitutes an act of "wounding."[67] It, of course, follows that any wound inflicted for purposes of healing is not encompassed by this prohibition.

Rabbi Weinberg (*No'am* IX, 215; *Seridei Esh* III, 350) observes that according to the previously cited explanations of *Hilkhot Roze'aḥ* 1:9 by R. Ezekiel Landau and R. Ḥayyim Soloveichik, abortion would not be sanctioned by Maimonides except when there exists an imminent threat to the life of the mother. Rabbi Weinberg adds, however, that in view of the fact that many authorities dispute Maimonides' position, "perhaps" the lenient ruling of R. Jacob Emden may be relied upon if continuation of pregnancy until term would be detrimental to the health of the mother.

In a similar vein, Rabbi Waldenberg notes (*Ẓiẓ Eli'ezer,* IX, 239) that "there is room for leniency" if the state of maternal health is very precarious or if necessary in order to secure relief from severe pain. As noted earlier, Rabbi Moses Jonah Zweig (*No'am,* VII, 48) rules that abortion on these grounds is permissible within the first forty days of gestation.

Among the authorities not previously cited who forbid destruction of the fetus other than in face of a definite threat to the life of the mother are: *Ko'ah Shor,* no. 21; *Levushei Mordekhai, Hoshen Mishpat,* no. 36; *Bet Shelomoh, Hoshen Mishpat,* no. 132; *Peri ha-Sadeh,* IV, no. 50; *Binyan David,* no. 47; *Avnei Zedek, Hoshen Mishpat,* no. 19; *Afarkasta de-Anya,* no. 169; and *Zur Ya'akov,* no. 141.

Preservation of Maternal Life During Parturition

The Mishnah, *Oholot* 7:6, is emphatic in its ruling against embryotomy once the major portion of the child has been delivered. The inferred presumption is that the abandonment of one life will assuredly save the other. There is, however, no specific statement of halakhic determination dealing with cases where non-interference would lead to the loss of both mother and child. The halakhic grounds which justify an embryotomy under such conditions, even subsequent to the commencement of parturition, are delineated by R. Israel Lipschutz, the author of *Tiferet Yisra'el,* in his commentary on this Mishnah. The issue hinges upon the applicability of a law recorded by Maimonides, *Hilkhot Yesodei ha-Torah* 5:5: ". . . if the heathen said to them, 'Give us one of your company and we shall kill him; if not we will kill all of you,' let them all be killed but let them not deliver to them [the heathens] a single Jewish soul. But if they specified [the victim] to them and said, 'Give us so and so or we shall kill all of you,' if he had incurred the death penalty as Sheba the son of Bichri, they may deliver him to them . . . but if he had not incurred the death penalty let them all be killed, but let them not deliver a single Jewish soul."

Maimonides' ruling is based upon the explication of the narrative of II Samuel 20:4–22 found in the Palestinian Talmud, *Terumot* 8:12. Joab, commander of King David's troops, had pursued Sheba the son of Bichri and beseiged him in the town of Abel and demanded that he be delivered to the king's forces. Otherwise Joab threatened to destroy the entire city. From the verse "Sheba the son of Bichri hath lifted up his hand against the king, against David" (20:21), Resh Lakish infers that acquiescence with this demand can be sanctioned only in instances where the victim's life is lawfully forfeit, as was the case with regard to Sheba the son of Bichri, who is described as being guilty of *lèse majesté;* in instances where the victim is innocent, all must suffer death rather than become accomplices to murder. R. Yohanan maintains that the question of guilt is irrelevant, but that the crucial element is rather the singling out of a specific individual. Members of a group have no right to select one of their number arbitrarily and deliver him to death in order to save themselves since the life of each individual is of inestimable value. However, once a specific person has been marked for death in any event, either alone if surrendered by his companions or together with the entire group if they refuse to comply, those who deliver him are not accounted as accessories. Maimonides' ruling is in accordance with the opinion of Resh Lakish.[68]

In a medical context, when confronted by the imminent loss of both mother and child, dismemberment of a partially delivered child having no possibility of survival in order to save the mother would be advocated by those authorities who require merely that the victim be "specified," since they do not require that he necessarily be guilty of a capital offense. However, according to Maimonides, the intended victim must be culpable as well and a newly born child is certainly guilty of no crime. Furthermore, this line of reasoning does not apply to the many cases where either the mother or child may be saved through the sacrifice of the other; in such situations the crucial element of "specification" is totally absent.

Yet another crucial discrepancy between our case and the paradigm instance of "specification" is stressed by R. Hayyim Sofer.[69] The provision regarding specification is a direct outgrowth of the law of pursuit. Sheba ben Bichri's refusal to surrender himself was the direct source of danger to his townspeople. This made him, in effect, a pursuer since it was within his power to remove the danger. Justification for turning him over to Joab was simply the application of the law of pursuit to this novel situation. The situation surrounding childbirth, argues R. Sofer, is not at all comparable. Since the birth process is not at all within the control of the child, he cannot be deemed a "pursuer" in permitting the genesis of a threat to the life of the mother. Since we are dealing with a natural process totally independent of human volition, the mother must be deemed as "pursued by Heaven." Even if the element of "specification" were present (i.e., the life of the mother could be saved by sacrificing the child but not vice versa), such "specification" would not render the partially born child a "pursuer" inasmuch as he cannot in this instance "surrender," even if he were capable of such choice.

R. Hayyim Sofer further asserts, on the basis of a contrary-to-fact hypothetical argument, that even if Halakhah were to sanction the taking of another's life in order to save one's own, this provision would be based solely on the consideration that an act of murder is inevitable in any event. However, death in childbirth, barring human interference, occurs through natural causes without any mortal becoming sullied by the crime of bloodshed. If so, "better two deaths than one murder." Accordingly, R. Hayyim Sofer refuses to grant permission to destroy the child in order to save the mother, even though its life is doomed in any event.

Presenting a second argument which would render this practice permissible, R. Israel Lipschutz reasons that Halakhah suspects that each newly born child may be premature and possibly incapable of survival and provides that the child's status remain in doubt until it demonstrates viability through survival for a minimum period of thirty days.[70] Therefore, argues R. Lipschutz, since there is an objective criterion for granting priority to the life of the mother, the usual principle "on what account is his blood sweeter than yours" does not apply and hence the child may be sacrificed in order to spare the life of the mother.[71]

This problem is discussed in the writings of several other authorities as well. In his commentary on the Mishnah, R. Akiva Eger[72] poses the question regarding the permissibility of killing a child in order to save the mother where failure to do so would result in the death of both. Quoting *Panim Me'irot,*[73] he concludes that the ultimate decision in this instance requires further deliberation. R. Moses Schick,[74] without citing R. Lipschutz's *Tiferet Yisra'el,* agrees with these conclusions in substance. However, noting a previously expressed opinion of *Ḥatam Sofer,*[75] he adds that facts ascertained solely through the testimony of medical practitioners can be accepted as establishing only a *safek,* i.e., as possibly being the case, but cannot be regarded as having been established with conclusive certainty. Since there remains an element of doubt, a decision on our part to terminate the life of the child is unwarranted. However, if the physician himself is confident of the certainty of his diagnosis and of his assessment of the medical prognosis, he may rely upon his own certainty and govern his own actions accordingly. R. Schick's responsum concludes with the statement that the matter requires further deliberation and that these views are not to be regarded as definitive decisions. In response to a similar query, R. David Hoffmann, citing the relevant sources, expresses his agreement with the opinion of *Tiferet Yisra'el.*[76]. R. Isaac Judah Schmelkes (*Teshuvot Beit Yizḥak,* II, *Yoreh De'ah,* no. 162) expresses some reservation but agrees that R. Schick's ruling may be relied upon, provided that the pertinent medical facts are established on the basis of the concurring opinions of two physicians of the Jewish faith who will appreciate the gravity of the potential transgression.

The position adopted by R. Joseph Saul Nathanson[77] is most engaging. Citing the decision recorded in *Bava Mezia* 62a,[78] "Your life takes precedence over the life of your fellow," this authority contends that the Mishnah's discussion of the treatment of a woman in "hard travail" and the restrictions placed upon efforts to preserve her life refer only to third parties.[79] An individual lacking personal involvement may not make one life subordinate to another, but as far as one's own life is concerned it takes precedence over the life of one's fellow. R. Joseph Saul Nathanson's view is actually an expression of an identical position cited by *Me'iri, Sanhedrin* (ed. Abraham Sofer, Frankfurt-am-Main, n.d.), p. 271, in the name of the "Sages of the Generations," who permit the mother herself to destroy the child even after final parturition has begun while forbidding others to do so. Rabbi Zweig dismisses this view as "the opinion of an individual" and hence having no standing in determination of Halakhah (*No'am* VII, 55).[80]

Maiming vs. Destruction of the Fetus

The law of pursuit provides that the life of the pursuer is forfeit only if his malevolent intention cannot be thwarted by otherwise disabling the pursuer. Thus, if it is possible to disable the aggressor by maiming or crippling him, his life may not be taken under the law of pursuit. R. Moses Samuel Horowitz[81] and R. Isaac Schorr (*Ko'ah Shor*, no. 20) both rule that this consideration applies to a fetus as well. Accordingly, when intrauterine amputation of a limb would suffice to save the mother without recourse to an embryotomy, destruction of the fetus cannot be sanctioned. R. Shelomo ha-Kohen of Vilna, author of the well-known *Heshek Shelomoh*, deems this conclusion incontravertible and concurs in this ruling.[82]

Indeed, this interesting ramification serves as the basis for a novel reinterpretation of Maimonides' position. Rabbi Horowitz and Rabbi Schorr, apparently without either having seen the other's work, both note the expression "for it is *as* one pursuing her." They infer that Maimonides does not really intend to invoke the law of pursuit. Instead, he relies on the implicit rationale that the fetus is not "a life." Yet one restrictive aspect of the law of pursuit is applicable; namely, that the fetus, even though it is not deemed to be "a life," cannot be destroyed if it is possible to save the mother by merely crippling her unborn child. This then, they declare, is the intention of the phrase "limb by limb" as used by the Mishnah—first one limb, then another is removed in an attempt to deliver the child. While preservation of maternal life is of paramount concern, care must be taken that no unnecessary harm be inflicted upon the fetus.

Interpreted in a similar manner, the further provision of the Mishnah, "but once the major portion has emerged one may not touch it" (the fetus), implies that even the maiming of a partially born child or amputation of a limb is forbidden in order to save the mother. R. Hayyim Sofer (*Mahaneh Hayyim, Hoshen Mishpat,* no. 50) draws such an inference and indicates that the rationale motivating the decision is the fact that the physician "cannot guarantee with certainty" that the child will survive the surgical procedure. However, if noninterference will result in the loss of both mother and child, R. Sofer permits maiming of the child in an attempt to save the life of the mother.

Abortion of Pregnancy on Psychiatric Grounds

The entire area of psychiatric problems and severe emotional disturbances and their bearing upon halakhic questions has as yet not been adequately explored. Guidelines are to be found in isolated references to various forms of mental illness scattered throughout responsa literature. The earliest references to mental disease sufficiently grave to imperil the life of the afflicted occurs in the *Issur ve-Heter he-Arukh*,[83] attributed to Rabbenu Jonah of Gerondi. *Issur ve-Heter he-Arukh* cites a specific query addressed to an earlier authority, Maharam, concerning an epileptic who sought advice concerning the permissibility of partaking of a forbidden food reported to possess medicinal properties capable of curing his disease. The decision, in which Nahmanides acquiesces, is in the affirmative, provided that the efficacy of the remedy has been established. This decision is predicated upon a determination that epilepsy constitutes a danger to life, since at times an epileptic may endanger himself by "falling into fire or water." R. Israel Meir Mizrahi[84] relies upon the decision of Nahmanides in ruling that insanity constitutes a danger to life and accordingly permits an abortion when it is feared that the mother may otherwise become mentally deranged. This position is also adopted by *Levushei Mordekhai, Hoshen Mishpat,* no. 39, who is cited by R. Waldenberg, *Ziz Eli'ezer,* IX, 327.[85] Similarly, R. Isaac Jacob Weiss, *Minhat Yizhak,* I, no. 115, and R. Moses Feinstein, *Iggerot Moshe, Even ha-Ezer,* I, no. 65, declare that mental derangement constitutes a danger to life.

Other authorities, however, apparently do not regard insanity (at least in all forms) as constituting a hazard to life. Thus when R. Moses Sofer[86] was asked whether it was permissible to have a mentally ill child admitted to an institution where he would be served forbidden foods, he discusses all aspects of the case without at all raising the question of *piku'ah nefesh* (danger to life). Rabbi Unterman, in an article contributed to *Ha-Torah ve-ha-Medinah* (IV, 27),[87] argues that the instinct for self-preservation is so deeply ingrained, and suicidal tendencies are so rare, that one cannot consider mental illnesses as falling under the category of diseases which imperil life.[88]

Abortion of a Bastard Fetus

R. Jair Bacharach was asked whether a dose of ecbolics could be administered to a Jewess who had become pregnant as the result of an adulterous relationship in order to induce the abortion of her bastard fetus. Noting that the customary prayer "Preserve this child to its father and to its mother" is omitted at the circumcision of the issue of an adulterous or incestuous union because "the proliferation of bastards in Israel" is not desirable, he concludes that while proliferation of such children may not be a social desideratum, and hence there is no obligation to offer prayer on their behalf, nevertheless there is no legal distinction between a bastard and a legitimate embryo which would sanction any overt action which might threaten its life (*Havvot Ya'ir,* no. 31). An identical query addressed to R. Jacob Emden (*She'elat Yavez,* I, no. 43) elicited a different response. Taking note of the earlier responsum in *Havvot Ya'ir,* R. Jacob Emden finds grounds to differentiate between the seduction of an unmarried maiden and an adulterous relationship with a married woman.[89] The latter, having committed a capital offense, is liable to the death penalty. Were we able to execute judgment in capital cases, the pregnant condition of the condemned would not warrant a delay in administering punishment. This is clearly established by the Mishnah (*Arakhin* 7a) even with regard to cases in which pregnancy occurs after commission of the crime. Since, in this case, the child was conceived in sin, there is all the more reason for immediate execution of the mother. R. Jacob Emden adds the rather astonishing opinion that, although we no longer administer capital punishment, nevertheless, one who has committed a crime punishable by death may commit suicide without fear of sin. R. Jacob Emden even deems self-immolation to be meritorious in such circumstances. R. Jacob Emden reasons that if the mother may destroy herself completely she may certainly destroy a part of her body. Hence he concludes there can be no prohibition against the destruction of a bastard fetus since its life is legally forfeit. From an observation added in the course of his discussion, it appears that R. Jacob Emden intended his remarks to apply only where formal warning of the nature of the transgression and its punishment was administered prior to the adulterous act, since capital punishment is not inflicted by the *Bet Din* in the absence of such warning.[90]

Rabbi Unterman[91] voices an obvious objection against the above decision. The Mishnah in *Arakhin* which provides for the execution of a pregnant woman is understood by the commentaries as having reference to situations where pregnancy was not detected until the verdict was announced; when pregnancy was known beforehand, the trial was delayed until after confinement in order to spare the life of the child. The status of an adulterous woman in our times is always that of a woman prior to trial. Accordingly, there is no justification for the destruction of a fetus illicitly conceived.

Rabbi Ben-Zion Uziel, in his *Mishpetei Uzi'el, Hoshen Mishpat,* III, no. 46, advances an original line of reasoning in substantiation of R. Jacob Emden's decision regarding the abortion of a bastard fetus. The Gemara (*Sotah* 37b) declares: "The whole section refers to none other than an adulterer and an adulteress—'Cursed is the man who makes a graven or molten image' (Deut. 27:15). Is it sufficient merely to pronounce such a person cursed? [His transgression is punishable not merely by a curse but by death.] Rather it refers to one who has engaged in immoral intercourse and begets a son who goes to live among the heathen and worships idols. Cursed be the father and mother of this person, for this is what they caused him to do.'' Rashi explains that since such a person is debarred from the assembly and cannot marry a Jewish woman of legitimate birth, his embarrassment causes him to mingle with heathens and his heathen associations lead him to idolatry. From this discussion one may deduce that while the act of adultery carries with it a statutory punishment irrespective of future developments, there is yet another "curse" incurred if the union leads to the birth of bastard progeny. Therefore, rules Rabbi Uziel, it is permissible to destroy the embryo in order not to incur this curse. It is of course self-understood that reference is only to cases of bastards falling under the "curse" and not to the progeny of an unmarried woman, for the Torah regards as a bastard only the issue of an adulterous or incestuous union. Rabbi Uziel further declares that only the parents themselves may abort the fetus. His reasoning is that only they incur the curse, hence only they may obviate the curse by destroying the fetus. An outsider who incurs no penalty does not experience the "grave need" deemed essential by R. Jacob Emden and has, therefore, no right to interfere with the development of the unborn child.

R. Moses Yekuthiel Kaufmann, author of *Lehem ha-Panim* (Furth, 5526), states unequivocally (*Kunteres Aharon,* no. 19, p. 58b) that it is forbidden to give a woman a drug for the purpose of aborting a bastard fetus.[92]

Abortion of an Abnormal Fetus

The status of abnormal and malformed human beings is well defined in Halakhah. Physical or mental abnormalities do not affect the human status of the individual. R. Judah he-Hasid[93] refers to the question of terminating the life of a monster-like child born with the teeth and tail of an animal. Indeed, the interlocutor raises the question only on basis of the fear aroused by reports that the creature would later "eat people." R. Eleazar Fleckeles of Prague[94] rules explicitly that the killing of even a grotesquely malformed child possessing animal features constitutes an act of murder. Challenging the questioner's view that the Talmud's suspension of the usual ritual impurity following the emission of similarly malformed or animal-like embryos indicates that upon birth a child so formed should not be classified as a human being, R. Fleckeles counters that this exclusion is limited to the laws of impurity applicable to miscarriages. The issue of a human mother, no matter how gravely deformed, enjoys human status and may not be destroyed either by overt act or by passively allowing it to die of starvation.

Rabbi Unterman,[95] in dealing with the question of abortion in cases where an expectant mother contracted German measles early in pregnancy, and Rabbi Moshe Yonah Zweig,[96] in discussing the deformities caused by thalidomide, both conclude that there is no distinction in the eyes of the law between normal and abnormal persons either with regard to the statutes governing homicide or with regard to those governing feticide. Rabbi Waldenberg (*Ziz Eli'ezer*, IX, 237) is the only authority who deems abnormality of the fetus to be justification for interruption of pregnancy and even he stipulates that the abortion must be performed in the early stages of pregnancy. Rabbi Waldenberg indicates that the difficulties engendered by the birth of an abnormal child may render abortion a "grave necessity" and therefore permissible according to the previously cited view of R. Jacob Emden. Rabbi Waldenberg originally permitted such termination of pregnancy within the first three months following conception provided there is as yet no fetal movement but has revised his position and now permits termination of pregnancy in such situations prior to the beginning of the last trimester.[97]

Abortions Under Noachide Law

Jewish law recognizes two distinct, divinely revealed codes of law. One of these codes is binding upon Jews as a result of the Sinaitic covenant; the second code, which is more limited in scope, encompassing the basic principles of moral behavior, is known as the Seven Commandments of the Sons of Noah. This latter code is viewed by Judaism as binding upon all non-Jews.

Noachides are specifically enjoined from destroying fetal life upon penalty of death (*Sanhedrin* 57b) on the basis of Genesis 9:6. This prohibition is recorded by Maimonides in his *Mishneh Torah, Hilkhot Melakhim* 9:4. Consequently, any aid extended to a gentile in the performance of an abortion is a violation of the precept "Thou shalt not place a stumbling block before the blind" (Lev. 19:14). This prohibition is clearly enunciated with regard to abortion of a fetus by R. Joseph Trani (*Teshuvot Maharit*, I, no. 97) and confirmed by his pupil, Rabbi Hayyim Benveniste (*Sheyarei Keneset ha-Gedolah, Tur, Hoshen Mishpat*, 425, no. 6). *Maharit*, however, notes that the Gemara (*Avodah Zarah* 6b) states that aid rendered to one transgressing a commandment is proscribed only if the sinner could not otherwise have fulfilled his desire. It is, for example, forbidden to bring a cup of wine to a Nazirite who is on the opposite side of the river and could not otherwise reach the wine; but if both the wine and the Nazirite are on the same side of the river and the Nazirite is capable of reaching the wine without assistance, any help extended does not fall under this prohibition. Such an act, while Biblically permitted, is banned by rabbinic edict legislating against "aiding transgressors." *Maharit* denies the applicability of the edict to aid rendered non-Jewish transgressors. Accordingly, *Maharit* rules that assistance in the performance of an abortion under these circumstances is forbidden only if no other physician is available; if others are available it is to be considered analagous to the case of both the Nazirite and the wine standing "on the same side of the river." There are nevertheless many authorities who agree that the rabbinic prohibition against "aiding transgressors" which applies even when both are "on the same side of the river" extends to aiding Noachide transgressors as well.[98] Furthermore, the author of *Mishneh le-Melekh* (*Hilkhot Malveh ve-Loveh* 4:2) argues that the availability and readiness of another individual to transport the wine over the river does not relieve the one who actually does so from culpability. The prohibition is deemed inoperative only if the transgression could be committed without "the placing of a stumbling block" by anyone else; when the transgression requires aid, the one who renders it is liable, according to this view, no matter how many others would have been willing to render similar aid.[99]

But may a Noachide destroy the life of an embryo in order to preserve the life of the mother? *Tosafot* (*Sanhedrin* 59a) poses the question but expresses doubt with regard to its resolution. The question seems to hinge upon the nature of the Noachide prohibition.[100] If, in extending the death penalty to the killing of a fetus under the Noachide Code, the Torah intends to indicate that with regard to Noachides fetal life is to be considered on a par with other human life, then, of course, the mother's life cannot be saved by a Noachide at the expense of the fetus. The law of pursuit cannot be invoked if the fetus is deemed "a life" under the Noachide dispensation, just as the law of pursuit does not apply in Jewish law after the commencement of birth, at which juncture the fetus is deemed "a life" according to the Sinaitic covenant.[101] On the other hand, the Torah may not deem the fetus to be "a life" even with regard to Noachides, but bans feticide under the Noachide code as a transgression totally unrelated to the concept of taking human life. If the Noachide prohibition is extraneous to the exhortation against homicide, it follows that the life of the mother would take precedence over that of the fetus. A virtually identical discussion establishing the prohibition against destruction of the fetus is presented by *Tosafot, Hullin* 33a, but without any suggestion whatsoever of the possibility that destruction of the fetus by a Noachide would be permissible under these circumstances. R. Isaac Schorr (*Ko'ah Shor,* no. 20, p. 32) concludes that since, at best, the matter remains in doubt the life of the fetus must remain inviolate.[102] He further advances a rather involved argument demonstrating that, regardless of the position adopted by *Tosafot,* there is no question that Maimonides forbids the destruction of a fetus by Noachides, even when the life of the mother is at stake. *Minhat Hinnukh*[103] advances yet another reason which precludes destruction of the fetus by a Noachide even if necessary in order to save the mother. According to this opinion, a Noachide may not transgress any provision of the Noachide Code in order to preserve a human life.[104]

Nevertheless, R. Isaac Schorr finds a basis upon which a non-Jewish physician might be requested to terminate the pregnancy of a Jewish woman. Requesting such aid should normally be discountenanced as a violation of "Thou shall not place a stumbling block before the blind." However, this commandment is no different from other negative prohibitions (excepting the three cardinal sins) which may be ignored when life is at stake. Since R. Moses Isserles (*Yoreh De'ah* 157:1) rules that this ban may be violated even if the "stumbling block" is the commission of one of the three cardinal sins, there is no barrier to requesting the non-Jewish physician to undertake such a procedure, if he is willing to do so, provided no Jewish physician is available. If a Jewish physician is available, his aid should be sought in order to obviate the necessity of "placing a stumbling block."[105]

A Final Caveat

In light of what may at times appear to be a harsh and forbidding stance, one might be tempted to conclude that Jewish law manifests an indifferent attitude toward the individual and his plight. It is important that we recognize that, quite to the contrary, Halakhah is motivated first and foremost by concern and solicitude for all living creatures. It is this extreme concern for man's inalienable right to life, both actual and potential, which permeates these many halakhic determinations.

A Jew is governed by such reverence for life that he trembles lest he tamper unmindfully with the greatest of all divine gifts, the bestowal or withholding of which is the prerogative of God alone. Although he be master over all within the world, there remain areas where man must fear to tread, acknowledging the limits of his sovereignty and the limitations of his understanding. In the unborn child lies the mystery and enigma of existence. Confronted by the miracle of life itself, man can only draw back in silence before the wonder of the Lord:

> Where wast thou when I laid the foundations of the earth?
> Declare, if thou hast the understanding . . .
> Have the gates of death been revealed unto thee?
> Or hast thou seen the gates of the shadow of death? . . .
> Declare, if thou knowest it all.[106]

As thou knowest not what is the way of the wind,

Nor how the bones do grow in the womb of her that is with child;
Even so thou knowest not the work of God
Who doeth all things.[107]

NOTES

1. *Emunah, Bittahon ve-Od* (Jerusalem, 5714), p. 21.
2. See below, n. 50.
3. This inference is not formulated explicitly by the *Tosafot* cited but is mentioned in passing by R. Jair Hayyim Bacharach in his *Teshuvot Havvot Ya'ir,* (Frankfort a. M., 5459), no. 31. The omission of this inference is perhaps intentional on the part of *Tosafot* since such omission is consistent with a distinction drawn by *Tosafot, Niddah,* 44a, to the effect that an embryo which has "torn itself loose" from its normal uterine position before the death of the mother enjoys inheritance rights with respect to the mother's property and passes on such rights to its heirs. This provision is based on the premise that the fetus' death is deemed to occur after that of the mother. One might therefore argue that "tearing itself loose" marks the stage at which the fetus is sufficiently viable to be accorded human status. Since the Mishnah refers to a woman who is in "hard travail," there is no evidence therefrom that an embryo in earlier stages of development, i.e., prior to having commenced the process of parturition, is accounted sufficiently human to render its destruction an offense.

Havvot Ya'ir endeavors to demonstrate that prenatal life is inviolate even at earlier stages of fetal development on the basis of the Talmudic discussion concerning the execution of an expectant mother who has incurred the death penalty. The Mishnah (*Arakhin* 7a) rules that the execution must be deferred until after the child's birth only if the convicted mother has already "sat on the birth stool," which the Gemara defines as being synonymous with the fetus' "tearing itself loose." Prior to this, execution is not delayed in order to preserve the unborn child. With regard to this inference the Gemara queries, *"Peshita! gufah he*—Of course! It [the fetus] is an organic part of her [the mother's] body." *Havvot Ya'ir* reasons that since the Gemara adds the phrase *gufah he* in formulating its question, one must conclude that the reason that the child is consigned to the same fate as the mother is that it is an organic part of her body. The logical inference is that were this rationale to be lacking, it would be forbidden to cause the death of the unborn fetus. For a conflicting inference which ignores this point, see R. Joseph Trani, *Teshuvot Maharit* (Fürth, 5528), I, no. 99.

For further discussion of the nature of the prohibition against feticide, see the sources cited by R. Hayyim Hezekiah Medini in his *Sedeh Hemed* (New York, 5722), I. 175 ff, *Kelalim, Ma'arekhet ha-Alef,* no. 52, and I, 304 f., *Sheyurei ha-Pe'ah, Ma'arekhet ha-Alef,* no. 19. See also the sources cited by R. Solomon Abraham Rezechte, *Bikkurei Shelomo* (Pietrokow, 5665), *Yoreh De'ah, Hashmatot,* no. 9.

4. Despite these two unequivocal statements, the language employed by *Tosafot, Niddah* 44b, led R. Zevi Hirsch Chajes to note in a gloss, *ad locum,* that *Tosafot* in *Niddah* expresses a contradictory opinion. Writing much earlier both *Havvot Ya'ir* in the above cited responsum and R. Jacob Emden in a gloss (*Niddah* 44b) state

without elaboration that *Tosafot* does not intend to express a permissive ruling but simply employs misleading phraseology. R. Jacob Emden adds in wonder, "Who is it that permits the killing of a fetus without reason?" See also the gloss of R. Solomon Eger *ad locum*. A close examination of the line of reasoning employed by *Tosafot* shows that the conclusion reached by *Maharaẓ Ḥajes* cannot be supported. *Tosafot* contends that the absence of statutory punishment with regard to the crime of feticide applies only to cases where the mother is alive at the time of destruction of the fetus; when, however, the mother's death precedes that of the fetus, *Tosafot* advances a tentative assertion to the effect that the fetus is independently viable and hence the killing of the fetus in such instances carries the full penalty for murder. If this is not the case and "it is permitted to kill the fetus," queries *Tosafot,* why is it then permissible to violate the Sabbath by carrying a knife through a public thoroughfare for the purpose of removing the fetus from the womb of its deceased mother? A literal reading indicates that, according to *Tosafot,* dispensation for the desecration of the Sabbath can be rightfully invoked only in order to preserve such lives which it is forbidden to destroy. For if the life in question may be destroyed deliberately, why then should the Sabbath be desecrated in order to save that which otherwise may be destroyed with impunity? Interpreted in this manner, there is no continuity whatsoever between this query and the previous assertion pertaining to the *penalty* for taking the life of an unborn child. Feticide might well *not* entail the punishment of homicide yet nevertheless constitute a moral offense, albeit an unpunishable one. Furthermore, *Tosafot's* refutation of this assumption is unclear if understood in the context of *Maharaẓ Ḥajes'* analysis. *Tosafot* negates the prior assumption by asserting that for the purpose of saving a life the Sabbath may be violated even if the life saved be that of one "whom it is permissible to kill." As evidence for this conclusion *Tosafot* cites the rule with regard to a *goses be-yedei adam* (one who has suffered a mortal wound, humanly inflicted), for the prolongation of whose life the Sabbath may be violated although "one who murders him is not culpable." According to *Maharaẓ Ḥajes'* understanding of the earlier remarks of *Tosafot,* the latter statement provides no substantiating evidence whatsoever. The status of a murderer of a *goses be-yedei adam* is clear: The killing is forbidden but carries no statutory punishment. Since it is forbidden to take his life, there is no question regarding the permissibility (according to *Tosafot,* but cf. *Teshuvot Shevut Ya'akov,* no. 13) of violating the Sabbath on his behalf; the absence of statutory punishment is deemed irrelevant. The issue in question, according to *Maharaẓ Ḥajes,* is solely that of the desecration of the Sabbath on behalf of a life (viz., that of a fetus) which might be destroyed with impunity. *Tosafot* endeavors to disprove the contention that it is somehow incongruous to sanction the desecration of the Sabbath in order to preserve that which there is not only no obligation to preserve but which may even be summarily destroyed. Indeed, the logic of this entailment is so strong that it is difficult to fathom its refutation. However, R. Solomon Drimer, *Teshuvot Bet Shelomo* (Lemberg, 1891), *Ḥoshen Mishpat,* no. 120, adopts a contrary view, reasoning that despite the prohibition against feticide, and despite a positive injunction to preserve the embryo, the Sabbath may be violated on behalf of an unborn child by application of the principle "Better to violate one Sabbath in order to observe many Sabbaths." If, on the other hand, we understand *Tosafot's* position in *Niddah* to be identical with that espoused by *Tosafot* in *Sanhedrin* and *Ḥullin,* the line of reasoning is most clear. In support of the assertion that the destruction of a fetus which has been preceded by death of the mother incurs the full penalty of murder, *Tosafot* endeavors to show that the desecration of the Sabbath is sanctioned only in order to save a life which it is not only forbidden to destroy but which, if unlawfully destroyed, is juridically punishable as a capital crime. This hypothesis is subsequently rejected by *Tosafot* with the argument that the killing of a *goses be-yedei adam* carries no such penalty, yet the Sabbath may be violated on his behalf. The conclusion, then, is that there is no evidence that the destruction of a fetus whose mother had preceded it in death carries a statutory punishment. That the taking of the life of a fetus is forbidden does not at all come into question according to this understanding of *Tosafot.* Cf. R. Moses Feinstein, *Iggerot Moshe, Yoreh De'ah,* II, no. 60, sec. 2.

According to any interpretation, the comparison by *Tosafot* of a fetus to a *goses be-yedei adam* defies comprehension. The absence of a statutory death penalty with regard to killing of a fetus is due to consideration of the embryo as not possessing independent animation in the degree requisite for consideration as a "life." The killing of a *goses* is not punishable because in the majority of instances the *goses* would die in any event. The Sabbath may be violated on his behalf because consideration of circumstances surrounding the "majority" of cases are irrelevant when a human life is at stake. Halakhah prescribes such measures even when chances that these measures may be efficacious are dim. The life of a *goses* is intrinsically human and hence the Sabbath is violated on his behalf even though chances of recovery are remote; at the same time his murderer cannot be put to death due to lack of definite assurance that the victim was viable. This does not provide demonstrative evidence contradictory to the hypothesis that provision for the rescue of a fetus through violation of the Sabbath *ipso facto* establishes that it is therefore a human life whose destruction is punishable. Cf. R. Jehiel Jacob Weinberg, *Seridei Esh* (Jerusalem, 5726), III, 350, n. 7. The approach offered in the name of Rabbi Sternbuch does not appear to resolve this perplexity.

5. *Teshuvot Ahi'ezer* (Vilna, 5699) III, 65, sec. 14. Although not adduced by *Ahi'ezer,* there is ample evidence that the principle "Is there anything which is forbidden to a Noachide yet permitted to a Jew?" establishes a Biblical prohibition. *Tosafot, Hullin* 33a, states explicitly with regard to *hazi shi'ur* (which is forbidden to Noachides) that the principle "Is there anything which is forbidden to a Noachide yet permitted to a Jew?" is consistent only with the opinion of R. Yohanan, who deems *hazi shi'ur* to be Biblically forbidden and in contradiction to the opinion of Resh Lakish, who deems *hazi shi'ur* to be rabbinically proscribed. Cf. R. Samuel Engel, *Teshuvot Maharash* (Varnov, 5696), V, no. 89, and R. Isaac Schorr, *Teshuvot Ko'ah Shor* (Kolomea, 5648), no. 20, page 33b; see also *Sedei Hemed,* I, 175; see also below, n.10.

6. However, cf. R. Samuel Strashun, *Mekorei ha-Rambam le-Rashash* (Jerusalem, 1957), p. 45, who writes that although feticide is Biblically forbidden "perhaps there is no punishment even 'at the hands of heaven.' "

7. Cf. below, n. 70.

8. This does not preclude recognition by Rabbenu Nissim of other considerations which would ban feticide under different circumstances on Biblical grounds. See below, n. 19 and n. 25. For a divergent interpretation of Rabbenu Nissim, see R. Moses Sternbuch, *Mo'adim u-Zemanim ha-Shalem,* I, no. 52.

9. *Ha-Pardes,* Nisan 5738; also published in *Sefer ha-Zikkaron le-Maran ha-Gri Abramsky* (Jerusalem, 5738). Against R. Feinstein's thesis it may be argued that the verse "they shall also both of them die" is cited as the source justifying deprival of the husband's proprietary interest in the unborn fetus. There is, then, no apparent need for Biblical sanction for deprival of the fetus' right to life.

10. Vol. VII, (Jerusalem, 5723), no. 48, p. 190; vol. VIII, (Jerusalem, 5725), no.

36, pp. 218-19 and vol. IX, (Jerusalem, 5727), no. 51, pp. 233-40; *Bikkurei Shelomo, Yoreh De'ah,* no. 10, sec. 2, and *Oraḥ Ḥayyim,* no. 33, sec. 5, also states that the prohibition is rabbinic in nature.

11. *Beit Yehudah (loc. cit.)* demonstrates that even indirect destruction of fetal life is forbidden on the basis of the Talmudic declaration (*Mo'ed Katan* 18a) that one who casts away his nail pairings is an evildoer since there is the danger that a pregnant woman may pass by and abort her unborn child. This is clearly an indirect cause and yet the perpetrator is deemed an evildoer.

12. This is contrary to the opinion of R. Waldenberg in his *Ẓiẓ Eli'ezer,* VIII, 219, who does not recognize any such distinction. R. Waldenberg, incidentally, does not note this distinction as drawn by *Teshuvot Ge'onim Batra'i.* Elsewhere, however, R. Waldenberg indicates that when termination of pregnancy is permissible, it is preferable to induce abortion by use of drugs if possible. See *Ẓiẓ Eli'ezer,* IX, 240. Cf. also R. Ovadiah Yosef, *Yabbi'a Omer* (Jerusalem, 5724), IV, *Even ha-Ezer,* no. 1, sec. 5. See also *Leḥem ha-Panim, Kunteres Aḥaron,* no. 19, who forbids drinking a "cup of roots" in order to kill the fetus. This prohibition is also cited by R. Shalom Schachne Tchernik, *Ḥayyim u-Verakhah le-Mishmeret Shalom,* no. 71 (p. 31a).

13. Cf. *Ẓiẓ Eli'ezer,* VIII, 219, and IX, 239.

14. R. Drimer similarly argues that the *a priori* principle "How do you know that your blood is sweeter than the blood of your fellow?" cannot be applied in assessing the value of fetal life. Cf. below n. 71.

15. This determination is based upon *Tosafot, Sanhedrin* 59b, and others who maintain that such practices are Biblically prohibited. For a comprehensive list of sources, see *Oẓar ha-Poskim* (Jerusalem, 5725), IX, 163-64, and R. Moses D. Tendler, *Tradition,* IX (1967), nos. 1-2, pp. 211-12. Regarding the question of whether Noachides are bound by the prohibition against onanism, see *Tosafot, Sanhedrin* 59b; *Mishneh le-Melekh, Hilkhot Melakhim* 10:7; R. Naphtali Ẓevi Judah Berlin, *Ha'amek She'elah* 165:2; and R. Joseph Rosen, *Teshuvot Ẓafenat Pa'ane'aḥ* (New York, 5714), no. 30.

16. R. Jacob Emden, *She'elot Yavez,* I (New York, 5721), no. 43, also cites this consideration. See also *Zekhuta de-Avraham,* cited by R. Meir Dan Plocki, *Ḥemdat Yisra'el* (Pietrokow, 5687), p. 175.

17. Cited by *Ḥemdat Yisra'el,* p. 175.

18. It is on the basis of *Havvot Ya'ir's* declaration that feticide is forbidden as a form of "destruction of the seed" and of the diminished severity of such an act when performed by a woman (according to Rabbenu Tam) that R. Waldenberg counsels that it is preferable to seek a female (Jewish) doctor to perform even those abortions which are halakhically permissible. See *Ẓiẓ Eli'ezer,* IX, 235.

19. Following this line of reasoning, feticide would be Biblically forbidden even according to Rabbenu Nissim, who does not consider destruction of a fetus to be a form of homicide.

20. *Ḥemdat Yisra'el,* pp. 175f.

21. See above, n. 15.

22. *Seridei Esh* (Jerusalem, 5726), III, no. 127, pp. 344f. This responsum was originally published as an article in *No'am,* IX (1966), pp. 193-215, and was reprinted subsequently in the third volume of *Seridei Esh* with a number of added notes.

23. *Teshuvot Maharit,* I, no. 97 and no. 99. R. Feinstein, however, writes that *Maharit* no. 99 is certainly a forged responsum [authored] by a mistaken student who recorded it in [*Maharit's*] name"; see below, n. 70.

24. Other authorities refute this evidence on the grounds that the fetus is an organic part of the mother and hence under identical sentence as the mother. Since it will die in any event, there is no reason why it cannot be put to death earlier in order to spare the mother dishonor. Cf. *Havvot Ya'ir*, no. 31; *She'elat Yavez*, no. 43; *Maharit*, I, no. 97; and R. Ben-Zion Uziel, *Mishpetei Uzi'el* (Jerusalem, 5657), III, *Hoshen Mishpat*, no. 46.

25. See n. 19. Cf. *Seridei Esh*, p. 349; and R. Moses Jonah Zweig, *No'am*, VIII (Jerusalem, 5725), 44 ff. Cf. however, *Ko'ah Shor*, no. 20, p. 34a, who argues that the prohibition of Deuteronomy 25:3 does not apply to the striking of a minor, much less to the injury of an embryo. The verse in question expressly refers to the punishment of forty stripes imposed by the *Bet Din* and admonishes the court not to administer more than the prescribed number of lashes. Other forms of physical assault are banned by implication: "If the Torah objects to the striking of a wicked man that he be not lashed more than in accordance with his wickedness, how much more so [does it object] to the striking of a righteous person" (Rambam, *Hilkhot Sanhedrin* 16:12). R. Schorr differs with *Maharit* and argues that only those who have reached their religious majority are included in this scriptural reference since only they are subject to the flagellation imposed by the *Bet Din*. However, R. Aryeh Lipschuetz, *Aryeh de-Bei Ila'i* (Przemysl, 5634), *Yoreh De'ah*, no. 6, advances this argument as conclusively demonstrating that *Maharit* is concerned with "wounding" of the mother rather than with injury of the fetus.

26. *Teshuvot Zafenat Pa'ane'ah*, no. 59. R. Ben Zion Uziel, *Mishpetei Uzi'el*, *loc. cit.*, explains *Tosafot's* mention of a ban against feticide as referring simply to the general obligation to be fruitful and multiply. One who does not engage in the fulfillment of this precept is accounted "as if he commits bloodshed" (*Yevamot* 63b). Although the context of the quotation deals with passive non-fulfillment of the *mitzvah,* this stricture is applicable all the more to an individual overtly seeking to prevent the development of an already existing life.

27. It is therefore significant that the Chief Rabbis of Israel (*J.T.A. Daily News Bulletin,* Dec. 7, 1974), the Chief Rabbi of France (*J.T.A. Daily News Bulletin,* Nov. 29, 1974), R. Moshe Feinstein (see above, n. 9) and the Union of Orthodox Rabbis of the United States and Canada (*Ha-Pardes,* Sivan 5736) have ruled that feticide is Biblically forbidden as an act of homicide.

28. Further grounds for this ruling are given by R. Unterman in his work *Shevet mi-Yehudah* (Jerusalem, 5715), I, 29. See below, n. 57.

29. It is, however, not entirely clear that feticide must be considered murder *per se* rather than an "appurtenance" of murder. While it is clear that killing a *terefah* is murder *per se,* that is so because the prohibition against such an act is derived from the prohibition "Thou shalt not kill." The prohibition against destroying a fetus, if derived from the principle "Is there anything which is forbidden to a Noachide yet permitted to a Jew" does not necessarily establish a prohibition which may be categorized as homicide itself. (See above, n. 5). The verse "Whoso sheddeth the blood of man *within man* shall his blood be shed (Gen. 9:6), which serves as an admonition against homicide in the Noachide Code, does not necessarily establish feticide as an act of homicide. (See above, p. 162). Rabbi Feinstein himself adds the comment that perhaps the prohibition is not "explicit" and hence the principle "Be killed and do not transgress" does not apply.

30. *Minhat Hinnukh* (Vilna, 5672), no. 296, part II, p. 218.

31. See, however, below, n. 71. Rabbi Feinstein expresses reservation with regard to whether or not the principle "How do you know that your blood is sweeter than the blood of your fellow?" applies to the killing of a fetus. See above, n. 9.

32. It is perhaps of interest to note that Aristotle (*De Historia Animalium,* VII, 3) declares that the male fetus is endowed with a rational soul on the fortieth day of gestation and the female on the eightieth. This distinction corresponds not only to the respective periods of impurity prescribed by Leviticus but to the opinion of R. Ishmael in the Mishnah, *Niddah* 30a, who is of the opinion that the prescribed periods of impurity correspond to the number of days required for the animation of the respective sexes and therefore declares that no impurity results from the miscarriage of a female embryo of less than eighty days. Aristotle's representation of animation as occurring on the fortieth or eightieth day, depending upon the sex of the fetus, was later incorporated in both Canon and Justinian law. See Rabbi Immanuel Jakobovits, *Jewish Medical Ethics* (New York, 1959), p. 175.

33. *Shakh, Hoshen Mishpat* 210:2; *Zafenat Pa'ane'ah,* no. 59; and R. Elchanan Wasserman, *Kovez Shi'urim,* II, no. 11, sec. 1.

34. Reference by the late Rabbi Zweig of Antwerp (*No'am,* VII, 53) to an opinion by *Havvot Ya'ir* to the effect that there is no prohibition during this period is erroneous. *Havvot Ya'ir,* in his introductory comments, calls attention to the fact that various stages of fetal development are recognized in different contexts, viz., forty days, three months, and independent movement of the fetal limbs, but quickly adds that it is not his desire to render judgment on the basis of "inclination of the mind or reasoning of the stomach." On the contrary, *Havvot Ya'ir's* failure to note such distinctions in the course of developing his own thesis portends his rejection of such a distinction.

It may be of interest to note that this misconstruction of *Havvot Ya'ir* is legend. *Sedei Hemed* cites with perplexity conflicting positions attributed to *Havvot Ya'ir* by other sources with regard to this question and notes in resignation that he does not have access to the responsa of *Havvot Ya'ir,* and hence cannot determine which quotation is correct. Upon reading these comments, R. Solomon Abraham Rezechte wrote to the author of *Sedei Hemed* that he has indeed seen the words of *Havvot Ya'ir* in the original and reports that the latter views the prohibition against feticide as binding during the early periods of pregnancy as well. See *Bikkurei Shelomo* (Pietrokow, 5665), no. 10, sec. 35. See also, below, n. 45.

R. Weinberg's summary declaration (p. 350) that such a prohibition does not exist according to the *Ba'al Halakhot Gedolot,* who permits desecration of the Sabbath in order to save an embryo even within this forty-day period, is contradictory to the reasoning of *Havvot Ya'ir,* as indicated by R. Weinberg himself (p. 339). R. Weinberg argues that *Havvot Ya'ir* fails to give consideration to the opinion of Nahmanides, who maintains that, despite the law against feticide, the Sabbath may not be violated on behalf of an unborn child. This allegation is readily refutable since *Havvot Ya'ir* argues merely that permission to violate the Sabbath in order to save a fetus logically entails a prohibition against destroying such a life, but not vice versa. It cannot be inferred from *Havvot Ya'ir* that the absence of such permission necessarily entails license to destroy the fetus.

35. *Torat ha-Adam, Sha'ar ha-Sakanah,* ed. R. Bernard Chavel, *Kitvei Ramban* (Jerusalem, 5724), II, 29; also cited by *Rosh* and *Ran* in their respective commentaries on *Yoma* 82a; see also *Korban Netanel, Yoma, Perek Yom ha-Kippurim,* no. 10.

36. See above, n. 34.

37. *Hemdat Yisra'el,* "Indexes and Addenda," p. 17.

38. *No'am,* VI, 4 f; *Shevet me-Yehudah,* I, 9 f.

39. *Teshuvot Maharit,* I, no. 99.

40. The authenticity of this quotation is highly questionable. R. Unterman (p. 8)

notes that he searched *Teshuvot ha-Rashba* in an unsuccessful attempt to locate this responsum. It seems probable that *Maharit's* quotation is culled from responsum no. 120 of vol. I in the published text (Bene-Berak, 5718). This responsum deals with the permissibility of rendering medical assistance to Noachide women so that they may be enabled to conceive. In language similar to that quoted by *Maharit,* mention is made of Ramban's actually having done so in return for financial compensation. However, no mention whatsoever is made of Ramban's having assisted in medical abortion. *Maharit* apparently had a variant textual version. Cf., also, R. Samuel Hubner, *Ha-Darom,* Tishri 5729, p. 33, who attempts to resolve the issue by suggesting an alternative punctuation of this quotation. R. Feinstein points to the absence of such a responsum in the works of Rashba as evidence that the responsum attributed to *Maharit* is itself a forgery; see above, n. 23.

41. See above, n. 15.

42. R. Unterman fails, however, to note the comments of R. Jacob Zevi Jalish in his *Melo ha-Ro'im, Sanhedrin* 57b, who expresses a contrary view. Examination of the phraseology of *Ḥemdat Yisra'el,* Part I, p. 108, indicates that R. Plocki also had such a distinction in mind. In cases of danger to the mother he permits abortion of embryos of less than forty days without further qualification and adds that there are grounds for permitting abortion at subsequent stages of development provided this procedure is performed by a Jewish physician.

43. The absence, in the Noachide Code, of a ban on feticide during the first forty days of gestation would, in the opinion of this writer, provide insight into what is otherwise considered an erroneous translation by the Septuagint of Exodus 21:22-23: "And if two men strive together and hurt a woman with a child so that her children depart and yet no harm *(ason)* follow, he shall surely be fined. . . . But if any harm follows, then thou shalt give life for life." Rabbinic exegesis regards the term "harm" as having reference to the death of the mother. Compensation is payable to the husband for the loss of his offspring only if the mother survives. Should the mother die as a result of this assault, the attacker is absolved from the payment of this fine. From these provisions the Gemara derives the principle that the commission of a capital crime, even if unintentional and hence not leading to the invocation of the statutory penalty, absolves the offender from the payment of any other compensation. The Septuagint, however, renders these verses as follows:

Ἐὰν δὲ μάχωνται δύο ἄνδρες καὶ πατάξωσι γυναῖκα ἐν γαστρὶ ἔχουσαν, καὶ ἐξέλθῃ τὸ παιδίον αὐτῆς μὴ ἐξεικονισμένον . . . And if two men strive and smite a woman with child, *and her child be born imperfectly formed,* he shall be forced to pay a penalty . . . Ἐὰν δὲ ἐξεικονισμένον ᾖ . . . But if it be perfectly formed, he shall give life for life

This reading understands the death penalty to which reference is made as being incurred for the killing of the fetus in cases where the fetus is *formed,* i.e., has already reached the fortieth day of gestation. It is clearly on the basis of this passage in the Septuagint that such a distinction is drawn by Philo (*De Spec. Legibus,* III, 108-10) and it was this reading of the Septuagint which influenced the attitude of the Church.Cf. Jakobovits, *op. cit.,* pp. 174, 179, 328, n. 43, and 333, n. 152. Samuel Poznanski, "Jakob ben Ephraim ein Antikaraischer Polemiker des X Jahrhunderts," *Gedenkbuch zur Errinerung an David Kaufmann,* ed. M. Brann and F. Rosenthal (Breslau, 1900), p. 186, suggests that the mistranslation is based on reading *ẓurah* for *ason.* On the basis of R. Unterman's thesis, the entire matter is quite readily resolved, particularly in light of the rabbinic tradition which states that modifications were intentionally introduced by the Jewish translators (see *Megillah* 9a). Addressed to gentiles, the translation may have been intended to incorporate ramifications of Noachide law. Since a Noachide incurs capital punishment for the destruction of a fetus, provided it is formed, he would be absolved from further punishment even in cases where the mother survives. An exhaustive interpretation of *ason,* then, signifies death of the mother if the attacker is a Jew, and either death of the mother or of a formed fetus if the attacker is a Noachide. The word *ason* as applied to a Noachide thus includes the death of a formed fetus and is rendered accordingly by the Septuagint. This interpretation is, of course, founded on the premise that the principle of absolution from the lesser of two simultaneously incurred punishments extends to Noachide law as well — a matter which bears further investigation. R. Joseph Babad is of the opinion that the principle *kim leh be-de-rabbah mineh* (imposition of the greater of two punishments to the exclusion of the lesser) does not apply to Noachides. See *Minḥat Ḥinnukh,* no. 34. However, there is basis for assuming that the question is the subject of controversy between Rashi and *Tosafot, Eruvin* 62a. Cf. *Encyclopedia Talmudit* (Tel Aviv, 5711), III, 354.

44. Rabbi Plocki's argument is predicated upon a faulty biological premise. Fertilization takes place in the Fallopian tube and subsequently the fertilized ovum descends into the uterus. A tampon inserted into the vagina does not penetrate beyond the cervical os. Contraception following cohabitation is designed to prevent sperm which have not already done so prior to insertion of the tampon from penetrating beyond the vagina. Thus there is no possibility of destroying an already fertilized ovum.

45. *Peri ha-Sadeh,* in turn, attributes this distinction to *Havvot Ya'ir.* In point of fact, this distinction, together with several others, was made by *Havvot Ya'ir* only by way of introduction. He concludes his prefatory remarks with the statement that it is not his goal to adjudicate such matters on the basis of *sevarat ha-keres* (an unfounded theory), but rather on the basis the "law of the Torah." At no point in his subsequent analysis does *Havvot Ya'ir* again refer to such a distinction. In fact, on the basis of *Havvot Ya'ir's* thesis that feticide is a form of *hashḥatat zera* such a distinction would be quite illogical. See above, n. 34.

46. R. Shaul Israeli, *Amud ha-Yemini,* no. 32, expresses a permissive view with regard to abortion of a deformed fetus during subsequent periods of pregnancy. His reasoning has, however, not been accepted by any recognized authority. The comments of R. Aryeh Leib Grossnass, *Lev Aryeh,* II, 205, do not serve to establish halakhic permissibility; see R. Moses Feinstein, *Iggerot Mosheh, Even ha-Ezer,* I, no. 62. For a recent, more permissive view expressed by Rabbi Waldenberg see J. David Bleich, *Contemporary Halakhic Problems* (New York, 1977), pp. 112–115, and below, n. 97. Cf. also R. Samuel Ḥayyim Katz, *Ha-Pardes,* Tammuz 5735.

47. R. Unterman's opinion was actually expressed much earlier in his *Shevet me-Yehudah,* I, 50.

48. See also R. Samuel Engel, *Teshuvot Maharash Engel,* VII, no. 85, who, after drawing a distinction between the first forty days and the subsequent periods of pregnancy, concludes with the statement, "but it is difficult to rely upon this."

49. See, however, R. Shelomo ha-Kohen of Vilna, who is of the opinion that such rescue of the mother, although permitted, is by no means obligatory. This scholar apparently maintains that the obligation to preserve a life is suspended when such life can be preserved only at the cost of another's life, even though such action involves no overt transgression. These views are recorded in a responsum addressed

to R. Moses Horowitz and incorporated by the latter in his *Yedei Moshe* (Pietrokow, 5658), no. 4, sec. 8.

50. *Yoreh De'ah* 194:10; *Siftei Kohen, loc. cit.,* no. 26; *Sidrei Taharah, loc. cit.* See also R. David Hoffman, *Melammed le-Ho'il* (Frankfort a. M., 5696), no. 69, and R. Meir Eisenstadt. *Teshuvot Panim Me'irot* (New York, 5722), III, no. 8.

51. The law of pursuit requires the bystander to disable the aggressor, by a fatal blow if necessary, in order to thwart the pursuer's intent to kill. See Rambam, *Hilkhot Roze'ah* 1:6.

52. *Noda bi-Yehudah, Mahadurah Tinyana* (Vilna, 5659), *Hoshen Mishpat,* no. 59.

53. *Havvot Ya'ir,* no. 31.

54. *Hiddushei R. Hayyim ha-Levi, Hilkhot Roze'ah* 1:9. Another version of R. Hayyim Soloveichik's exposition of Rambam's position appears in *Moriah,* Sivan, 5739.

55. *Even he-Azel* (Jerusalem, 5696), II, *Hilkhot Roze'ah,* 1:9. Cf. also *Iggerot Moshe, Yoreh De'ah,* II, no. 60, sec. 2. See also R. Jehiel Jacob Weinberg, *Seridei Esh,* III, 343.

56. P. 26ff. A similar explanation is offered by R. Nahum Rabinovitch, *Ha-Darom* (5729), no. 28, pp. 19f. For yet another interpretation of Rambam (albeit one which does not affect our discussion), see R. Isaac Judah Shmelkes, *Teshuvot Beit Yizhak* (New York, 5720), *Yoreh De'ah,* II, no. 162. See also R. Zweig, *No'am,* VII, 52.

57. The principle "Be killed but do not transgress" applies only to actual homicide but imposes no obligation in face of coercion to prevent fulfillment of the obligation to rescue the life of one's fellowman. Since, according to R. Unterman, killing a fetus does not fall within the category of murder but is inherently contraindicated by the obligation to preserve fetal life, it follows that there is no obligation to refrain from destroying a fetus at the cost of one's own life.

58. *Teshuvot Ahi'ezer,* II, no. 72.

59. *Seridei Esh,* III, 342; cf. also R. Meir Dan Plocki, *Hemdat Yisra'el, Maftehot ve-Hosafot,* p. 32, who makes much the same point.

60. Cf., however, R. Chaim Ozer Grodzinski, *Teshuvot Ahi'ezer,* I, no. 23, sec. 2, who declares that the law of pursuit applies not only in cases of certainty but also in cases of "estimation *(umdena),* i.e. when a prognosis of mortality is based upon "the estimation of the physicians."

61. R. Feinstein forbids an abortion unless in the opinion of the physicians it is "nearly certain" that otherwise the mother will die; see above, n. 9.

62. The same opinion is recorded by R. David Dov Meisels, *Binyan David* (Ouhel, 5692), no. 47, in the name of *Avnei Zedek, Hoshen Mishpat,* no. 19.

63. *Levushei Mordekhai, Mahadurah Tinyana* (Budapest, 5684), *Yoreh De'ah,* no. 87.

64. A similar interpretation of Rambam is offered by *Mishpetei Uzi'el,* III, 211.

65. *She'elat Yavez,* no. 43. This opinion was apparently accepted by R. Shlomoh Kluger, whose views are recorded in *Zehuta de-Avraham,* no. 60, and by *Ziz Eli'ezer,* VII, 190; VIII, 219; IX, 237. R. Waldenberg stipulates (IX, 240) that consent of the husband must be obtained in such instances since he is deemed to possess proprietory rights with regard to the unborn child. R. Waldenberg further stipulates (VII, 190) that determination of medical necessity must be made by an Orthodox physician or at the very minimum by a "concerned physician who relates to the laws of the Torah with honor and concern." *Binyan David,* no. 60, requires the concurring opinions of two medical practitioners, neither of whom is aware of the diagnosis of his colleague. R. Ovadiah Yosef, *Yabbi'a Omer,* IV, *Even ha-Ezer,*

no. 1, sec. 10, rules that an abortion for the purpose of preserving maternal health may be performed only within the first three months of pregnancy; see above n. 34 and n. 45.

66. See also *Torat Ḥesed, Even ha-Ezer,* no. 42, sec. 32; *Yabbi'a Omer,* IV, no. 1, sec. 8. R. Feinstein points out that R. Jacob Emden himself did not render a definitive ruling permitting abortion in such circumstances. The phraseology employed by R. Jacob Emden is "*Yesh ẓad le-hakel le-ẓorekh gadol* — there is ground for leniency in case of great need." The term "there is ground for leniency," argues R. Feinstein, implies that there are "more grounds to forbid."

67. *Teshuvot Maharit,* I, no. 97. This will serve in a measure to resolve the apparent discrepancy between responsa nos. 97 and 99 which is pointed out by *Sedei Ḥemed,* p. 175. In no. 99 R. Trani states that there is no ban based upon the prohibition against destruction of human life; not mentioned is the prohibition against flagellation to which reference is made in no. 97. The latter prohibition is, of course, inoperative when indicated for therapeutic purposes. The author of *Teshuvot Binyan David* (no. 60), however, regards *Maharit* as permitting abortions only when the mother's life is in danger. It seems that *Paḥad Yiẓḥak* must also have understood this to be the intention of R. Trani since he records the decision of *Maharit* yet, in the same paragraph as previously noted, denies the propriety of an abortion in case of danger to the mother resulting from causes other than the pregnancy *per se.* Cf. also, *Yabbi'a Omer,* IV, *Even ha-Ezer,* no. 1, sec. 6–8. For other attempts to resolve the problems surrounding these two responsa of *Maharit* see *Teshuvot Aryeh de-Bei Ila'i, Yoreh De'ah,* no. 19, and *Ẕiẓ Eli'ezer* IX, 234, and *Yabbi'a Omer* IV, no. 1, sec. 7.

68. Rosh and Ran, however, both rule in accordance with the opinion of R. Yoḥanan; R. Moses Isserles, *Yoreh De'ah* 157:1, cites both views without offering a definitive ruling.

69. *Teshuvot Maḥaneh Ḥayyim* (Munkacs, 5635), *Ḥoshen Mishpat,* no. 50.

70. A similar reservation concerning the status of an unborn child was voiced by R. Isaiah Pick (as evidenced by the responsum addressed to him by R. Ezekiel Landau, *Noda bi-Yehudah,* II, *Ḥoshen Mishpat,* no. 59), who apparently was of the opinion that the general ruling that all infants are considered to be viable does not apply to embryos, since the generalization is based upon observation that such is the case in the preponderant number of instances. The establishment of such a "majority" is especially limited to experience associated with born children. No such observation is permissible with regard to unborn children. Hence this principle, argues R. Pick, must be limited and considered as encompassing only born infants, i.e., stating only that the majority of fully delivered infants are viable. Cf. also the previously cited commentary of R. Elijah Mizraḥi on Exodus 21:12.

71. An identical distinction is made by R. Isaiah Pick in a communication addressed to R. Landau and quoted by the latter in his *Noda bi-Yehudah,* II, *Ḥoshen Mishpat,* no. 59, and by R. Judah Rosanes, *Parashat Derakhim, Derush* 17. A similar distinction with regard to *terefah* is made by *Minḥat Ḥinnukh,* no. 296. See also *Ẕiẓ Eli'ezer,* X, no. 25, chap. 5, sec. 4.

The view expressed by R. Lipschutz concerning the inapplicability of this principle is somewhat problematic in light of *Kesef Mishneh's* analysis of *Yesodei ha-Torah* 5:5. The Gemara, *Pesaḥim* 25b, states that the principle "be killed but do not transgress" as applied to an act of homicide is an *a priori* principle based upon reason alone. If so, questions *Kesef Mishneh,* what is the basis for the extension of the ruling "be killed but do not transgress" to a situation in which the victim is singled out and the entire group warned that, if the specified individual is not delivered, all will perish? In such cases the dictates of reason would indicate that it is preferable by far to sacrifice a single life rather than to suffer the loss of the entire group. *Kesef Mishneh* concludes that the Sages possessed a tradition extending this principle even to cases in which the *a priori* reason advanced does not apply. See also *Aḥi'ezer,* II, no. 16, sec. 5. The distinction both with regard to fetal life and *terefah* as drawn by the above cited authorities is rejected by *Noda bi-Yehudah, loc. cit.*

72. *Tosafot R. Akiva Eger, Oholot* 6:17, no. 17.

73. R. Meir Eisenstadt, *Teshuvot Panim Me'irot* (New York, 5722), III, no. 8.

74. *Teshuvot Maharam Schick* (New York, 5721), *Yoreh De'ah,* no. 155.

75. This principle is established by R. Moses Sofer, *Teshuvot Ḥatam Sofer* (New York, 5718), *Yoreh De'ah,* no. 158. The credence given to even a single witness in matters of halakhic proscription extends only to testimony of observed events. Diagnosis and treatment of medical conditions necessarily contain an element of subjective judgment; hence the judgment of a medical practitioner constitutes a *safek* rather than a certainty. As such, it cannot provide sufficient basis for sanctioning that which is forbidden in cases of "doubt." Elsewhere (*Yoreh De'ah,* nos. 173 and 175) *Ḥatam Sofer* states that medical testimony is indeed sufficient to demonstrate that certain physiological processes do occur. Nevertheless such testimony cannot establish that a specific physiological process is actually taking place in a given patient since such diagnosis involves a subjective judgment.

76. *Melammed le-Ho'il, Yoreh De'ah,* no. 69.

77. *Teshuvot Sho'el u-Meshiv* (New York, 5714), I, no. 22, p. 13.

78. Due to a printer's error, the text appears to read *Baba Meẓi'a* 71 rather than 62a.

79. See *Teshuvot Tiferet Ẓevi, Oraḥ Ḥayyim,* no. 14.

80. R. Moses Jonah Zweig, *No'am,* VII, 48, errs in ascribing an identical view to the *Maḥaneh Ḥayyim.* In point of fact, R. Sofer employs the phraseology of a contrary-to-fact conditional, viz., if feticide were at all permissible it would be permissible only if performed by the mother itself. R. Zweig judiciously notes that *Maḥaneh Ḥayyim* was not available to him. Apparently he was forced to rely upon secondary sources, a fact which explains the reason for his inaccuracy.

81. *Yedei Moshe* (Pietrokow, 5658), no. 4, sec. 8. *Yedei Moshe* was originally published as an appendix to *Sefer ha-Parnes* (Vilna, 5651), authored by R. Moses Parnes.

82. This responsum is included in *Yedei Moshe.* The reference is to no. 5, sec. 8, of that work.

83. *Issur ve-Heter he-Arukh* (Vilna, 5651), no. 59, sec. 35. Cf. also *Haggahot Maimuniyyot, Hilkhot Ma'akhalot Assurot* 14:15.

84. *Peri ha-Areẓ,* III, *Yoreh De'ah* (Jerusalem 5665), no. 21. Cf. *Piskei Teshuvah,* ed. R. Abraham Pieterkovsky (Pietrokow, 5693), II, no. 261.

85. See also *Ẓiẓ Eli'ezer,* IV, no. 13, sec. 3. Cf. *Teshuvot ha-Rashba ha-Meyuḥasot le-ha-Ramban,* no. 281; *Magen Avraham, Oraḥ Ḥayyim* 554:8 and *Peri Megadim,* ad loc.; *Teshuvot Admat Kodesh,* I, *Yoreh De'ah,* no. 6; *Peri ha-Areẓ,* III, *Yoreh De'ah,* no. 2; *Birkei Yosef, Shiyurei Berakhah, Yoreh De'ah* 155:2; *Levushei Mordekhai,* I, *Hoshen Mishpat,* no. 39 and IV, no. 68; *Teshuvot Neẓer Mata'ai,* I, no. 8; and R. Judah Leib Graubart, *Havallim ba-Ne'imim,* IV, no. 13.

86. *Teshuvot Ḥatam Sofer, Oraḥ Ḥayyim,* no. 83. A careful reading of this responsum indicates that, contrary to R. Unterman's assumption, *Ḥatam Sofer* may be discussing a case of mental retardation rather than a form of mental illness. Cf. *Iggerot Moshe, Oraḥ Ḥayyim,* II, no. 88; *Shevet Sofer, Even ha-Ezer,* no. 21; and *Bet Yiẓḥak, Even ha-Ezer.* no. 39, sec. 6.

87. See also *idem, Shevet me-Yehudah,* I, 49, and 297.

88. At the same time R. Unterman, *Ha-Torah ve-ha-Medinah,* IV, 29, and *Shevet me-Yehudah,* I, 49 and I, 64, sanctions desecration of the Sabbath in order to effect a cure in cases of insanity. R. Unterman maintains that the principle "Better to violate a single Sabbath in order that many Sabbaths be observed" is applicable in such instances. Cf., however, R. Eliezer Waldenberg, *Ramat Raḥel,* no. 28. R. Unterman's position is contradicted by *Hatam Sofer, Oraḥ Ḥayyim,* no. 83, who maintains that this principle does not apply in the case of a person who, at the time of the contemplated desecration of the Sabbath, is exempt from observing Sabbath restrictions. According to *Hatam Sofer,* there is no obligation to effect a change in the status of such an individual. Cf., also, *Magen Avraham, Oraḥ Ḥayyim* 340:29, to whom this is a matter of doubt.

89. Abortion of a pregnancy resulting from rape, even in the case of a married woman, would not be sanctioned by R. Emden according to this line of reasoning. R. Waldenberg, *Ẓiẓ Eli'ezer,* IX, 237, cites a responsum of *Rav Pe'alim,* I, *Even ha-Ezer,* no. 4, who argues that the psychological and sociological difficulties involved in the rearing of such a child constitute "great pain" and "grave need" which R. Emden recognizes as sufficient grounds for termination of a pregnancy.

90. R. Jacob Emden's remarks, even with this qualification, remain perplexing. A person guilty of a capital transgression, even if a formal warning has been administered and the act committed in the presences of witnesses, may not be executed other than upon the verdict of a *Bet Din.* A person who kills such a transgressor prior to the pronouncement of guilt by the *Bet Din* is guilty of a capital offense. See above, n. 9.

91. *No'am,* VI, 3. He further cites the opinion of *Yeshu'ot Malko* to the effect that the Sabbath may be violated in order to save the life of a fetus even if the mother belongs to the class of those liable to death on whose behalf the Sabbath may not be violated. Cf. *Mishpetei Uzi'el, Hoshen Mishpat,* III, 57.

92. Although termination of a pregnancy resulting from rape is not sanctioned by most authorities, postcoital contraception prior to fertilization of the ovum presents a different halakhic question. Immediate removal of the semen by means of a suction device operated by a female would be warranted according to some authorities, particularly if the rapist is a non-Jew. Cf. R. Eliezer Ḥayyim Deutsch, *Peri ha-Sadeh,* IV, no. 50; and R. Jeruchem Judah Perilman (known as the *Minsker Gadol*), *Or Gadol,* no. 31.

93. *Sefer Ḥasidim* (Jerusalem, 5720), no. 186.

94. *Teshuvah me-Ahavah* (Prague, 5669), I, no. 53. Halakhic literature on this topic was reviewed by R. Immanuel Jakobovits, *Tradition,* V (Spring 1963), 268 ff., and *Tradition,* VI (Spring-Summer 1964), 114 ff.

95. *No'am,* VI, 1–11.

96. *Ibid.,* VII, 36–56.

97. See above, notes 45 and 46. The grave question of aborting a defective fetus was re-examined by Rabbi Waldenberg in the Adar 5736 issue of *Assia* and in *Ẓiẓ Eli'ezer,* XIII, no. 102, Rabbi Waldenberg now notes that the distinction frequently attributed to *Ḥavvot Ya'ir* is spurious. There is thus no source for a distinction between the first trimester and later stages of pregnancy. Since in *Ẓiẓ Eli'ezer* Rabbi Waldenberg permitted abortion of a defective fetus only during the first trimester, at which time such an abortion is purportedly sanctioned also by the weight of *Havvot Ya'ir's* opinion, it might be concluded that, subsequent to discovery that there exists no authority who views the prohibition as inoperative during the first trimester, permission to abort an abnormal fetus should be withheld. Rabbi Waldenberg, however, reaches the opposite conclusion. In this

recent responsum he relies entirely upon the opinions of R. Emden and *Maharit* and permits abortion of a Tay-Sachs fetus during later stages of pregnancy as well. In doing so Rabbi Waldenberg rules contrary to his own previously expressed position. Rabbi Waldenberg's presently held view is that abortion of a defective fetus may be sanctioned until the end of the second trimester of pregnancy provided that the abortion itself poses no danger to the mother. He refuses to permit abortion beyond this period because a seven-month abortus may be viable. He further recommends that, if possible, the abortion should be performed by a female physician since, according to many authorities, women are not bound by the prohibition against "destruction of the seed " Rabbi Waldenberg's position is strongly contested by Rabbi Moshe Feinstein, *Ha-Pardes,* Nisan 5738; see above, note 9. Responses by Rabbi Waldenberg appear in Abraham S. Abraham, *Lev Avraham* (Jerusalem, 5738), II, 26–27 and Abraham Steinberg, *Hilkhot Rofim u-Refu'ah* (Jerusalem, 5738), pp. 30–46.

98. Cf. *Sedei Hemed,* II, 298.

99. Cf. *Sedei Hemed,* II, 303–304.

100. See below, n. 104. *Ko'ah Shor* explains the *safek* of *Tosafot* in yet another manner. Since a Noachide is not commanded to "sanctify the Name," he may commit idolatry for the sake of preserving his life. R. Schorr argues that this dispensation extends to murder as well and infers that it is the extension of this provision to encompass murder which was the subject of *Tosafot's* "doubt." However, *Mishneh le-Melekh, Hilkhot Melakhim* 10:2, states explicitly that the taking of another's life in order to save one's own is forbidden even to Noachides, since with regard to homicide this injunction is not derived from the commandment to "sanctify the Name" but upon the *a priori* principle "Why is your blood sweeter than that of your fellow?" The author's grandson raises this point in a note (p. 35a) appended to this responsum of *Ko'ah Shor* but fails to cite *Mishneh le-Melekh.* See, however, *Pithei Teshuvah, Yoreh De'ah,* 155:4, who discusses the question of whether or not the principle "and you shall live by them" applies to Noachides. See also *Perashat Derakhim, Derush* 2. The "doubt" expressed by *Tosafot* may possibly be explained in another manner: Since under Jewish law feticide is not a capital crime it may be deduced that fetal life is not equal in worth to maternal life. The life of the mother is thus "sweeter" than the life of the fetus. For this reason the life of the fetus may "perhaps" be sacrificed in order to preserve the life of the mother.

101. Furthermore, since the law of pursuit must be invoked if the fetus is deemed to be "a life," performance of an abortion by a Noachide would be precluded by those authorities who maintain that the law of pursuit is not operative in the Noachide Code. Cf. *Teshuvot Ben Yehudah,* no. 21; and *Sedei Hemed,* II, 14, no. 44. However, *Minhat Hinnukh,* no. 296, and *Ko'ah Shor,* p. 32b, argue that the law of pursuit extends to Noachides, as well as indeed seems to be indicated by the language of Rambam, *Hilkhot Melakhim* 9:4; see also R. Hayyim Soloveichik, *Hiddushei Rabbenu Hayyim ha-Levi al ha-Rambam, Hilkhot Roze'ah* 1:9.

102. See R. Aryeh Leib Grossnass, *Ha-Pardes, Shevat* 5732, and *Lev Aryeh,* II, no. 32, who suggests that the "doubt" expressed by *Tosafot* is limited to the destruction of the fetus of a Jewish mother in order to save her life, but does not extend to the abortion of a non-Jewish fetus.

103. *Minhat Hinnukh,* no. 296.

104. The Gemara, *Sanhedrin* 74b, states that a Noachide may commit any transgression in private, including idolatry, in order to preserve his own life. The Gemara also discusses the question of whether or not he is permitted to do so in

public, since he is not explicitly commanded to "sanctify the Name." There is no explicit reference in the Gemara with regard to violations in order to preserve the life of another. *Ko'aḥ Shor,* p. 33a, adopts a view diametrically opposed to that of *Minḥat Ḥinnukh* and asserts that a Noachide may transgress any commandment, including the three cardinal sins, in order to save the life of his fellow. See above, n. 100.

105. When it is necessary to employ a non-Jew for this purpose, *Teshuvot Maharash,* V, no. 89, counsels that it is preferable to transmit the request to the non-Jewish physician through another gentile. This determination is based upon *Avodah Zarah* 14a, which rules that one need not avoid making accessible a "stumbling block" to one who in turn will place it before the blind. This indirect procedure thus circumvents the transgression of "placing a stumbling block."

106. Job 38:4–5, 17–18.

107. Eccles. 11:5.

10
Tay-Sachs Disease: To Screen Or Not To Screen
FRED ROSNER

Medical Aspects

History   In 1881, the British ophthalmologist Warren Tay first described degeneration of the macular region of the eye in a one-year-old child. Six years later, the American neurologist Bernard Sachs published the clinical and pathological findings.[1-4] Sachs noted the familial nature of the condition, which he called amaurotic familial idiocy. There are six different types, including infantile, late infantile, and adult forms.

Clinical Manifestations   For purposes of this paper, the term Tay-Sachs disease refers to the congenital disorder that occurs primarily but not exclusively in Jewish families from Eastern Europe. The disease is characterized by weakness beginning at about six months of age, progressive mental and motor deterioration, blindness, paralysis, dementia, seizures, and death usually by three years of age. The "cherry-red spot" in the macula of the eye is the clinical sign most frequently associated with Tay-Sachs disease.

  Pathologically, there is a ballooning of nerve cells throughout the nervous system due to accumulation of lipid material. By electron microscopy, cytoplasmic nerve cell lipid bodies are visible. The lipid that accumulates is ganglioside GM_2 and the specific enzymatic defect responsible for the widespread deposition of this lipid is the absence of hexosaminidase A. The diagnosis of Tay-Sachs disease requires the identification of the accumulated lipid material and documentation of the specific enzymatic defect.[5]

Genetics The inheritance of Tay-Sachs disease follows laws of Mendelian genetics. The transmission appears to be autosomal recessive, since both parents of patients are clinically normal, sex ratios are equal, and both parents have enzyme levels that are intermediate between those of patients and normal controls. Thus a child who inherits one recessive gene from only one parent is a carrier or has the trait, but is clinically completely normal. Only a child who inherits two Tay-Sachs genes, one from each parent, will have the fatal disease. If two carriers marry, there is a 25% chance with each pregnancy that the child will have the disease and a 50% chance that the child, like the parents, will be a carrier. There is also a 25% chance that the child will be totally free of the disease as well as of the carrier state. If a carrier marries a noncarrier, none of the children can have the fatal disease, but half the children will be carriers.

Concerning the gene frequency, it has been estimated that one in 30 Ashkenazi Jews and one in 300 non-Jews is a carrier of the Tay-Sachs gene. If a Jew (one in 30 risk) marries another Jew (one in 30 risk), the chance that both husband and wife are carriers is one in 900. Therefore, one in 900 Jewish couples is at risk for having children with Tay-Sachs disease. For such a couple, each pregnancy has a 25% chance of producing a child with the fatal disease. Hence, the incidence of Tay-Sachs disease in the Jewish population (assuming there is no intermarriage with non-Jews) is one in 3600 births. The disease is 100 times less common in non-Jews. In view of the high rates of intermarriage between Jews and non-Jews in the United States, the incidence of Tay-Sachs births is probably much less than one in 3600. One expert has calculated that 30 children with Tay-Sachs disease are born annually in North America.[4] There is also a debate in the medical literature as to whether the incidence of Tay-Sachs disease is increasing[6] or not.[7]

Detection of Carriers Since hexosaminidase A is deficient in all tissues of patients with Tay-Sachs disease, and since carriers, on the average, have 50% of normal hexosaminidase A activity, the assay for this enzyme can be performed on serum,[4] fibroblasts,[8] or other easily available tissue including leukocytes and tears.[9] The test exploits the different thermal stabilities of the two hexosaminidases: hexosaminidase A is heat labile, whereas hexosaminidase B remains unchanged by heat at 50°C. This serum heat inactivation test is currently in use in many medical centers, some of which employ semiautomated methodology.[10] Electrophoretic separation of the two hexosaminidases can also be achieved.[9]

Amniocentesis and Prenatal Diagnosis Intrauterine diagnosis of Tay-Sachs disease in an unborn fetus is now possible by a procedure called transabdominal amniocentesis, in which a small quantity of amniotic fluid, which bathes the developing embryo, is removed from the mother's uterus. The fetal cells in this fluid are grown in the laboratory and tested for the presence or absence of hexosaminidase A. Amniotic fluid itself or un-cultured cells can also be used for enzyme assay.[11-15] The incidence of unfavorable side effects of amniocentesis to mother or fetus is low and accidents of major significance are unusual.

There are pitfalls in the prenatal diagnosis of even major chromosomal abnormalities by amniocentesis.[16] Specifically, in regard to Tay-Sachs disease antenatal diagnosis is not always correct. Uncultured amniotic fluid cells may have decreased hexosaminidase A activity even in normal fetuses.[13,14] Furthermore, some members of families in which Tay-Sachs has appeared have no detectable enzyme activity but seem to be healthy. In such families, the absence of the enzyme in amniotic fluid cells of cultures may be uninterpretable.[15] In spite of these and other technological problems, the results of amniocentesis in large numbers of patients provide accurate prenatal diagnosis in most instances.[17]

The overwhelming majority of publications in the medical literature fail to address the moral, ethical, social, psychological, and religious in-dications and contraindications for amniocentesis for the prenatal diagnosis of Tay-Sachs disease. I will discuss these later in this essay.

The "Cure" of Tay-Sachs Disease   Amniocentesis to detect the disease and screening programs to detect the carrier state of Tay-Sachs will be un-necessary if and when the cure for this disease is developed. One cannot properly speak of cure when discussing a genetic disorder. However, since the specific enzymatic deficiency in Tay-Sachs disease is now known, it seems theoretically possible to prepare, purify, and administer this enzyme as replacement therapy to patients afflicted with the disease. The situation may be analogous to supplying insulin to a diabetic. The disease may not be cured, but the clinical symptomatology may be controlled and the patient enabled to lead a nearly normal life. Preliminary attempts at such replacement therapy for Tay-Sachs disease seem to be forthcoming in the not too distant future.

Screening for Tay-Sachs Carriers

The medical literature[18-38] and lay press[39-40] have recently become replete with articles and letters and debates concerning the screening of large populations of Jewish people for the carrier state of Tay-Sachs disease and the performance of amniocentesis for the prenatal detection of the fatal disease. Many private organizations and governmental agencies have published pamplets and other descriptive material relating to various aspects of Tay-Sachs disease.[41] The Director of the British Tay-Sachs Foundation, in two identical letters in the *British Medical Journal*[31] and *Lancet,*[32] offered screening for the carrier state and amniocentesis for prenatal diagnosis of the disease.

With rare exceptions, the articles, pamphlets, booklets, and letters relating to Tay-Sachs disease not only offer but recommend abortion if the amniocentesis reveals an affected child. Some authors even state that selective feticide has rabbinical approval,[33] a contention that I strongly dispute.[36] To eliminate Tay-Sachs disease by "selective termination of affected pregnancies"[42] is not acceptable in Judaism. Although local rabbinical support for Tay-Sachs screening programs may be active and even overwhelming, such support is usually limited to detecting the carrier state and does not include the performance of amniocentesis with the sole aim of abortion if the fetus is found to have Tay-Sachs disease. The heated discussions on this point in the medical literature[18-23, 25-36] have already been alluded to. A more detailed look at the traditional Jewish position is presented later in this paper.

There are causes other than religious ones to make one think twice before undertaking mass screening programs. Kuhr presented the reasons that led an advisory committee of physicians in Dayton, Ohio, to decide against organizing a mass screening program for Tay-Sachs disease.[25] Dr. Kuhr's letter, entitled "Doubtful Benefits of Tay-Sachs Screening," was followed by an angry outcry from other members of the medical community.[26-28] The major reason for the decision of the advisory committee was the potential psychic burden on the young people discovered to be heterozygotes. Kuhr further pointed out a study of the behavior of physicians and clients in a voluntary program of testing for the Tay-Sachs gene in which a 15% anxiety reaction to the discovery of the carrier state is mentioned.[24,29]

Another group of physicians specifically discourages unmarried people from being tested because of the possible social problems that carrier identification might create.[43] What are the psychological problems created by the information that one is a carrier for a fatal genetic disease? Should a known carrier refuse to marry a mate who has not been tested? Should two carriers break up an engagement or a marriage if they learn they are both carriers as a result of a screening program? Should a young person inquire about the Tay-Sachs status of a member of the opposite sex prior to meeting that individual on a social level? When does a person who knows he is a carrier tell this fact to the girl that he expects to marry? Should one sacrifice primary prevention of Tay-Sachs disease by mate selection to avoid psychosocial consequences, as some advocate?[43] Is this method of disease prevention the most attractive aspect of genetic screening for recessives, as others state?[25]

One must remember that 29 of 30 people tested for the carrier state are found to be free of the Tay-Sachs gene. It is certainly desirable for these 29 of each 30 tested to have peace of mind. Is the anxiety of the 30th person on learning that he or she is a carrier sufficiently great to warrant not testing at all? Obviously not! However, one cannot minimize the possible psychosocial trauma to such an individual.

The social stigma of being a carrier of the Tay-Sachs gene is not fully appreciated. Misinformed and/or uninformed people may look at carriers in the same manner as patients with epilepsy and leprosy were looked at half a century ago, i.e., as individuals afflicted with a "taboo" disease, to be shunned and ostracized from normal social contact. Discrimination against carriers of Tay-Sachs disease may also occur in a variety of areas, if the experience of sickle cell screening is repeated. Individuals found to have sickle cell trait have been dismissed from their jobs. Several life insurance companies charge higher premiums for individuals with sickle cell trait or refuse to insure them at all. Several airlines reject flight attendants from employment in that capacity if they have sickle cell trait. The United States Air Force does not train black recruits with sickle cell trait to become pilots. Job seeking is thus made more difficult for carriers of this hemoglobinopathy. The National Association of Sickle Cell Clinics has compiled a list of 21 major insurance companies that discriminate against blacks and others with sickle cell trait. Maryland is the first state to have passed a law banning discrimination in employment, life, accident, and health insurance against those who possess the sickle cell trait.

Is this fate also to be suffered by people who, on screening, are found to be carriers of the Tay-Sachs gene? Total confidentiality in screening might avoid such problems and should be an essential part of all such programs.

The selection of target groups to be screened for the Tay-Sachs gene, the planning, organization, and implementation of such screening events, the educational activities that must precede screening, the laboratory aspects of the testing, and the referral of people for counseling are beyond the scope of this essay. Suffice it to say that compliance with screening for Tay-Sachs disease[24] is dependent not only on the motivation of the client, his or her perception of the susceptibility to and seriousness of the inherited condition, the possible consequences of noncompliance and the potential benefits from participation, but also on the moral, ethical, and religious background of the Jewish people who are the clients at risk.

If the purpose of Tay-Sachs screening is to provide eligible clients with genetic counseling about reproductive and mating options, few will argue against screening. If the purpose, however, is to introduce couples at risk to the benefits of prenatal diagnosis by amniocentesis with the specific intent of recommending abortion of affected fetuses, a procedure that may be contrary to the religious dictates of the client, then screening should not be performed. The religious teachings of the Jewish people must be considered if co-operation from the rabbinate and compliance from the clients is to be obtained in any screening program. A plan for the screening of heterozygotes for Tay-Sachs disease in Israel specifically includes the rabbinate, although the portion of the plan that dictates abortion for homozygote fetuses is obviously not acceptable to either of the Chief Rabbis.[38]

There is little doubt that screening for hypertension and diabetes and other common conditions, which, although not curable, can be controlled by medical therapy, is highly desirable and should be done. There is less certainty that the benefits of Tay-Sachs screening outweigh the disadvantages, although a qualified affirmative answer on this matter is my position. It is not sufficient to know whether screening is feasible and/or effective; it is also important to know whether it is moral.

Legal Aspects

Some bitter lessons were learned from the laws passed in regard to sickle cell screening. Georgia has a law that requires sickle cell screening of all newborns unless the parents object on religious grounds. In California, all black people admitted to hospitals must be screened by law. In Illinois, mandatory premarital screening for sickle cell trait was enacted "if the physician indicates that it is needed." In New York, premarital testing only of blacks is required. Many other states have passed mandatory screening laws but few, if any, enforce them.

Most of the above-mentioned laws were challenged on constitutional grounds. Obligatory screening of any age group for any genetic disease seems to be an unconstitutional invasion of the rights of the individual. As a result, many of the laws pertaining to sickle cell screening have been or are being repealed or amended. In some states, such as Virginia and Kentucky, premarital screening is now voluntary, the mandatory provision of the original law having been amended.

In the famous Jacobsen decision in 1905, the United States Supreme Court upheld the law of mandatory smallpox vaccination on the basis of the needs of society to protect its citizens from smallpox. However, neither sickle cell disease nor Tay-Sachs disease is a contagious illness and, therefore, does not constitute a danger to others. Although there may be a financial burden on society to care for such patients and/or to support the screening, education, and counseling of potential carriers of either disease, mandatory screening laws still seem to be unconstitutional when weighed against the right of individual privacy.

Discriminatory screening along racial or ethnic lines is also unconstitutional. To pass a law mandating sickle cell screening *only* for blacks or Tay-Sachs screening *only* for Jews is clearly discriminatory and underinclusive. Screening must be offered to all, although not all ethnic or racial groups need participate in the screening if they so choose.

If any law is to be passed in regard to Tay-Sachs disease, it must indicate that screening is completely voluntary and that the results will remain confidential. Not only is the preservation of confidentiality an essential component of the doctor-patient relationship and a patient's constitutional right, but a repetition of discriminatory practices that occurred in the sickle cell screening experience must be avoided. Finally, any proposed law concerning Tay-Sachs screening may *not* require abortion, sterilization, or prohibition of marriage but must preserve the fundamental rights of marriage or procreation.

The Jewish View

Rabbi Moses Feinstein, dean of American orthodox rabbis, was asked whether or not it is advisable for a boy or girl to be screened for Tay-Sachs disease, and if it is proper, at what age should the test be performed. He was further asked whether screening should be performed as part of a publicized screening program or only as a private test. His written responsum of 1973 states that "... it is advisable for one preparing to be married, to have himself tested. It is also proper to publicize the fact, via newspapers and other media, that such a test is available. It is clear and certain that absolute secrecy must be maintained to prevent anyone from learning the results of such a test performed on another. The physician must not reveal these to anyone . . . these tests must be performed in private, and, consequently, it is not proper to schedule these tests in large groups as, for example, in Yeshivas, schools, or other similar situations . . ."[44]

Rabbi Feinstein also points out that most young people are quite sensitive to nervous tension or psychological stress and, therefore, young men (below age 20) or women (below age 18) not yet contemplating marriage should not be screened for Tay-Sachs disease. Finally, Rabbi Feinstein points out that abortion of a defective fetus after amniocentesis is a forbidden act in Jewish law.

Rabbi J. David Bleich, writing in the official journal of the Rabbinical Council of America, indicates that the elimination of Tay-Sachs disease is, of course, a goal to which all concerned individuals subscribe.[45] The Jewish legal ramifications of the testing program appear in another article by Rabbi Bleich in the summer 1972 issue of the Hebrew periodical *Or ha-Mizraḥ*. He points out that "... the obligation with regard to procreation is not suspended simply because of the statistical probability that some children of the union may be deformed or abnormal. While the couple may quite properly be counseled with regard to the risks of having a Tay-Sachs child, it should be stressed that failure to bear natural children is not a halakhically viable alternative.

"Of at least equal if not graver concern is the proposal that fetal monitoring be performed with a view toward termination of the pregnancy if the fetus be identified as a victim of Tay-Sachs disease.

"The fear that a child may be born physically malformed or mentally deficient does not in itself justify recourse to abortion . . . Since the sole available medical remedy following diagnosis of severe genetic defects is abortion of the fetus, which is not sanctioned by Halakhah in such instances, amniocentesis, under these conditions, does not serve as an aid in treatment of the patient and is not halakhically permissible . . ."

Rabbi Bleich concludes that screening programs for the detection of carriers of Tay-Sachs disease "are certainly to be encouraged." He suggests that the most propitious time for such screening is childhood or early adolescence, since early awareness of a carrier state, particularly as part of a mass screening program, is advantageous.

At its 70th anniversary biennial convention during the Thanksgiving weekend of 1974, the Union of Orthodox Jewish Congregations of America adopted a resolution concerning Tay-Sachs screening that essentially echoes the opinion of Rabbi Bleich cited above. The Union suggests that "the Orthodox community can extend support to programs of genetic screening *only* when competent halakhic guidance is provided for all participants." The Union called upon its constituent synagogues to work for such programs in every Jewish community but emphasized that all Tay-Sachs screening programs must be accompanied by adequate and competent rabbinic counseling.

The Association of Orthodox Jewish Scientists issued a statement in 1973 outlining its position in regard to Tay-Sachs screening as follows: "We endorse voluntary screening of young adults of an age in which marriage has become a serious consideration but before definite marital commitments have been made. The screening of younger individuals, years before marriage, yields no immediate benefits and might result in a longer period of anxiety in carriers than is warranted. We feel that all screening must be linked to both genetic and religious personal counseling. Emotionally immature individuals may be traumatized psychologically if they learn of their carrier state, and these individuals must be provided with the opportunity for additional professional psychological support. Genetic counseling must be in consonance with Torah principles.

"The Association is unalterably opposed to amniocentesis, whose natural and logical consequence is abortion. It likewise feels that screening of married couples or those whose marriage is imminent and who are not committed to disruption of their mutual marital commitments, were both partners to be discovered to be Tay-Sachs carriers, is unwise, again because virtually the only consequences would be abortion, or a childless marriage. We are also concerned that any program be absolutely voluntary, and that the nature of any educational drive be informational rather than coercive. There must also be absolute assurance that the confidentiality of all carriers will be safeguarded.'' (Personal communication from the President of the A.O.J.S.)

The various objections to amniocentesis and abortion in Jewish law are predicated on considerations surrounding the fetus. Extreme emotional stress in the mother leading to suicidal intent might constitute one of the situations in which abortion might be sanctioned by even the most orthodox rabbi. If a woman who suffered a nervous breakdown following the birth (or death) of a child with Tay-Sachs disease becomes pregnant again, and is so distraught with the knowledge that she may be carrying another child with the fatal disease that she threatens suicide, Jewish law might allow amniocentesis. If this procedure reveals an unaffected fetus, the pregnancy continues to term. If the result of the amniocentesis indicates a homozygous fetus with Tay-Sachs disease, rabbinic consultation regarding the decision of whether or not to perform an abortion should be obtained.

The rabbinic consultant to the orthodox Sha'arei Zedek Hospital in Jerusalem, Rabbi Eliezer J. Waldenberg, stated that, if amniocentesis reveals an affected fetus, abortion is permitted up to the seventh month of pregnancy because of the "great need," which consists of the enormous mental anguish of the mother in knowing the fatal outcome awaiting her diseased child in a few years.[46]

Other more lenient rulings are cited by Jakobovits in a recently published article.[47] These rulings have been emphatically rejected by other leading rabbinic authorities.[48] No general rule of permissiveness or prohibition can be enunciated in regard to abortion in Jewish law. Each case must be individualized and evaluated on the basis of its merits taking into consideration all the prevailing medical, psychological, social, and religious circumstances.

Concluding Note

A research group on ethical, social, and legal issues in genetic counseling and genetic engineering of the Institute of Society, Ethics, and the Life Sciences recently proposed a set of principles for guiding the operation of genetic screening programs to focus attention on the problems of stigmatization, confidentiality, breaches of individual rights to privacy, and freedom of choice in childbearing. Some of the principles include "the need for well planned program objectives, involvement of the communities immediately affected by the screening, absence of compulsion, provision of counseling services, an understanding of the relation of screening to realizable or potential therapies, and well formulated procedures for protecting the rights of individual and family privacy." This research group pointed out that widespread genetic screening may produce ethical, psychologic, and sociomedical problems for which physicians and the public may be unprepared.[49]

In the past several years, screening for sickle cell trait has become widespread. There are some, however, who believe that "screening for sickle cell trait *per se* now seems unjustified, except for genetic counseling purposes, which, as many would now agree, should be undertaken only at the specific request of high-risk individuals who are able to grasp the implications. However, even judiciously conducted screening and genetic counseling may still produce psychosocial side effects that are yet to be fully assessed."[50] Efforts to educate, test, and counsel for the sickle cell gene have shown features that can arouse anxiety, fear, and apprehension; generate guilt, resentent, and frustration; inhibit the development of personal self-esteem and racial pride; destroy families; and reactivate neglect of the sickle cell problem.[51] There have been no systematic studies to date of these factors in relation to either sickle cell disease or Tay-Sachs disease.

The birth of a child with a serious congenital deformity or mental deficiency or a lethal metabolic error, such as Tay-Sachs disease, is a terrible shock to any parents. The personal decisions involved are very difficult: whether to marry; whether to have children; whether to have a further child; whether to adopt a child. For the general Jewish population, not only must medical, genetic, and psychological factors be considered in any given case, but the religious attitude of Judaism toward such matters as abortion, contraception, amniocentesis, genetic screening, and procreation, to name but a few, must be taken into account. Hence, rabbinic consultation and advice should be sought concomitantly with the medical-genetic counseling. One can inform and educate the Jewish community about Tay-Sachs screening, but such a program will truly achieve its goal only when the community wants it and is willing to work for it.

It seems desirable to screen a limited population that would be followed closely to observe all the psychological and social implications as well as the genetic accomplishments of the screening. In this way, the scientific and religious approaches might coincide and any ultimate conclusion would be based on fact instead of speculation. There is no reason to be stampeded by those professional enthusiasts whose interests are founded on mass screening.

NOTES

1. Volk, B. W., ed., *Tay-Sachs Disease,* New York, Grune and Stratton, 1964.

2. Wilkins, R. H., and Brody, I. A., "Tay-Sachs Disease," *Arch. Neurol.,* 1969, *20,* 103–111.

3. Schneck, L., Volk, B. W., and Saifer, A., "The Gangliosidoses," *Amer. J. Med.,* 1969, *46,* 245–263.

4. O'Brien, J. S., "Tay-Sachs Disease: From Enzyme to Prevention," *Federation Proc.,* 1973, *32,* 191–199.

5. Öhman, R., Ekelund, H., and Svennerholm, L., "The Diagnosis of Tay-Sachs Disease," *Acta Pediatr. Scand.,* 1971, *60,* 399–406.

6, Shaw, R. F., and Smith, A. P., "Is Tay-Sachs Disease Increasing?" *Nature,* 1969, *224,* 1214–1215.

7. Myrianthopoulos, N. C., Naylor, A. F., and Aronson, S. M., "Tay-Sachs Disease Is Probably Not Increasing," *Nature,* 1970, *227,* 609.

8. O'Brien J. S., "Diagnosis of Tay-Sachs," *Nature,* 1969, *224,* 1038.

9. Carmody, P. J., Rattazzi, M. C., and Davidson, R. G., "Tay-Sachs Disease—the Use of Tears for the Detection of Heterozygotes," *New Eng. J. Med.,* 1973, *289,* 1072–1074.

10. Kaback, M. M., and Zeiger, R. S., "Heterozygote Detection in Tay-Sachs Disease: A Prototype Community Screening Program for the Prevention of Recessive Genetic Disorders," *Adv. Exp. Med. Biol.,* 1972, *19,* 613–632.

11. O'Brien, J. S., Okada, S., Fillerup, D. L., Veath, M. L., Adornato, B., Brenner, P. H., and Leroy, J. G., "Tay-Sachs Disease: Prenatal Diagnosis," *Science,* 1971, *172,* 61–64.

12. Navon, R., and Padeh, B., "Prenatal Diagnosis of Tay-Sachs Genotypes," *Brit. Med. J.,* 1971, *4,* 17–20.

13. Schneck, L., Adachi, M., and Volk, B. W., "The Fetal Aspects of Tay-Sachs Disease," *Pediatrics,* 1972, *49,* 342–351.

14. Saifer, A., Schneck, L., Perle, G., Valenti, C., and Volk, B. W., "Caveats of Antenatal Diagnosis of Tay-Sachs Disease," *Amer. J. Obst. Gynec.,* 1973, *115,* 553–555.

15. Nadler, H. L., "Prenatal Diagnosis of Inborn Defects: A Status Report," *Hosp. Pract.,* 1975, *10,* 41–51.

16. Kardon, N. B., Chernay, P. R., Hsu, L. Y., Martin, J. L., and Hirschhorn, K., "Pitfalls in Prenatal Diagnosis Resulting from Chromosomal Mosaicism," *J. Ped.,* 1972, *80,* 297–299.

17. Milunsky, A., "Prenatal Diagnosis of Tay-Sachs Disease," *Lancet,* 1973, *2,* 1442.

18. Rosner, F., "Amniocentesis in Tay-Sachs Disease," *J. Am. Med. Assoc.,* 1974, *228,* 829.

19. Jackson, L. G., Glazerman, L. R., Faust, H. S., and Nimoityn, P., "Screening for Carriers of Tay-Sachs Disease," *J. Am. Med. Assoc.,* 1974, *229,* 640.

20. Pearlmutter, F. A., "Tay-Sachs Disease," *J. Am. Med. Assoc.,* 1974, *230,* 38.

21. Schwartz, H., "Amniocentesis in Tay-Sachs Disease," *J. Am. Med. Assoc.,* 1975, *231,* 1229.

22. Roberts, E. J., "Amniocentesis in Tay-Sachs Disease," *loc. cit.,* 1230–1231.

23. Orleans, J., "Amniocentesis in Tay-Sachs Disease," *loc. cit.,* 1231.

24. Beck, E., Blaichman, S., Scriver, C. R., and Clow, C. L., "Advocacy and

Compliance in Genetic Screening. Behavior of Physicians and Clients in a Voluntary Program of Testing for the Tay-Sachs Gene," *New Eng. J. Med.,* 1974, *291,* 1166–1170.

25. Kuhr, M. D., "Doubtful Benefits of Tay-Sachs Screening," *New Eng. J. Med.,* 1975, *292,* 371.

26. Beck, E., Blaichman, S., Scriver, C. R., and Clow, C. L., "Doubtful Benefits of Tay-Sachs Screening," *loc. cit.,* 371.

27. Schneck, L., Saifer, A., and Volk, B. W., "Benefits of Tay-Sachs Screening," *loc. cit.,* 758.

28. Jackson, L. G., Nimoityn, P., Faust, H. S., and Glazerman, L. R., "Benefits of Tay-Sachs Screening," *loc. cit.,* 758–759.

29. Kuhr, M. D., "Tay-Sachs Screening," *loc. cit.,* 1300.

30. Kaback, M. M., "Heterozygote Screening—A Social Challenge," *New Eng. J. Med., ,*1973, *289,* 1090–1091.

31. Evans, P., "Testing for Tay-Sachs Carriers," *Brit. Med. J.,* 1973, *3,* 408.

32. _____, "Testing for Tay-Sachs Heterozygotes," *Lancet,* 1973, *2,* 391.

33. Edwards, J. H. "Testing for Tay-Sachs Heterozygotes," *loc. cit.,* 1143.

34. Evans, P. R., Ellis, R. B., and Masson, P. K., "Testing for Tay-Sachs Heterozygotes," *loc. cit.,* 1143–1144.

35. Ellis, R. B., Ikonne, J. V., Patrick, A. D., Stephens, R., and Willcox, P., "Prenatal Diagnosis of Tay-Sachs Disease," *op. cit.,* 1144–1145.

36. Rosner, F., "Screening for Tay-Sachs Disease," *Lancet,* 1974, *1,* 359.

37. Jackson, L. G., "Heterozygote Detection for Autosomal Recessive Genetic Diseases. Community Aspects of the Tay-Sachs Experience," *Clin. Ped.,* 1974, *13,* 307–309.

38. Padeh, B., "A Screening Program for Tay-Sachs Disease in Israel," *Israel J. Med. Sci.,* 1973, *9,* 1330–1334.

39. Seligmann, J., "Jewish Diseases," *Newsweek,* May 26, 1975, p. 57.

40. Edelson, E., "The Jewish Disease," *New York Daily News,* Nov. 9, 1971.

41. "Tay-Sachs. The Killer Is Cornered," New York, National Tay-Sachs and Allied Diseases Assoc.; "What You Should Know about Tay-Sachs Disease and How to Protect against This Fatal Illness," New York State Department of Health; "Tay-Sachs Facts. What Every Family Should Know about This Fatal Childhood Illness," California Tay-Sachs Disease Prevention Program. "Tay-Sachs Disease and Birth Defects Prevention," National Foundation—March of Dimes, White Plains, N.Y. "Operation Gene Screen," Albert Einstein College of Medicine, New York, and National Genetics Foundation.

42. Glazermann, L. R., "Screening for Genetic Disease," *New Eng. J. Med.,* 1973, *289,* 754–755.

43. Kaback, M. M., Zeiger, R. S., Reynolds, L. W., et al., "Tay-Sachs Disease: A Model for the Control of Recessive Genetic Disorders," *Proceedings of the Fourth International Conference on Tay-Sachs Disease,* Vienna, Sept. 2–8, 1973. Amsterdam, Excerpta Medica, 1974, 248–262.

44. Copy kindly provided by Rabbi Feinstein's son-in-law, Rabbi Dr. Moses D. Tendler.

45. Bleich, J. D., "Tay-Sachs Disease," *Tradition,* 1972, 13, 145–148.

46. Waldenberg, E. J., "Medico-Halakhic Aspects of Tay-Sachs Disease," *Assia* (Jerusalem) #13 Adar 2–5736 (March, 1976), pp. 8–10 (Hebrew).

47. Jakobovits, I., "Tay-Sachs Disease and the Jewish Community," *Proc. Assn. Orthodox Jewish Scientists,* 1977 Vol. 5, pp. 1–4.

48. Feinstein, M., Unpublished responsum; Bleich, J. D., *Contemporary*

Halakhic Problems, New York, Ktav 1977, pp. 112–114 and p. 346, n. 42.

49. Lappé, M., Gustafson, J. M., and Roblin, R., "Ethical and Social Issues in Screening for Genetic Disease," *New Eng. J. Med.,* 1972, *286,* 1129–1132.

50. Mamman, I., "Screening for Sickling," *Lancet,* 1975, *1,* 1030.

51. Whitten, C. F. and Fischhoff, J., "Psychosocial Effects of Sickle Cell Disease," *Arch. Int. med.,* 1974, *133,* 681–689.

11
Transsexual
Surgery
J. DAVID BLEICH

Transsexuals are persons who are born with the anatomy of one sex but suffer from an identification with the other sex which in many instances is total and lifelong. It is claimed by some scientists doing research in this area that this abnormality is the result of hormone disturbances which are quite likely prenatal in origin. In a rapidly increasing number of cases transsexualism is now being treated medically by a combination of hormone therapy and sex-change surgery. While such operations were performed in Europe on an intermittent basis as early as 1930, sex-change operations have become prevalent in our country only since the late 1960s. There are an estimated ten thousand transsexuals in the United States, of whom approximately fifteen hundred have changed their sex by means of surgery. Public awareness of this phenomenon has been heightened by the recent publication of *Conundrum,* an autobiography by Jan (formerly James) Morris, in which the author discusses his own transsexualism with skill and sensitivity.

The growing acceptance of transsexual surgery has made the question of sex-change a topical halakhic issue. A number of rather cursory items dealing with this topic, which are noteworthy primarily on account of the sources cited, have appeared in the 5733 volume of *No'am* and in the Kislev-Tevet and Tammuz-Av 5733 issues of *Ha-Ma'or.* These articles do not treat the unique halakhic problems of hermaphrodites or of individuals born with ambiguous genitalia.

Sex-change operations involving the surgical removal of sexual organs are clearly forbidden on the basis of the explicit Biblical prohibition. "And that which is mauled or crushed or torn or cut you shall not offer unto the Lord; nor should you do this in your land" (Lev. 22:24). Sterilization of women is also prohibited, as recorded in *Even ha-Ezer* 5:11.

Reprinted from *Tradition* (Spring, 1974). Copyright © 1974 by the Rabbinical Council of America.

Rabbi Meir Amsel (*Ha-Ma'or,* Kislev-Tevet 5733) notes that yet another prohibition is also applicable to sex-change procedures, a consideration which may extend as well to hormone treatment for purposes of sex-change. The commandment "A woman shall not wear that which pertains to a man, nor shall a man put on a woman's garment" (Deut. 22:5) is not limited to the wearing of apparel associated with the opposite sex but encompasses any action uniquely identified with the opposite sex, proscribing, for example, shaving of armpits or dyeing of hair by a male. A procedure designed to transform sexual characteristics violates the very essence of this prohibition.

Once a sexual transformation has actually been effected, a host of practical halakhic questions arise. The resolution of these questions hinges upon the crucial conceptual problem of whether or not a change of sex has indeed occurred from the point of view of Halakhah. It should be emphasized that while sexual organs can be removed, medical science is (at least as yet) incapable of substituting functional reproductive organs of the opposite sex. Sex-change procedures involve the construction of simulated sexual organs devoid of reproductive powers.

The most obvious halakhic questions concern the sexual status of such individuals with regard to marriage and divorce and with regard to their status *vis-à-vis* the respective obligations of men and women in the performance of *mitzvot.* A related question is discussed by *Teshuvot Besamim Rosh,* a work of questionable authenticity commonly attributed to Rabbenu Asher. *Besamim Rosh,* no. 340, questions whether a man whose genitalia have been completely removed need divorce his wife in order to dissolve their marriage or whether a divorce is unnecessary since the male has been sexually transformed, and hence "a new body has appeared and is comparable to a woman's." *Besamim Rosh* reaches no definitive conclusion with regard to whether or not a divorce is necessary in the event that the operation is performed subsequent to entry into a valid marriage. However, *Besamim Rosh* strongly asserts that, regardless of an individual's sexual status with regard to other matters, once the male sexual organs have been removed the person in question is no longer competent to contract a valid marriage as a man.[1] Although not stated explicitly, it may be assumed, according to *Besamim Rosh,* that such a person is also unqualified to contract a marriage as a woman since true female genital organs remain absent even subsequent to successful completion of the surgical procedure.

For *Besamim Rosh* sexual identity, insofar as marriage is concerned, depends entirely upon the presence of genital organs. No mention is made of the presence or absence of secondary sexual characteristics and indeed it is not difficult to understand why they are deemed irrelevant. Hence, despite the comments of Rabbi Amsel, who asserts that secondary sexual characteristics play a role in sexual identification, there is no evidence that the transformation of secondary sexual characteristics affects sexual status in any way.

One contemporary authority has ruled, without citing the ambivalent attitude of *Besamim Rosh,* that no divorce is necessary in order to permit the remarriage of a woman whose husband has undergone a sex-change operation. Rabbi Eliezer Waldenberg, *Ẕiẕ Eli'ezer,* X, no. 25, chap. 26, sec. 6, argues that if the person in question can no longer contract a marriage as a male (as indeed is the stated position of *Besamim Rosh*), the emergence of such a condition automatically terminates any existing marriage. The Gemara, *Yevamot* 49b, declares that although a husband is obliged to divorce an adulterous wife and is not permitted to remarry her, nevertheless, should he subsequently enter into such a marriage, the marriage is, *post factum,* deemed valid and must be dissolved by means of a divorce. Rashi and *Nemukei Yosef, ad locum,* explain that the marriage, when contracted, must be deemed valid, as evidenced by the fact that the original marriage is not automatically terminated upon the commission of adultery by the wife. The clear inference is that if Halakhah recognizes the continued existence of a previously contracted marriage despite a change in pertinent circumstances, a newly contracted marriage under the same circumstances is also valid. Conversely, if under the new circumstances a marriage cannot be contracted, it follows that an already existing marriage must be deemed to have been terminated automatically upon emergence of the new situation.[2] Unlike *Besamim Rosh,* Rabbi Waldenberg is of the opinion that the surgical removal of male sexual organs effects a change in sexual identity in the eyes of Halakhah. Rabbi Waldenberg, however, cites no evidence whatsoever for this view.

There is at least one early source which apparently declares that a male cannot acquire the status of a woman by means of surgery. Rabbi Abraham Hirsch (*No'am* 5733) cites the comments of Rabbenu Ḥananel, quoted by Ibn Ezra in his commentary on Leviticus 18:22. Rabbenu Ḥananel declares that intercourse between a normal male and a male in whom an artificial vagina has been fashioned by means of surgery constitutes sodomy. This would appear to be the case, according to Rabbenu Ḥananel, even if the male genitalia were removed.[3]

The corollary to this question arises with regard to a woman who has acquired the sexual characteristics of a male as a result of transsexual surgery. A nineteenth-century author, R. Joseph Palaggi, *Yosef et Eḥav* 3:5, opines that no divorce is necessary in order to dissolve a marriage contracted prior to such transformation. This author goes beyond the position of *Besamim Rosh,* who, as noted, did not reach a definitive conclusion in his discussion of the parallel question with regard to sex change in a male. In opposition to R. Palaggi's view it may, however, be argued that gender is irreversibly determined at birth and that sex, insofar as Halakhah is concerned, cannot be transformed by surgical procedures. This position is particularly cogent in view of the fact that fertile organs of the opposite sex cannot be acquired by means of surgery. The view that sexual identity cannot be changed by means of surgery would appear to be the position of Rabbenu Ḥananel. According to Rabbenu Ḥananel, this principle would appear to govern all halakhic questions pertaining to sexual identity.

Parenthetically, it is of interest to note that various courts in the United States have ruled that, in the eyes of the law, surgery to transform genitalia has no effect upon the gender of the person upon whom such procedures are performed (*Anonymous* v. *Anonymous,* 67 Misc. 2d 982; *Baker* v. *Nelson,* 291 Minn. 310, 191 N.W. 2d 185; 409 U.S. 810, 93 Supreme Court, 37; *Jones* v. *Hallahan,* Ky., 501, S.W. 2d 588). Recently, a justice of the New York State Supreme Court ruled that a woman who underwent surgery to become a man and subsequently married could not seek a divorce since a valid marriage had, in fact, never existed. The decision states that a marriage contract entered into by individuals of the same sex, one of whom has undergone sex-reversal surgery, has no validity either in fact or in law (*New York Law Journal,* April 30, 1974, p. 17, col. 4).

Another interesting question arises with regard to circumcision. In female-to-male transformations a simulated male organ is often created by means of skin grafts and silicone forms. In some cases this effect is achieved by freeing the clitoris from its connective tissue. There is no question that this newly fashioned organ need not be circumcised. This is abundantly clear from the conclusion reached by *She'elat Yaveẓ,* I, no. 171, in the discussion of a similar question arising with regard to a congenital defect. *Yosef et Eḥav* cites the comments of *Yad Ne'eman,* who maintains that circumcision would be unnecessary even if the new organ were physiologically similar to that of a male in every respect. In the opinion of the latter authority, the phraseology employed by Scripture, "un-circumcised male" (Gen. 17:13), applies solely to an individual who is a male at the time of birth.

A peripheral halakhic question which arises in cases of sexual trans-formation concerns which of the blessings included in the morning service should be recited by an individual who has undergone a transsexual procedure. Is the person in question to recite the blessing "Who has not made me a woman" or the blessing "Who has made me in accordance with His will"? The question is a compound one involving two separate issues. The first question is identical with the issue previously discussed: Is the individual's gender deemed to have been changed or is it deemed to have remained unchanged? Secondly, assuming that surgical transformation is to be recognized as indeed having effected a transformation from the point of view of Halakhah, there exists a halakhic controversy with regard to whether the blessings to be recited each morning are determined by the individual's status at birth or by his status at the time the blessings are pronounced. This difference of opinion is reflected in the controversy with regard to the recitation of the blessing "Who has not made me a gentile" by a proselyte. Rambam maintains that since the convert was born a gentile, it follows that he cannot truthfully pronounce the blessing "Who has not *made* me a gentile." Rashi disagrees and maintains that the blessing is fundamentally an expression of thanksgiving for being bound by the commandments of the Torah incumbent upon members of the Jewish faith and hence may be pronounced by the proselyte, since at the time of the recitation of the blessing he is indeed a Jew and subject to all *mitzvot*. The blessings "Who has not made me a woman" and "Who has made me in accordance with His will" reflect the differing status of men and women with regard to the performance of *mitzvot*. Hence, if the surgical transformation effects a change in the eyes of Halakhah, the proper blessing should, according to the opinion of Rashi, reflect the changed status, whereas, according to the opinion of Rambam, the usage "Who has made" or "Who has not made" in this context would express a falsehood.

It has been suggested that the entire question may be obviated by composing a text which would be more appropriate to such situations. According to this view, the proper blessings would be "Who has transformed me into a male" and "Who has transformed me in accordance with His will." Quite apart from the unwarranted assumption regarding divine approbation implied by this phraseology, it may be objected that in the absence of any liturgical formulation pertaining to "transformation" the proposed texts do not constitute rabbinically ordained formulae and hence cannot serve as valid substitutes for statutory blessings.

Although Judaism does not sanction the reversal of sex by means of surgery, transsexualism is a disorder which should receive the fullest measure of medical and psychiatric treatment consistent with Halakhah. Transsexuals should be encouraged to undergo treatment to correct endocrine imbalances, where medically indicated, and to seek psychiatric guidance in order to alleviate the grave emotional problems which are frequently associated with this tragic condition.

NOTES

1. R. Aryeh Leib Grossnass, *Lev Aryeh,* II, no. 49, takes exception to both the reasoning and the ruling of *Besamim Rosh*. R. Grossnass does, however, express doubt with regard to the necessity for a bill of divorce on the basis of *Minhat Ḥinnukh,* no. 203, but contends that for all other purposes, transsexual surgery has no effect upon sexual identity insofar as Halakhah is concerned.

2. This argument was originally advanced by *Minḥat Ḥinnukh,* no. 203, in explanation of an intriguing position taken by *Terumat ha-Deshen,* no. 102. *Terumat ha-Deshen* questions whether the wife of the prophet Elijah was permitted to remarry. According to tradition, Elijah neither died nor divorced his wife but ascended to heaven bodily. *Terumat ha-Deshen* rules that Scripture forbids man to cohabit with "the wife of his fellow" but does not forbid the wife of an angel. (Cf., however, R. Solomon Kluger, *Ḥokhmat Shelomo, Even ha-Ezer,* no. 17, who differs. See also R. Elchanan Wasserman, *Koveẓ Shi'urim,* II, no. 28.) *Minḥat Ḥinnukh* explains, on the basis of the previous argument, that since an angel cannot contract a marriage, a marriage to a man who becomes an angel is automatically terminated. (For a different explanation, see *Teshuvot Mahari Asad, Even ha-Ezer,* no. 4. See also *Lev Aryeh,* II, no. 49.)

R. Waldenberg, *Ẓiẓ Eli'ezer,* X, no. 25, chap. 26, sec. 6, and XI, no. 78, maintains that surgical reversal does effect a change in sexual identity in the eyes of Halakhah. He therefore argues that just as cohabitation is forbidden with the wife of his fellow but not with the wife of an angel, so also the concept of the wife of his fellow excludes the concept of the wife of a woman.

3. It might be argued against R. Hirsch that citation of Rabbenu Ḥananel is not conclusive in showing that Halakhah does not recognize reversal of sexual identity. The situation depicted by Rabbenu Ḥananel, after all, refers to a homosexual act with a male in whom an artificial orifice has been constructed; Rabbenu Ḥananel clearly does not describe a situation in which sex reversal has also been undertaken by means of removal of the male genitalia. Nevertheless, in context, the argument has not lost its cogency. If surgical changes in sexual identity are recognized for purposes of Halakhah, it would stand to reason that just as male-female changes effect a change in sexual identity, the construction of female organs, when unaccompanied by removal of male organs, should similarly be recognized as effecting a change in sexual identity from male to hermaphrodite. Rabbenu Ḥananel, as is evident from the text of these remarks, does not view penetration of the female organ of a hermaphrodite by a male as constituting a homosexual act (although he does allow for such a position in subsequent remarks). Yet, according to Rabbenu Ḥananel, intercourse via the artifically constructed vagina does constitute sodomy. This, then, indicates that the individual is regarded as a male rather than a hermaphrodite. Therefore it follows that if surgical procedures do not effect a change in status from male to hermaphrodite, such procedures cannot create a change of status from male to female in the eyes of Halakhah.

12
Judaism and the Modern Attitude to Homosexuality

NORMAN LAMM

Popular wisdom has it that our society is wildly hedonistic, with the breakdown of family life, rampant immorality, and the world, led by the United States, in the throes of a sexual revolution. The impetus of this latest revolution is such that new ground is constantly being broken, while bold deviations barely noticed one year are glaringly more evident the year following and become the norm for the "younger generation" the year after that.

Some sex researchers accept this portrait of a steady deterioration in sex inhibitions and of increasing permissiveness. Opposed to them are the "debunkers" who hold that this view is mere fantasy and that, while there may have been a significant leap in verbal sophistication, there has probably been only a short hop in actual behavior. They point to statistics which confirm that now, as in Kinsey's day, there has been no reported increase in sexual frequencies along with the alleged de-inhibition to rhetoric and dress. The "sexual revolution" is, for them, largely a myth. Yet others maintain that there is in Western society a permanent revolution against moral standards, but that the form and style of the revolt keeps changing.

The determination of which view is correct will have to be left to the sociologists and statisticians—or, better, to historians of the future who will have the benefit of hindsight. But certain facts are quite clear. First, the complaint that moral restraints are crumbling has a two or three thousand year history in Jewish tradition and in the continuous history of Western civilization. Second, there has been a decided increase at least in the area of sexual attitudes, speech, and expectations, if not in practice. Third, such social and psychological phenomena must sooner or later beget changes in

Reprinted from *Encyclopaedia Judaica Yearbook 1974*. Copyright © 1974 by Keter Publishing House Jerusalem Ltd.

mores and conduct. And finally, it is indisputable that most current attitudes are profoundly at variance with the traditional Jewish views on sex and sex morality.

Of all the current sexual fashions, the one most notable for its militancy, and which most conspicuously requires illumination from the sources of Jewish tradition, is that of sexual deviancy. This refers primarily to homosexuality, male or female, along with a host of other phenomena such as transvestism and transsexualism. They all form part of the newly approved theory of the idiosyncratic character of sexuality. Homosexuals have demanded acceptance in society, and this demand has taken various forms—from a plea that they should not be liable to criminal prosecution, to a demand that they should not be subjected to social sanctions, and then to a strident assertion that they represent an "alternative life-style" no less legitimate than "straight" heterosexuality. The various forms of homosexual apologetics appear largely in contemporary literature and theater, as well as in the daily press. In the United States, "gay" activists have become increasingly and progressively more vocal and militant.

Legal Position

Homosexuals have, indeed, been suppressed by the law. For instance, the Emperor Valentinian, in 390 C.E., decreed that pederasty be punished by burning at the stake. The sixth-century Code of Justinian ordained that homosexuals be tortured, mutilated, paraded in public, and executed. A thousand years later, Gibbon said of the penalty the Code decreed that "pederasty became the crime of those to whom no crime could be imputed." In more modern times, however, the Napoleonic Code declared consensual homosexuality legal in France. A century ago, anti-homosexual laws were repealed in Belgium and Holland. In this century, Denmark, Sweden and Switzerland followed suit and, more recently, Czechoslovakia and England. The most severe laws in the West are found in the United States, where they come under the jurisdiction of the various states and are known by a variety of names, usually as "sodomy laws." Punishment may range from light fines to five or more years in prison (in some cases even life imprisonment), indeterminate detention in a mental hospital, and even to compulsory sterilization. Moreover, homosexuals are, in various states, barred from the licensed professions, from many professional societies, from teaching, and from the civil service—to mention only a few of the sanctions encountered by the known homosexual.

More recently, a new leniency has been developing in the United States and elsewhere with regard to homosexuals. Thus, in 1969, the National

Institute of Mental Health issued a majority report advocating that adult consensual homosexuality be declared legal. The American Civil Liberties Union concurred. Earlier, Illinois had done so in 1962, and in 1971 the state of Connecticut revised its laws accordingly. Yet despite the increasing legal and social tolerance of deviance, basic feelings toward homosexuals have not really changed. The most obvious example is France, where although legal restraints were abandoned over 150 years ago, the homosexual of today continues to live in shame and secrecy.

Statistics

Statistically, the proportion of homosexuals in society does not seem to have changed much since Professor Kinsey's day (his book, *Sexual Behavior in the Human Male,* was published in 1948, and his volume on the human female in 1953). Kinsey's studies revealed that hard-core male homosexuals constituted about 4–6% of the population: 10% experienced "problem" behavior during a part of their lives. One man out of three indulges in some form of homosexual behavior from puberty until his early twenties. The dimensions of the problem become quite overwhelming when it is realized that, according to these figures, of 200 million people in the United States some ten million will become or are predominant or exclusive homosexuals, and over 25 million will have at least a few years of significant homosexual experience.

The New Permissiveness

The most dramatic change in our attitudes to homosexuality has taken place in the new mass adolescent subculture—the first such in history—where it is part of the whole new outlook on sexual restraints in general. It is here that the fashionable Sexual Left has had its greatest success on a wide scale, appealing especially to the rejection of Western traditions of sex roles and sex typing. A number of different streams feed into this ideological reservoir from which the new sympathy for homosexuality flows. Freud and his disciples began the modern protest against traditional restraints, and blamed the guilt that follows transgression for the neuroses that plague man. Many psychoanalysts began to overemphasize the importance of sexuality in human life, and this ultimately gave birth to a kind of sexual messianism. Thus, in our own day Wilhelm Reich identifies sexual energy as "vital energy *per se*" and, in conformity with his Marxist ideology, seeks to harmonize Marx and Freud. For Reich and his followers, the sexual revolution is a *machina ultima* for the whole Leninist liberation in all spheres of life and society. Rebellion against restrictive moral codes has become, for them, not merely a way to hedonism but a form of sexual mysticism: orgasm is seen not only as the pleasurable climactic release of internal sexual pressure, but as a means to individual creativity and insight as well as to the reconstruction and liberation of society. Finally, the emphasis on freedom and sexual autonomy derives from the Sartrean version of Kant's view of human autonomy.

It is in this atmosphere that pro-deviationist sentiments have proliferated, reaching into many strata of society. Significantly, religious groups have joined the sociologists and ideologists of deviance to affirm what has been called "man's birthright of unbounded ambisexuality." A number of Protestant churches in America, and an occasional Catholic clergyman, have pleaded for more sympathetic attitudes toward homosexuals. Following the new Christian permissiveness espoused in *Sex and Morality* (1966), the report of a working party of the British Council of Churches, a group of American Episcopalian clergymen in November 1967 concluded that homosexual acts ought not to be considered wrong, *per se*. A homosexual relationship is, they implied, no different from a heterosexual marriage: but must be judged by one criterion—"whether it is intended to foster a permanent relation of love." Jewish apologists for deviationism have been prominent in the Gay Liberation movement and have not hesitated to advocate their position in American journals and in the press. Christian groups began to emerge which catered to a homosexual clientele, and Jews were not too far behind. This latest Jewish exemplification of the principle of *wie es sich christelt, so juedelt es sich* will be discussed at the end of this essay.

Homosexual militants are satisfied neither with a "mental health" approach nor with demanding civil rights. They are clear in insisting on society's recognition of sexual deviance as an "alternative life-style," morally legitimate and socially acceptable.

Such are the basic facts and theories of the current advocacy of sexual deviance. What is the classical Jewish attitude to sodomy, and what suggestions may be made to develop a Jewish approach to the complex problem of the homosexual in contemporary society?

Biblical View

The Bible prohibits homosexual intercourse and labels it an abomination: "Thou shalt not lie with a man as one lies with a woman: it is an abomination" (Lev. 18:22). Capital punishment is ordained for both transgressors in Lev. 20:13. In the first passage, sodomy is linked with buggery, and in the second with incest and buggery. (There is considerable terminological confusion with regard to these words. We shall here use "sodomy" as a synonym for homosexuality and "buggery" for sexual relations with animals.)

The city of Sodom had the questionable honor of lending its name to homosexuality because of the notorious attempt at homosexual rape, when the entire population—"both young and old, all the people from every quarter"—surrounded the home of Lot, the nephew of Abraham, and demanded that he surrender his guests to them "that we may know them" (Gen. 19:5). The decimation of the tribe of Benjamin resulted from the notorious incident, recorded in Judges 19, of a group of Benjamites in Gibeah who sought to commit homosexual rape.

Scholars have identified the *kadesh* proscribed by the Torah (Deut. 23:18) as a ritual male homosexual prostitute. This form of heathen cult penetrated Judea from the Canaanite surroundings in the period of the early monarchy. So Rehoboam, probably under the influence of his Ammonite mother, tolerated this cultic sodomy during his reign (I Kings 14:24). His grandson Asa tried to cleanse the Temple in Jerusalem of the practice (I Kings 15:12), as did his great-grandson Jehoshaphat. But it was not until the days of Josiah and the vigorous reforms he introduced that the *kadesh* was finally removed from the Temple and the land (II Kings 23:7). The Talmud too (*Sanhedrin,* 24b) holds that the *kadesh* was a homosexual functionary. (However, it is possible that the term also alludes to a heterosexual male prostitute. Thus, in II Kings 23:7, women are described as weaving garments for the idols in the *batei ha-kedeshim* [houses of the *kadesh*]: the presence of women may imply that the *kadesh* was not necessarily homosexual. The Talmudic opinion identifying the *kadesh* as a homosexual prostitute may be only an *asmakhta*. Moreover, there are other opinions in Talmudic literature as to the meaning of the verse: see Onkelos, Lev. 23:18, and Naḥmanides and *Torah Temimah, ad loc.*)

Talmudic Approach

Rabbinic exegesis of the Bible finds several other homosexual references in the scriptural narratives. The generation of Noah was condemned to eradication by the Flood because they had sunk so low morally that, according to Midrashic teaching, they wrote out formal marriage contracts for sodomy and buggery—a possible cryptic reference to such practices in the Rome of Nero and Hadrian (Lev. R. 18:13).

Of Ham, the son of Noah, we are told that "he saw the nakedness of his father" and told his two brothers (Gen. 9:22). Why should this act have warranted the harsh imprecation hurled at Ham by his father? The rabbis offer two answers: one, that the text implied that Ham castrated Noah: second, that the Biblical expression is an idiom for homosexual intercourse (see Rashi, *ad loc.*). On the scriptural story of Potiphar's purchase of Joseph as a slave (Gen. 39:1), the Talmud comments that he acquired him for homosexual purposes, but that a miracle occurred and God sent the angel Gabriel to castrate Potiphar (*Sotah* 13b).

Post-Biblical literature records remarkably few incidents of homosexuality. Herod's son Alexander, according to Josephus (Wars, I, 24:7), had homosexual contact with a young eunuch. Very few reports of homosexuality have come to us from the Talmudic era (TJ *Sanhedrin* 6:6, 23c: Jos. Ant., 15:25–30).

The incidence of sodomy among Jews is interestingly reflected in the Halakhah on *mishkav zakhur* (the Talmudic term for homosexuality: the Bible uses various terms—thus the same term in Num. 31:17 and 35 refers to heterosexual intercourse by a woman, whereas the expression for male homosexual intercourse in Lev. 18:22 and 20:13 is *mishkevei ishah*). The Mishnah teaches that R. Judah forbade two bachelors from sleeping under the same blanket, for fear that this would lead to homosexual temptation (*Kiddushin* 4:14). However, the Sages permitted it *(ibid.)* because homosexuality was so rare among Jews that such preventive legislation was considered unnecessary (*Kiddushin* 82a). This latter view is codified as Halakhah by Maimonides (*Yad, Issurei Bi'ah* 22:2). Some 400 years later, R. Joseph Caro, who did not codify the law against sodomy proper, nevertheless cautioned against being alone with another male because of the lewdness prevalent "in our times" (*Even ha-Ezer* 24). About a hundred years later, R. Joel Sirkes reverted to the original ruling, and suspended the prohibition because such obscene acts were unheard of amongst Polish Jewry (*Bayit Hadash* to *Tur, Even ha-Ezer* 24). Indeed, a distinguished contemporary of R. Joseph Caro, R. Solomon Luria, went even further and declared homosexuality so very rare that, if one refrains from sharing a blanket with another male as a special act of piety, one is guilty of self-righteous pride or religious snobbism (for the above and additional authorities, see *Ozar ha-Posekim,* IX, 236–238).

Responsa

As is to be expected, the responsa literature is also very scant in discussions of homosexuality. One of the few such responsa is by the late R. Abraham Isaac Ha-Kohen Kook, when he was still the rabbi of Jaffa. In 1912 he was asked about a ritual slaughterer who had come under suspicion of homosexuality. After weighing all aspects of the case, R. Kook dismissed the charges against the accused, considering them unsupported hearsay.

Furthermore, he maintained the man might have repented and therefore could not be subject to sanctions at the present time.

The very scarcity of halakhic deliberations on homosexuality, and the quite explicit insistence of various halakhic authorities, provide sufficient evidence of the relative absence of this practice among Jews from ancient times down to the present. Indeed, Prof. Kinsey found that, while religion was usually an influence of secondary importance on the number of homosexual as well as heterosexual acts by males, Orthodox Jews proved an exception, homosexuality being phenomenally rare among them.

Jewish law treated the female homosexual more leniently than the male. It considered lesbianism as *issur,* an ordinary religious violation, rather than *arayot,* a specifically sexual infraction, regarded much more severely than *issur.* R. Huna held that lesbianism is the equivalent of harlotry and disqualified the woman from marrying a priest. The Halakhah is, however, more lenient, and decides that while the act is prohibited, the lesbian is not punished and is permitted to marry a priest (*Sifra* 9:8: *Shab.* 65a: *Yev.* 76a). However, the transgression does warrant disciplinary flagellation (Maimonides, *Yad, Issurei Bi'ah* 21:8). The less punitive attitude of the Halakhah to the female homosexual than to the male does not reflect any intrinsic judgment on one as opposed to the other, but is rather the result of a halakhic technicality: there is no explicit Biblical proscription of lesbianism, and the act does not entail genital intercourse (Maimonides, *loc. cit.*).

The Halakhah holds that the ban on homosexuality applies universally, to non-Jew as well as to Jew (*Sanh.* 58a: Maimonides, *Melakhim* 9:5, 6). It is one of the six instances of *arayot* (sexual transgressions) forbidden to the Noachide (Maimonides, *ibid*).

Most halakhic authorities — such as Rashba and Ritba — agree with Maimonides. A minority opinion holds that pederasty and buggery are "ordinary" prohibitions rather than *arayot* — specifically sexual infractions which demand that one submit to martyrdom rather than violate the law — but the Jerusalem Talmud supports the majority opinion. (See D. M. Krozer, *Devar Ha-Melekh,* I, 22, 23 (1962), who also suggests that Maimonides may support a distinction whereby the "male" or active homosexual partner is held in violation of *arayot,* whereas the passive or "female" partner transgresses *issur,* an ordinary prohibition.)

Reasons for Prohibition

Why does the Torah forbid homosexuality? Bearing in mind that reasons proferred for the various commandments are not to be accepted as determinative, but as human efforts to explain immutable divine law, the rabbis of the Talmud and later Talmudists did offer a number of illuminating rationales for the law.

As stated, the Torah condemns homosexuality as *to'evah,* an abomination. The Talmud records the interpretation of Bar Kapparah who, in a play on words, defined *to'evah* as *to'eh attah bah.* "You are going astray because of it" (*Nedarim* 51a). The exact meaning of this passage is unclear, and various explanations have been put forward.

The *Pesikta (Zutarta)* explains the statement of Bar Kapparah as referring to the impossibility of such a sexual act resulting in procreation. One of the major functions (if not the major purpose) of sexuality is reproduction, and this reason for man's sexual endowment is frustrated by *mishkav zakhur* (so too *Sefer ha-Ḥinnukh,* no. 209).

Another interpretation is that of the *Tosafot* and R. Asher ben Jeḥiel (in their commentaries to *Ned.* 51a) which applies the "going astray" or wandering to the homosexual's abandoning his wife. In other words, the abomination consists of the danger that a married man with homosexual tendencies may disrupt his family life in order to indulge his perversions. Saadiah Gaon holds the rational basis of most of the Bible's moral legislation to be the preservation of the family structure (*Emunot ve-De'ot* 3:1: cf. *Yoma* 9a). (This argument assumes contemporary cogency in the light of the avowed aim of some gay militants to destroy the family, which they consider an "oppressive institution.")

A third explanation is given by a modern scholar, Rabbi Baruch Ha-Levi Epstein (*Torah Temimah* to Lev. 18:22), who emphasizes the unnaturalness of the homosexual liaison: "You are going astray from the foundations of the creation." *Mishkav zakhur* defies the very structure of the anatomy of the sexes, which quite obviously was designed for heterosexual relationships.

It may be, however, that the very variety of interpretations of *to'evah* points to a far more fundamental meaning, namely, that an act characterized as an "abomination" is *prima facie* disgusting and cannot be further defined or explained. Certain acts are considered *to'evah* by the Torah, and there the matter rests. It is, as it were, a visceral reaction, an intuitive disqualification of the act, and we run the risk of distorting the Biblical judgment if we rationalize it. *To'evah* constitutes a category of objectionableness *sui generis:* it is a primary phenomenon. (This lends additional force to Rabbi David Z. Hoffmann's contention that *to'evah* is used by the Torah to indicate the repulsiveness of a proscribed act, no matter how much it may be in vogue among advanced and sophisticated cultures: see his *Sefer Va-yikra,* II, p. 54.).

Jewish Attitudes

It is on the basis of the above that an effort must be made to formulate a

Jewish response to the problems of homosexuality in the conditions under which most Jews live today, namely, those of free and democratic societies and, with the exception of Israel, non-Jewish lands and traditions.

Four general approaches may be adopted:

1) *Repressive.* No leniency toward the homosexual, lest the moral fiber of the rest of society be weakened.

2) *Practical.* Dispense with imprisonment and all forms of social harassment, for eminently practical and prudent reasons.

3) *Permissive.* The same as the above, but for ideological reasons, viz., the acceptance of homosexuality as a legitimate alternative "life-style."

4) *Psychological.* Homosexuality, in at least some forms, should be recognized as a disease and this recognition must determine our attitude toward the homosexual.

Let us now consider each of these critically.

Repressive Attitude   Exponents of the most stringent approach hold that pederasts are the vanguard of moral malaise, especially in our society. For one thing, they are dangerous to children. According to a recent work, one third of the homosexuals in the study were seduced in their adolescence by adults. It is best for society that they be imprisoned, and if our present penal institutions are faulty, let them be improved. Homosexuals should certainly not be permitted to function as teachers, group leaders, rabbis, or in any other capacity where they might be models for, and come into close contact with, young people. Homosexuality must not be excused as a sickness. A sane society assumes that its members have free choice, and are therefore responsible for their conduct. Sex offenders, including homosexuals, according to another recent study, operate "at a primate level with the philosophy that necessity is the mother of improvisation." As Jews who believe that the Torah legislated certain moral laws for all mankind, it is incumbent upon us to encourage all societies, including non-Jewish ones, to implement the Noachide laws. And since, according to the Halakhah, homosexuality is prohibited to Noachides as well as to Jews, we must seek to strengthen the moral quality of society by encouraging more restrictive laws against homosexuals. Moreover, if we are loyal to the teachings of Judaism, we cannot distinguish between "victimless" crimes and crimes of violence. Hence, if our concern for the moral life of the community impels us to speak out against murder, racial oppression, or robbery, we must do no less with regard to sodomy.

This argument is, however, weak on a number of grounds. Practically, it fails to take into cognizance the number of homosexuals of all categories, which, as we have pointed out, is vast. We cannot possibly imprison all offenders, and it is a manifest miscarriage of justice to vent our spleen only on the few unfortunates who are caught by the police. It is inconsistent, because there has been no comparable outcry for harsh sentencing of other transgressors of sexual morality, such as those who indulge in adultery or incest. To take consistency to its logical conclusion, this hard line on homosexuality should not stop with imprisonment but demand the death sentence, as is Biblically prescribed. And why not the same death sentence for blasphemy, eating a limb torn from a live animal, idolatry, robbery—all of which are Noachide commandments? And why not capital punishment for Sabbath transgressors in the State of Israel? Why should the pederast be singled out for opprobrium and be made an object lesson while all others escape?

Those who might seriously consider such logically consistent, but socially destructive, strategies had best think back to the fate of that Dominican reformer, the monk Girolamo Savonarola, who in 15th-century Florence undertook a fanatical campaign against vice and all suspected of venal sin, with emphasis on pederasty. The society of that time and place, much like ours, could stand vast improvement. But too much medicine in too strong doses was the monk's prescription, whereupon the population rioted and the zealot was hanged.

Finally, there is indeed some halakhic warrant for distinguishing between violent and victimless (or consensual and non-consensual) crimes. Thus, the Talmud permits a passer-by to kill a man in pursuit of another man or of a woman when the pursuer is attempting homosexual or heterosexual rape, as the case may be, whereas this is not permitted in the case of a transgressor pursuing an animal to commit buggery or on his way to worship an idol or to violate the Sabbath, (*Sanh.* 8:7, and v. Rashi to *Sanh.* 73a, s.v. *al ha-behemah*).

Practical Attitude   The practical approach is completely pragmatic and attempts to steer clear of any ideology in its judgments and recommendations. It is, according to its advocates, eminently reasonable. Criminal laws requiring punishment for homosexuals are simply unenforceable in society at the present day. We have previously cited the statistics on the extremely high incidence of pederasty in our society. Kinsey once said of the many sexual acts outlawed by the various states, that, were they all enforced, some 95% of men in the United States would be in jail. Furthermore, the special prejudice of law enforcement authorities against homosexuals — rarely does one hear of police entrapment or of jail sentences for non-violent heterosexuals — breeds a grave injustice: namely, it is an invitation to blackmail. The law concerning sodomy has been called "the blackmailer's charter." It is universally agreed that prison does little to help the homosexual rid himself of his peculiarity. Certainly, the failure of rehabilitation ought to be of concern to civilized men. But even if it is not, and the crime be considered so serious that incarceration is deemed advisable even in the absence of any real chances of rehabilitation, the casual pederast almost always leaves prison as a confirmed criminal. He has been denied the company of women and forced into the society of those whose sexual expression is almost always channeled to pederasty. The casual pederast has become a habitual one: his homosexuality has now been ingrained in him. Is society any safer for having taken an errant man and, in the course of a few years, for having taught him to transform his deviancy into a hard and fast perversion, then turning him loose on the community? Finally, from a Jewish point of view, since it is obviously impossible for us to impose the death penalty for sodomy, we may as well act on purely practical grounds and do away with all legislation and punishment in this area of personal conduct.

This reasoning is tempting precisely because it focuses directly on the problem and is free of any ideological commitments. But the problem with it is that it is too smooth, too easy. By the same reasoning one might, in a *reductio ad absurdum* do away with all laws on income tax evasion, or forgive, and dispense with all punishment of Nazi murders. Furthermore, the last element leaves us with a novel view of the Halakhah: if it cannot be implemented in its entirety, it ought to be abandoned completely. Surely the Noachide laws, perhaps above all others, place us under clear moral imperatives, over and above purely penological instructions? The very practicality of this position leaves it open to the charge of evading the very real moral issues, and for Jews the halakhic principles, entailed in any discussion of homosexuality.

Permissive Attitude   The ideological advocacy of a completely permissive attitude toward consensual homosexuality and the acceptance of its moral legitimacy is, of course, the "in" fashion in sophisticated liberal circles. Legally, it holds that deviancy is none of the law's business; the homosexuals' civil rights are as sacred as those of any other "minority group." From the psychological angle, sexuality must be emancipated from the fetters of guilt induced by religion and code-morality, and its idiosyncratic nature must be confirmed.

Gay Liberationists aver that the usual "straight" attitude toward homosexuality is based on three fallacies or myths: that homosexuality is an illness; that it is unnatural; and that it is immoral. They argue that it cannot be considered an illness, because so many people have been shown to practice it. It is not unnatural, because its alleged unnaturalness derives from the impossibility of sodomy leading to reproduction, whereas our overpopulated society no longer needs to breed workers, soldiers, farmers, or hunters. And it is not immoral, first, because morality is relative, and secondly, because moral behavior is that which is characterized by "selfless, loving concern."

Now, we are here concerned with the sexual problem as such, and not with homosexuality as a symbol of the whole contemporary ideological polemic against restraint and tradition. Homosexuality is too important — and too agonizing — a human problem to allow it to be exploited for political aims or entertainment or shock value.

The bland assumption that pederasty cannot be considered an illness because of the large number of people who have or express homosexual tendencies cannot stand up under criticism. No less an authority than Freud taught that a whole civilization can be neurotic. Erich Fromm appeals for the establishment of *The Sane Society* — because ours is not. If the majority of a nation are struck down by typhoid fever, does this condition, by so curious a calculus of semantics, become healthy? Whether or not homosexuality can be considered an illness is a serious question, and it does depend on one's definition of health and illness. But mere statistics are certainly not the *coup de grâce* to the psychological argument, which will be discussed shortly.

The validation of gay life as "natural" on the basis of changing social and economic conditions is an act of verbal obfuscation. Even if we were to concur with the widely held feeling that the world's population is dangerously large, and that Zero Population Growth is now a desideratum, the anatomical fact remains unchanged: the generative organs are structured for generation. If the words "natural" and "unnatural" have any meaning at all, they must be rooted in the unchanging reality of man's sexual apparatus rather than in his ephmeral social configurations.

Militant feminists along with the gay activists react vigorously against the implication that natural structure implies the naturalness or unnaturalness of certain acts, but this very view has recently been confirmed by one of the most informed writers on the subject. "It is already pretty safe to infer from laboratory research and ethological parallels that male and female are wired in ways that relate to our traditional sex roles . . . Freud dramatically said that anatomy is destiny. Scientists who shudder at the dramatic, no matter how accurate, could rephrase this: anatomy is functional, body functions have profound psychological meanings to people, and anatomy and function are often socially elaborated" (Arno Karlen, *Sexuality and Homosexuality,* p. 501).

The moral issues lead us into the quagmire of perennial philosophical disquisitions of a fundamental nature. In a way, this facilitates the problem for one seeking a Jewish view. Judaism does not accept the kind of thoroughgoing relativism used to justify the gay life as merely an alternate life-style. And while the question of human autonomy is certainly worthy of consideration in the area of sexuality, one must beware of the consequences of taking the argument to its logical extreme. Judaism clearly cherishes holiness as a greater value than either freedom or health. Furthermore, if every individual's autonomy leads us to lend moral legitimacy to any form of sexual expression he may desire, we must be ready to pull the blanket of this moral validity over almost the whole catalogue of perversions described by Krafft-Ebing, and then, by the legerdemain of granting civil rights to the morally non-objectionable, permit the advocates of buggery, fetishism, or whatever to proselytize in public. In that case, why not in the school system? And if consent is obtained before the death of one partner, why not necrophilia or cannibalism? Surely, if we declare pederasty to be merely idiosyncratic and not an "abomination," what right have we to condemn sexually motivated cannibalism — merely because most people would react with revulsion and disgust?

"Loving, selfless concern" and "meaningful personal relationships" — the great slogans of the New Morality and the exponents of situation ethics — have become the litany of sodomy in our times. Simple logic should permit us to use the same criteria for excusing adultery or any other act heretofore held to be immoral; and indeed, that is just what has been done, and it has received the sanction not only of liberals and humanists, but of certain religionists as well. "Love," "fulfillment," "exploitative," "meaningful" — the list itself sounds like a lexicon of emotionally charged terms drawn at random from the disparate sources of both Christian and psychologically-oriented agnostic circles. Logically, we must ask the next question: what moral depravities can not be excused by the sole criterion of "warm, meaningful human relations" or "fulfillment," the newest semantic heirs to "love?"

Love, fulfillment, and happiness can also be attained in incestuous contacts—and certainly in polygamous relationships. Is there nothing at all left that is "sinful," "unnatural," or "immoral" if it is practiced "between two consenting adults?" For religious groups to aver that a homosexual relationship should be judged by the same criteria as a heterosexual one — i.e., "whether it is intended to foster a permanent relationship of love" — is to abandon the last claim of representing the "Judeo-Christian tradition."

I have elsewhere essayed a criticism of the situationalists, their use of the term "love," and their objections to traditional morality as exemplified by the Halakhah as "mere legalism" (see my *Faith and Doubt,* chapter IX, p. 249 ff.). Situationalists, such as Joseph Fletcher, have especially attacked "pilpulistic Rabbis" for remaining entangled in the coils of statutory and legalistic hairsplitting. Among the other things this typically Christian polemic reveals is an ignorance of the nature of Halakhah and its place in Judaism, which never held that the law was the totality of life, pleaded again and again for supererogatory conduct, recognized that individuals may be disadvantaged by the law, and which strove to rectify what could be rectified without abandoning the large majority to legal and moral chaos simply because of the discomfiture of the few.

Clearly, while Judaism needs no defense or apology in regard to its esteem for neighborly love and compassion for the individual sufferer, it cannot possibly abide a wholesale dismissal of its most basic moral principles on the grounds that those subject to its judgments find them repressive. All laws are repressive to some extent—they repress illegal activities — and all morality is concerned with changing man and improving him and his society. Homosexuality imposes on one an intolerable burden of differentness, of absurdity, and of loneliness, but the Biblical commandment outlawing pederasty cannot be put aside solely on the basis of sympathy for the victim of these feelings. Morality, too, is an element which each of us, given his sensuality, his own idiosyncracies, and his immoral proclivities, must take into serious consideration before acting out his impulses.

Psychological Attitudes   Several years ago I recommended that Jews regard homosexual deviance as a pathology, thus reconciling the insights of Jewish tradition with the exigencies of contemporary life and scientific information, such as it is, on the nature of homosexuality (*Jewish Life,* Jan-Feb. 1968). The remarks that follow are an expansion and modification of that position, together with some new data and notions.

The proposal that homosexuality be viewed as an illness will immediately be denied by three groups of people. Gay militants object to this view as an instance of heterosexual condescension. Evelyn Hooker and her group of psychologists maintain that homosexuals are no more pathological in their personality structures than heterosexuals. And psychiatrists Thomas Szasz in the U.S. and Ronald Laing in England reject all traditional ideas of mental sickness and health as tools of social repressiveness or, at best, narrow conventionalism. While granting that there are indeed unfortunate instances where the category of mental disease is exploited for social or political reasons, we part company with all three groups and assume that there are a significant number of pederasts and lesbians who, by the criteria accepted by most psychologists and psychiatrists, can indeed be termed pathological. Thus, for instance, Dr. Albert Ellis, an ardent advocate of the right to deviancy, denies there is such a thing as a well-adjusted homosexual. In an interview, he has stated that whereas he used to believe that most homosexuals were neurotic, he is now convinced that about 50% are borderline psychotics, that the usual fixed male homosexual is a severe phobic, and that lesbians are even more disturbed than male homosexuals (see Karlen, *op. cit.,* p. 223 ff.).

No single cause of homosexuality has been established. In all probability, it is based on a conglomeration of a number of factors. There is overwhelming evidence that the condition is developmental, not constitutional. Despite all efforts to discover something genetic in homosexuality, no proof has been adduced, and researchers incline more and more to reject the Freudian concept of fundamental human biological bisexuality and its corollary of homosexual latency. It is now widely believed that homosexuality is the result of a whole family constellation. The passive, dependent, phobic male homosexual is usually the product of an aggressive, covertly seductive mother who is overly rigid and puritanical with her son — thus forcing him into a bond where he is sexually aroused, yet forbidden to express himself in any heterosexual way — and of a father who is absent, remote, emotionally detached, or hostile (I. Bieber *et al. Homosexuality,* 1962).

Can the homosexual be cured? There is a tradition of therapeutic pessimism that goes back to Freud but a number of psychoanalysts, including Freud's daughter Anna, have reported successes in treating homosexuals as any other phobics (in this case, fear of the female genitals). It is generally accepted that about a third of all homosexuals can be completely cured: behavioral therapists report an even larger number of cures.

Of course, one cannot say categorically that all homosexuals are sick — any more than one can casually define all thieves as kleptomaniacs. In order to develop a reasonable Jewish approach to the problem and to seek in the concept of illness some mitigating factor, it is necessary first to establish the main types of homosexuals. Dr. Judd Marmor speaks of four categories. "Genuine homosexuality" is based on strong preferential erotic feelings for members of the same sex. "Transitory homosexual behavior" occurs among adolescents who would prefer heterosexual experiences but are denied such opportunities because of social, cultural, or psychological reasons. "Situational homosexual exchanges" are characteristic of prisoners, soldiers, and others who are heterosexual but are denied access to women for long periods of time. "Transitory and opportunistic homosexuality" is that of delinquent young men who permit themselves to be used by pederasts in order to make money or win other favors, although their primary erotic interests are exclusively heterosexual. To these may be added, for purposes of our analysis, two other types. The first category, that of genuine homosexuals, may be said to comprehend two subcategories: those who experience their condition as one of duress or uncontrollable passion which they would rid themselves of if they could, and those who transform their idiosyncrasy into an ideology, i.e., the gay militants who assert the legitimacy and validity of homosexuality as an alternative way to heterosexuality. The sixth category is based on what Dr. Rollo May has called "the New Puritanism," the peculiarly modern notion that one must experience all sexual pleasures, whether or not one feels inclined to them, as if the failure to taste every cup passed at the sumptuous banquet of carnal life means that one has not truly lived. Thus, we have transitory homosexual behavior not of adolescents, but of *adults* who feel that they must "try everything" at least once or more than once in their lives.

A Possible Halakhic Solution

This rubric will now permit us to apply the notion of disease (and, from the halakhic point of view, of its opposite, moral culpability) to the various types of sodomy. Clearly, genuine homosexuality experienced under duress (Hebrew: *ones*) most obviously lends itself to being termed pathological, especially where dysfunction appears in other aspects of the personality. Opportunistic homosexuality, ideological homosexuality, and transitory adult homosexuality are at the other end of the spectrum, and appear most reprehensible. As for the intermediate categories, while they cannot be called illness, they do have a greater claim on our sympathy than the three types mentioned above.

In formulating the notion of homosexuality as a disease, we are not asserting the formal halakhic definition of mental illness as mental incompetence, as described in TB *Hag.* 3b, 4a, and elsewhere. Furthermore, the categorization of a prohibited sex act as *ones* (duress) because of uncontrolled passions is valid, in a technical halakhic sense, only for a married woman who was ravished and who, in the course of the act, became a willing participant. The Halakhah decides with Rava, against the father of Samuel, that her consent is considered duress because of the passions aroused in her (*Ket.* 51b). However, this holds true only if the act was initially entered into under physical compulsion (*Kesef Mishneh* to *Yad, Sanh.* 20:3). Moreover, the claim of compulsion by one's erotic passions is not valid for a male, for any erection is considered a token of his willingness (*Yev.* 53b; Maimonides, *Yad, Sanh.* 20:3). In the case of a male who was forced to cohabit with a woman forbidden to him, some authorities consider him guilty and punishable, while others hold him guilty but not subject to punishment by the courts (*Tos., Yev.* 53b: *Hinnukh,* 556; *Kesef Mishneh, loc. cit.: Maggid Mishneh* to *Issurei Bi'ah,* 1:9). Where a male is sexually aroused in a permissible manner, as to begin coitus with his wife, and is then forced to conclude the act with another woman, most authorities exonerate him (Rabad and *Maggid Mishneh,* to *Issurei Bi'ah, in loc.*). If, now, the warped family background of the genuine homosexual is considered *ones,* the homosexual act may possibly lay claim to some mitigation by the Halakhah. (However, see *Minhat Hinnukh,* 556, end; and M. Feinstein, *Iggerot Moshe* (1973) on *YD,* no. 59, who holds, in a different context, that any pleasure derived from a forbidden act performed under duress increases the level of prohibition. This was anticipated by R.

Joseph Engel, *Atvan de-Oraita,* 24.) These latter sources indicate the difficulty of exonerating sexual transgressors because of psycho-pathological reasons under the technical rules of the Halakhah.

However, in the absence of a Sanhedrin and since it is impossible to implement the whole halakhic penal system, including capital punishment, such strict applications are unnecessary. What we are attempting is to develop guidelines, based on the Halakhah, which will allow contemporary Jews to orient themselves to the current problems of homosexuality in a manner articulating with the most fundamental insights of the Halakhah in a general sense, and consistent with the broadest world-view that the halakhic commitment instills in its followers. Thus, the aggadic statement that "no man sins unless he is overcome by a spirit of madness" (*Sot.* 3a) is not an operative halakhic rule, but does offer guidance on public policy and individual pastoral compassion. So in the present case, the formal halakhic strictures do not in any case apply nowadays, and it is our contention that the aggadic principle must lead us to seek out the mitigating halakhic elements so as to guide us in our orientation to homosexuals who, by the standards of modern psychology, may be regarded as acting under compulsion.

To apply the Halakhah strictly in this case is obviously impossible; to ignore it entirely is undesirable, and tantamount to regarding Halakhah as a purely abstract, legalistic system which can safely be dismissed where its norms and prescriptions do not allow full formal implementation. Admittedly, the method is not rigorous, and leaves room for varying interpretations as well as exegetical abuse, but it is the best we can do.

Hence there are types of homosexuality that do not warrant any special considerateness, because the notion of *ones* or duress (i.e., disease) in no way applies. Where the category of mental illness does apply, the act itself remains *to'evah* (an abomination), but the fact of illness lays upon us the obligation of pastoral compassion, psychological understanding, and social sympathy. In this sense, homosexuality is no different from any other anti-social or anti-halakhic act, where it is legitimate to distinguish between the objective act itself, including its social and moral consequences, and the mentality and inner development of the person who perpetrates the act. For instance, if a man murders in a cold and calculating fashion for reasons of profit, the act is criminal and the transgressor is criminal. If, however, a psychotic murders, the transgressor is diseased rather than criminal, but the objective act itself remains a criminal one. The courts may therefore treat the perpetrator of the crime as they would a patient, with all the concomitant compassion and concern for therapy, without condoning the act as being morally neutral. To use halakhic terminology, the objective crime remains a *ma'aseh averah,* whereas the person who transgresses is considered innocent on the grounds of *ones.* In such cases, the transgressor is spared the full legal consequences of his culpable act, although the degree to which he may be held responsible varies from case to case.

An example of a criminal act that is treated with compassion by the Halakhah, which in practice considers the act pathological rather than criminal, is suicide. Technically, the suicide or attempted suicide is in violation of the law. The Halakhah denies to the suicide the honor of a eulogy, the rending of the garments by relatives or witnesses to the death, and (according to Maimonides) insists that the relatives are not to observe the usual mourning period for the suicide. Yet, in the course of time, the tendency has been to remove the stigma from the suicide on the basis of mental disease. Thus, halakhic scholars do not apply the technical category of intentional (la-da'at) suicide to one who did not clearly demonstrate, before performing the act, that he knew what he was doing and was of sound mind, to the extent that there was no hiatus between the act of self-destruction and actual death. If these conditions are not present, we assume that it was an insane act or that between the act and death he experienced pangs of contrition and is therefore repentant, hence excused before the law. There is even one opinion which exonerates the suicide unless he received adequate warning (hatra'ah) before performing the act, and responded in a manner indicating that he was fully aware of what he was doing and that he was lucid (J. M. Tykocinski, Gesher ha-Ḥayyim, I, ch. 25, and Encyclopaedia Judaica, 15:490).

Admittedly, there are differences between the two cases: pederasty is clearly a severe violation of Biblical law, whereas the stricture against suicide is derived exegetically from a verse in Genesis. Nevertheless, the principle operative in the one is applicable to the other: where one can attribute an act to mental illness, it is done out of simple humanitarian considerations.

The suicide analogy should not, of course, lead one to conclude that there are grounds for a blanket exculpation of homosexuality as mental illness. Not all forms of homosexuality can be so termed, as indicated above, and the act itself remains an "abomination." With few exceptions, most people do not ordinarily propose that suicide be considered an acceptable and legitimate alternative to the rigors of daily life. No sane and moral person sits passively and watches a fellow man attempt suicide because he "understands" him and because it has been decided that suicide is a "morally neutral" act. By the same token, in orienting ourselves to certain types of homosexuals as patients rather than criminals, we do not condone the act but attempt to help the homosexual. Under no circumstances can Judaism suffer homosexuality to become respectable. Were society to give its open or even tacit approval to homosexuality, it would invite more aggressiveness on the part of adult pederasts toward young people. Indeed, in the currently permissive atmosphere, the Jewish view would summon us to the semantic courage of referring to homosexuality not as "deviance," with the implication of moral neutrality and non-judgmental idiosyncracy, but as "perversion" — a less clinical and more old-fashioned word, perhaps, but one that is more in keeping with the Biblical *to'evah*.

Yet, having passed this moral judgment, we cannot in the name of Judaism necessarily demand that we strive for the harshest possible punishment. Even where it was halakhically feasible to execute capital punishment, we have a tradition of leniency. Thus, R. Akiva and R. Tarfon declared that had they lived during the time of the Sanhedrin, they never would have executed a man. Although the Halakhah does not decide in their favor (*Mak.*, end of ch. I), it was rare indeed that the death penalty was actually imposed. Usually, the Biblically mandated penalty was regarded as an index of the severity of the transgression, and the actual execution was avoided by strict insistence upon all technical requirements — such as *hatra'ah* (forewarning the potential criminal) and rigorous cross-examination of witnesses, etc. In the same spirit, we are not bound to press for the most punitive policy toward contemporary lawbreakers. We are required to lead them to rehabilitation (*teshuvah*). The Halakhah sees no contradiction between condemning a man to death and exercising compassion, even love, toward him (*Sanh.* 52a). Even a man on the way to his execution was encouraged to repent (*Sanh.* 6:2). In the absence of a death penalty, the tradition of *teshuvah* and pastoral compassion to the sinner continues.

I do not find any warrant in the Jewish tradition for insisting on prison sentences for homosexuals. The singling-out of homosexuals as victims of society's righteous indignation is patently unfair. In Western history, anti-homosexual crusades have too often been marked by cruelty, destruction, and bigotry. Imprisonment in modern times has proven to be extremely haphazard. The number of homosexuals unfortunate enough to be apprehended is infinitesimal as compared to the number of known homosexuals; estimates vary from one to 300,000 to one to 6,000,000! For homosexuals to be singled out for special punishment while all the rest of society indulges itself in every other form of sexual malfeasance (using the definitions of Halakhah, not the New Morality) is a species of double-standard morality that the spirit of Halakhah cannot abide. Thus, the Mishnah declares that the "scroll of the suspected adulteress" (*megillat sotah*) — whereby a wife suspected of adultery was forced to undergo the test of "bitter waters" — was cancelled when the Sages became aware of the ever-larger number of adulterers in general (*Sot.* 9:9). The Talmud bases this decision on an aversion to the double standard: if the husband is himself an adulterer, the "bitter waters" will have no effect on his wife, even though she too be guilty of the offense (*Sot.* 47b). By the same token, a society in which heterosexual immorality is not conspicuously absent has no moral right to sit in stern judgment and mete out harsh penalties to homosexuals.

Furthermore, sending a homosexual to prison is counterproductive if punishment is to contain any element of rehabilitation or *teshuvah*. It has rightly been compared to sending an alcoholic to a distillery. The Talmud records that the Sanhedrin was unwilling to apply the full force of the law where punishment had lost its quality of deterrence; thus, 40 (or four) years before the destruction of the Temple, the Sanhedrin voluntarily left the precincts of the Temple so as not to be able, technically, to impose the death sentence, because it had noticed the increasing rate of homicide (*Sanh.* 41a, and elsewhere).

There is nothing in the Jewish law's letter or spirit that should incline us toward advocacy of imprisonment for homosexuals. The Halakhah did not, by and large, encourage the denial of freedom as a recommended form of punishment. Flogging is, from a certain perspective, far less cruel and far more enlightened. Since capital punishment is out of the question, and since incarceration is not an advisable substitute, we are left with one absolute minimum: strong disapproval of the proscribed act. But we are not bound to any specific penological instrument that has no basis in Jewish law or tradition.

How shall this disapproval be expressed? It has been suggested that, since homosexuality will never attain acceptance anyway, society can afford to be humane. As long as violence and the seduction of children are not involved, it would be best to abandon all laws on homosexuality and leave it to the inevitable social sanctions to control, informally, what can be controlled.

However, this approach is not consonant with Jewish tradition. The repeal of anti-homosexual laws implies the removal of the stigma from homosexuality, and this diminution of social censure weakens society in its training of the young toward acceptable patterns of conduct. The absence of adequate social reproach may well encourage the expression of homosexual tendencies by those in whom they might otherwise be suppressed. Law itself has an educative function, and the repeal of laws, no matter how justifiable such repeal may be from one point of view, does have the effect of signaling the acceptability of greater permissiveness.

Some New Proposals

Perhaps all that has been said above can best be expressed in the proposals that follow.

First, society and government must recognize the distinctions between the various categories enumerated earlier in this essay. We must offer medical and psychological assistance to those whose homosexuality is an expression of pathology, who recognize it as such, and are willing to seek help. We must be no less generous to the homosexual than to the drug addict, to whom the government extends various forms of therapy upon request.

Second, jail sentences must be abolished for all homosexuals, save those who are guilty of violence, seduction of the young, or public solicitation.

Third, the laws must remain on the books, but by mutual consent of judiciary and police, be unenforced. This approximates to what lawyers call "the chilling effect," and is the nearest one can come to the category so well known in the Halakhah, whereby strong disapproval is expressed by affirming a halakhic prohibition, yet no punishment is mandated. It is a category that bridges the gap between morality and law. In a society where homosexuality is so rampant, and where incarceration is so counter-productive, the hortatory approach may well be a way of formalizing society's revulsion while avoiding the pitfalls in our accepted penology.

For the Jewish community as such, the same principles, derived from the tradition, may serve as guidelines. Judaism allows for no compromise in its abhorrence of sodomy, but encourages both compassion and efforts at rehabilitation. Certainly, there must be no acceptance of separate Jewish homosexual societies, such as — or especially — synagogues set aside as homosexual congregations. The first such "gay synagogue," apparently, was the "Beth Chayim Chadashim" in Los Angeles. Spawned by that city's Metropolitan Community Church in March 1972, the founding group constituted itself as a Reform congregation with the help of the Pacific Southwest Council of the Union of American Hebrew Congregations some time in early 1973. Thereafter, similar groups surfaced in New York City and elsewhere. The original group meets on Friday evenings in the Leo Baeck Temple and is searching for a rabbi — who must himself be "gay". The membership sees itself as justified by "the Philosophy of Reform Judaism." The Temple president declared that God is "more concerned in our finding a sense of peace in which to make a better world, than He is in whom someone sleeps with" (cited in "Judaism and Homosexuality," *C.C.A.R. Journal,* Summer 1973, p. 38; five articles in this issue of the Reform group's rabbinic journal are devoted to the same theme, and most of them approve of the Gay Synagogue).

But such reasoning is specious, to say the least. Regular congregations and other Jewish groups should not hesitate to accord hospitality and membership, on an individual basis, to those "visible" homosexuals who qualify for the category of the ill. Homosexuals are no less in violation of Jewish norms than Sabbath desecrators or those who disregard the laws of *kashrut*. But to assent to the organization of separate "gay" groups under Jewish auspices makes no more sense, Jewishly, than to suffer the formation of synagogues that cater exclusively to idol worshipers, adulterers, gossipers, tax evaders, or Sabbath violators. Indeed, it makes less sense, because it provides, under religious auspices, a ready-made clientele from which the homosexual can more easily choose his partners.

In remaining true to the sources of Jewish tradition, Jews are commanded to avoid the madness that seizes society at various times and in many forms, while yet retaining a moral composure and psychological equilibrium sufficient to exercise that combination of discipline and charity that is the hallmark of Judaism.

Mental Health and Drugs

13
Psychiatry, Psychotherapy and Halakhah: A Torah Perspective on the Philosophy of Behavior Change

MOSHE HALEVI SPERO

Introduction

Jewish professionals have accepted the responsibility of scrutinizing the various sciences in the interests of synthesizing the philosophies and practices of the former with the Torah *weltanschauung*. For this effort to be worthwhile it must involve more than purely historical searches for the scientific underpinnings of Jewish religious practices or for the Talmudic precursors of scientific practices and beliefs; though such endeavors are also not without heuristic benefit.[1] Useful syntheses must grapple with the genuine halakhic issues which have arisen in such encounters. In search for such synthesis in the field of the behavioral sciences, this chapter will examine the specialty of psychotherapy in terms of several of the critical halakhic and ethico-moral issues which present themselves for the Jewish individual — practitioner or patient.

For the purposes of this examination, the terms psychiatry, psychology and psychotherapy will be used interchangeably though not in ignorance of certain basic differences among these terms which should be pointed out to the lay reader. *Psychiatry* is a medical profession; its practitioners are MDs specializing in the treatment of minor to severe behavioral, emotional or psychosomatic pathology who are trained in the use of (though may not exclusively utilize) medical techniques of behavior change.[2] It is out of the field of psychiatry that the "healing" or psychotherapeutic role — the infamous "medical model" of current debate — emerged for all future mental health professions. *Clinical psychology,* an outgrowth of the empirical advances of general psychology but modeled after the psychiatric role, deals with the non-medical treatment of psychopathology — its practitioners are PhDs — and specializes in the testing and measurement of behavioral, some neurological and learning disorders.[3] *Psychiatric social work,* historically directly linked with the psychiatric profession, also treats psychopathology, though in certain settings its practice may be more circumscribed.[4] Practitioners in all three professions may cross-specialize in the specific treatment and diagnosis of children, adults, families or groups. Thus, for all intents and purposes, in numerous applications, there is little difference between the three specialties.

The matter of a clinician's *psychological orientation;* i.e., what *model* of behavior dynamics and development governs one's understanding and approach to psychopathology, its etiology and treatment, is a complex one. One may uphold through training and practice classical or Freudian psychoanalysis, neo- and post-Freudian schools of analysis, Adlerian, Gestalt, client-centered, transactional, existential, and behavioral, biodynamic or social learning doctrines, or any compatible combination of two or more of the above. The tendency to equate the specialized technique of psychoanalysis with the whole of psychiatry is an historically based misconception. Sigmund Freud was a physician and many analytic training schools currently insist that their trainees be physicians, yet there are also presently many excellent lay analysts (MSWs or PhDs), or psycho*dynamically* oriented clinicians, and even many behavioral psychiatrists.[5] (The possibility of lay analysis was already recognized by Freud and encouraged by his daughter, Anna, a lay child analyst of her own acclaim.[6]) In view of these many divergent models, and in order to present an analysis which is of most use, I will address myself to the broadest and most widely accepted usages of terms such as psychiatry and psychotherapy.

In fact, in considering the dynamic relationship between psychotherapy and Halakhah, my presumption is that psychotherapy is the basic focus of all three mental health disciplines previously mentioned, and is defined as the process of bringing about behavioral/emotional change.[7] In using this term, I will generally intend psychotherapies such as the so-called talking cure, relationship therapy, insight-oriented therapy, and operant conditioning procedures known as behavior modification or behavioral therapy which constitute the most frequently utilized modes of intervention for the majority of 'psychological' disturbances. There are other, strictly medical psychiatric techniques which amount practically to psychotherapy insofar as they bring about behavioral/emotional change, such as ECT (electroconvulsive or "shock" therapy), psychosurgery (lobotomies, topectomies, leukotomies, etc.), sex-reassignment surgery, psychopharmacological treatment and others. Although each of these techniques merits separate discussion which space here cannot allow, much of our general examination of the philosophy of psychotherapy will apply equally to the ultimate goals and outcomes of the medical techniques as well as to the nonmedical psychotherapies.[8]

The reader will discern from the above that, unlike other medical specialties, and perhaps unlike many of the general sciences, the *philosophies* of psychiatric or psychological change and their underlying *values* and assumptions are as much our concern in this sort of halakhic analysis as are practical techniques, if only because these values and philosophies are often indicted as being in great conflict with Torah values. We shall see that psychotherapy or certain psychotherapies in specific are denounced for their various commitments to the denial of guilt and sin, of the role and usefulness of religion, for their upholding psychological determinism, etc.[9] The issue of interest here, more specifically, is whether or not one needs to and, then, can one prudently separate allegedly undesirable underlying philosophy from "pure" technique and still be left with an entity which has therapeutic viability and yet is consistent with halakhic standards? The need for a Torah-analysis is brought forth clearly in the following comment, "One must admit that the very nature of psychotherapy, the doctor-patient intimacy, the shaping and modifying of behavior, and the total involvement in the life of another, puts the therapist in a position wherein he must deal with the patient's behavior relevant to Halakhah, and is in a position to evoke in the patient behavior that is halakhically correct."[10]

Unfortunately, despite these and many other areas needing study and development to create a synthetic approach to Judaism and psychotherapy, the concerned individual has up until most recently been confronted with an unjustifiable lacuna in traditional Jewish scholarship on the matter. The creation of the *Journal of Psychology and Judaism* in 1976 has been a significant development of relevance.[11] A recent issue of the AOJS's *Intercom* was devoted entirely to the subject of mental health.[12] Indeed, "The most neglected field in the development of Jewish law on medical subjects is no doubt psychiatry."[13] Synthetic approaches forwarded to date by some non-orthodox Jewish authors are either imprecise psychiatrically (or just too general, as is the fault with many of the traditional studies as well) or evince limited conceptions of Jewish philosophy and Halakhah, and are thus of little use for the orthodox practitioner or patient.[14] One can speculate, with just cause, that this dearth of research is a manifestation of the effects of a strong, emotional reaction of hostility and discomfort on the part of the Jewish community to Freudian and later psychoanalytic attitudes about religion, guilt and sin — which a significant and vocal portion of the orthodox community has projected unthinkingly upon all forms of psychotherapy or psychiatry. This is evinced, in part, by the endless searches made by some observant professionals for the "Torah psychology" as opposed to investing energy into studying the basic compatabilities between the two.[15] It is certainly proven by the many followers of the view expressed more than thirty years ago by Rabbi Twerski of Slotopoli-Chertkov that psychology is in our day what philosophy was in the times of the Rambam: a major peril to the intellectual and spiritual existence of the Jewish people![16] In view of the above, another project of this paper will be to see just how justified and productive such an overgeneralized reaction is.

I

It has been argued that psychotherapy cannot exist divorced from any distinct view of human nature and of man's effective ability to change,[17] several implications of which I have discussed elsewhere.[18] Clearly this assertion must be so as long as psychotherapy addresses itself to the uniquely human psyche, to problems inherent in human nature, to bio*social* adjustment; so long as it deals with the boundaries of human freedom and understanding, human interrelations, etc.[19] Even the behavioral therapies which theoretically view man as being not markedly different than animal inasmuch as the behavior of both species is seen as governed by the universal principles of operant conditioning — which, despite B. F. Skinner's humanitarian protestations to the contrary, tends to deny the reality of man *qua* man — is nonetheless *a* view of human nature.[20]

Psychotherapy's view of man is not irrelevant to a study concerned with Halakhah and psychiatric philosophy. First, the quality of a healthy religion is based in part on the degree to which it addresses itself to not only the transcendental but also the mundane physical and psychic needs of its believers. It follows from this definition that religion can be expected to be therapeutic in one capacity or another inasmuch as relative mental adjustment is a prerequisite for the exercise of free will necessary for true religious commitment. That this is also the case with Judaism follows from the implications of the Biblical concepts *derakheha darkhei no'am, be-khol derakhav da-ehu* and *va-ḥai bahem*.[21] Second, in view of a burgeoning tendency to look to psychotherapy and some of its fadistic offshoots as potential solutions for many of society's human and cosmic problems and as routes to personal transcendence — roles which until now have traditionally been those of religion — one must give thought to the nature of such solutions and to the types of new worlds that might develop, guided by a purely 'psychiatric' or existential perception of human nature, in the light of Torah teachings. Third, even "pure" technique is inextricably tied to a philosophy of change insofar as the justification and construction of technique is concerned. This much is certainly the case with regard to the deterministic assumptions of behavioral or psychoanalytic experiments, understandings of symptom development, and the outcomes of therapy. The case has also been made that both Freud and Skinner, and certainly the respective schools of psychotherapy which have since developed from the original theorizations of these two innovators, were greatly influenced by the prevalent climates of philosophical opinion in their times.[22] These influences may or may not have been consistent with Torah norms, and if they are not — and if they are believed to inhere in pure technique — might be construed as contaminating variables in an otherwise acceptable system.

These issues are all critical ones which the subsequent discussions will hopefully shed light on. Two crucial aspects of the interconnectedness between psychotherapeutic philosophy and technique can be isolated for our consideration: (1) the role of the assumption of non-judgementalness in therapeutic practice (the philosophical position of value neutrality) and the potential difficulties this assumption can pose for the religious patient; and (2) the psychiatric view of religion and its correlates in relation to treating disturbed religious clients. Each of these implications will be discussed in turn.

II

Modern psychotherapy and psychiatry have strained to eradicate from their systems such value-laden terms as "mental illness," "mental patient," and even some of its psychiatric diagnostic nomenclature — e.g., minimal brain dysfunction (MBD), hyperactivity, homosexuality—in deference to the discomfort and stigma often caused by social responses to these labels.[23] However, for the most part, psychotherapy must involve value assumptions.[24] For example, a patient clearly comes to the professional to obtain help in either removing an inappropriate or undesirable behavioral/emotional pattern or adding a missing, more appropriate behavior. "Undesirable" "inappropriate," "appropriate," etc., all refer to value investments. Indeed, the general therapeutic goal of "adjustment" always implies working either with some negatively valued deficiency or surficiency which also represents the phenomenological perception a therapist must accept for the sake of "beginning where the client is."[25] Others, though admitting to the above, still view psychotherapy as essentially non-judgemental in that it never seeks to label a client and his behavior or beliefs "bad" or "wrong" nor considers him to *blame* for his condition. Of course, this in no way releases the patient from *responsibility* over his or her actions, as A. Amsel seems to think,[26] but seeks only to assert that the therapist, though in an influential position vis-a-vis the client, does not judge the client. That is, the therapist does not deny the importance of the role of moral educator but rather disclaims it as the *therapeutic* role.

Nonetheless, while this is a substantial qualification of the non-judgemental viewpoint, there can still be no doubt that the institution of psychotherapy is based, in part, on a consensus agreement *and a value judgement* that a circumscribed set of behavior/emotional variations are non-normal and non-functional from the standpoint of the society one has chosen to live in. Thus, even psychiatric *relativism* becomes no less a bona fide philosophical position involving, at some juncture, the imposition of values. Psychiatry definitely confers positive value upon alleviation of suffering reinforcing freedom from fetishized and ritualized neurotic behavior, freedom from irrational motives leading to self-harm or harm to others, freedom to find satisfactory levels of adjustment in marital, sexual and interfamilial patterns of interaction.[27]

It should be clear by now that psychotherapy operates with value judgements. Only once this is recognized can legitimate grounds be had for suspecting potential disagreement between the values of the former and the Torah viewpoint.

There are many areas of such conflict: the belief in sin and commitment to the reality of guilt *versus* a belief that guilt and sin-consciousness is neurotogenic; the belief that non-heterosexual relationships are perversions *versus* the belief that one is entitled to pursue alternative ambisexual life-styles; the laws of *z'ni'ut* (modesty) and *taharat ha-mishpaḥah* (laws of family purity and sexual conduct) *versus* some of the "now" philosophies of certain radical therapies and even some techniques of sex therapy; the belief in free will *versus* the doctrine of psychic determinism, and others. With regard to every one of the above oppositionals discussed, I believe that conflict need not actualize if approached synthetically, and that psychiatry can and often does subscribe to halakhically compatible views. Note, therefore, that when I imply that many of these 'conflicts' are actually pseudo-problems I do not mean that the conflicts suggested can never arise, or that there are no professionals who provoke actual conflict in these and other neutral areas. I mean that I do not believe that psychotherapy, in principle, need be in conflict in the areas to be discussed.

A.

One area of potential conflict which must be shown to be exaggerated out of proportion in view of modern trends in psychiatry and psychotherapy is the general psychiatric view of religion. The sources of contention most often referred to in this regard are the classical Freudian psychoanalytic and some neo-analytic views of religion. Whether these specific examples constitute ample grounds for the frequently-asserted generalization that psychiatry is out to destroy religious commitment or that psychoanalytic doctrine can never be looked to for therapeutic value because of this one onerous aspect of its original formulation is beside the point. One has to examine the psychiatric or the specific psychoanalytic world-view, compare it to the Jewish religious world-view, and ascertain whether any halakhic compatibility, in principle, can be forthcoming.

First, in what particular ways would, say, the Freudian view of religion ever come into conflict with Judaism? By either one of two ways: either in direct confrontation as a values conflict between a Jewish patient and a psychoanalytically-oriented therapist — which will need to be explained — or, on a broader scale, through a confrontation between the Jewish individual and culture *versus* another influential culture that is permeated with Freudian dogma or with the tenets of any therapeutic system which is considered to be antithetical to Judaism.

As far as the latter consideration is concerned, one is forced to admit that it is in this manner of confrontation that a faulty philosophy can do its greatest damage, yet not necessarily through the fault of the philosophy itself. That is, while one might wish to claim that a generation of children has been 'ruined' by having been brought up on the dubious principles of neo-Freudian perscriptions for mothering, etc., one more realistically has to lay a great proportion of the blame on the too-eager caseworkers who overexaggerate and generalize various analytic beliefs or upon non-psychiatric social philosophers who modify and twist Freudian clinical doctrine into strange social doctrines for which it was never intended. Just why people need "psychotherapeutic religions" to guide their lives and ease their insecurities will be brought up at the conclusion of this essay. Suffice it for this part of the discussion that my proposed synthesis and any halakhic discussion of therapeutic principles apply to the latters' clinical applications and clinical outlook in therapeutically advised circumstances.

The first consideration is now relevant. The Freudian view of religion — in an admittedly superficial presentation — as a development from primal, oedipally-based aggressive rebellion of sons against fathers, etc., was a theoretical opinion arrived at late in Freud's scientific career.[28] It was a case of Freud's force-feeding a given social institution — religion — into a presumedly universal and timeless theoretical outlook; *the theoretical outlook itself, however, in no way called for* this careless treatment of religion. This, among other things, has motivated most of Freud's biographers and explanators to look for an explanation of the psychoanalytic view of religion somewhere in the deeper recesses of Freud's own mind. This theoretical opinion, on the other hand, becomes a value *conflict* should a Freudian analyst feel that a client's analysis is not complete until the latter has sufficient 'insight' to recognize his religious commitments as neurotically based. We have a conflict here because the psychotherapist is confronting the client's original conception of religion, as an aspect of the moral or ontological domain, with the analyst's own conception of religion as a pseudo-moral affair belonging to the psychiatric domain. In truth, there are many clinicians who apparently cannot bracket their hostilities toward religion which they conceive of as an atavism along the continuum of universal psychological development. Moreover, keeping in mind our second consideration, had this outgrowth of psychoanalytic doctrine fully indoctrinated culture and society, which it obviously has not, then it would indeed have been an intellectual and spiritual disaster.

However, it is most encouraging to note that, precisely because this anti-religious bias is not a necessary component of the psychoanalytic system of psychology, that analyst and certainly other psychodynamically-oriented therapists have thoughtfully reappraised this view and have promoted more tolerant views demanding the preservation of the transcendant value and worth of mature religion. It may not be too partisan to observe that to the degree that the motive behind Freud's many ill-advised animadversions about religion was the message that blind faith is a poor basis for ethics and is potentially unwholesome,[29] similar sentiments can be found in the halakhic framework; e.g., "The simpleton cannot be pious," "Do not perform the *mitzvot* unthinkingly (lit., by rote)," "He who speculates on Divine beliefs stands higher than the simple believer."[30] Indeed, though not a halakhic issuance, recall Rabbi Mendel of Kotzk's castigation of blindly accepted religion, "Any God which the simple peasant claims to understand cannot be my God."[31]

Whether or not Freud can be made out to appear partially justified in at least his own personal psychoanalytic crusade, insofar as the modern psychiatric world-view is concerned, it is currently recognized that psychotherapy must deal with the whole life of the client and with the various means by which man lives out his existence. At the same time, psychiatry cannot dictate the terms in which man may be at peace with himself and others. "For the psychiatrist to interfere with the patient's religion is unethical. It is wrong to assume that anything which presents itself in the guise of religion is unstable, and the reverse is also false."[32] One perceptive analyst put it, "If we suggest that religion represents a reasonable reaching out on man's part for a socially acceptable and integrative solution for . . . his dependency needs, consistent with the current stage of human development, then no issue can be taken with his religious participation . . . In my opinion, therefore, the retention of religious beliefs and practices would not itself warrant the conclusion that an analysis has not been successfully concluded."[33] Though the above author's preconceptions about religion are quite transparent, it would appear that psychoanalysis need no longer be considered opposed in principle to religious commitment.

B.

A practical issue which emerges from the foregoing is who determines what defines "mature" and "immature" religion? There are cases where even the orthodox professional may justifiably question the maturity of certain individual's types of religious commitment, such as the allegedly neurotic religion of some *ba'alei teshuvah* (penitents) who undergo "crisis conversion" to cover up or augment deeper intrapsychic conflicts or latent, unresolved adolescent rebellion, etc. I have shown elsewhere how such neurotic religion can often retard religious as well as psychic growth.[34] Can neurotic religion in such patients, and in more severe cases where less conscious control over both religious as well as emotional aspects of personality are exhibited, ever be sacrificed in the interests of preserving mental health — with the hopes that the more mature patient can and will seek out anew more mature levels of religious commitment and expression? Supposing such a calculation can be legitimately considered from the halakhic standpoint, can such a decision ever be given over to a non-observant professional? These seem to be the real issues over which much thought must be given.

The issue can be expanded to include the following consideration: is one ever correct in viewing penitence, the process of *teshuvah,* as a successful piece of psychotherapy in its own right? This question is moot precisely in view of the many such individuals who present the rabbi or observant therapist with leaps-of-faith precipitated by psychological crises of an *a*religious nature.

In response, there is no doubt that, although religious practice can be expected, as a latent function of religion, to bring about certain therapeutic benefits, on the other hand, to *substitute* it for psychotherapy, when psychotherapy is what is really indicated, is to require the wrong thing from religion. Like other expressions of life, Judaism requires a balance between activity and passivity, between man's life urges and catabolic urges. Judaism represents courage, imagination and creativity, but also comfort, security and relaxation. This understanding lies behind the rabbinic conception of the continuous struggle between the two *yeẓarim,* or character passions of man.[35] Maintaining this balance becomes a difficult task when still unresolved psychic crises involving religion — such as one's past troubles with parents or other authority figures which may now be transferred to God — make additional demands of the penitent's personality.

Menninger and Pruyser have demonstrated the complexity of this problem. "Some people *with or without mental disorder,* feel greatly helped by a deep sense of trust in the intentions of the Divine or of nature toward them, or in people in general . . . which imbues them with a sense of optimism about the goodness of life which, in the case of patients, is therapeutically useful . . . Some people, *with or without mental disorder,* have a deep sense of distrust and chronic disappointment in other people, their God, or in nature or culture generally, which makes them cynical, angry, bitter, lonely, withdrawn, etc. In the case of patients, this basic value system is therapeutically a great liability. Some people, *with or without mental disorder,* experience a deep sense of meaninglessness, boredom . . . as if no value can be found worth living for or aiming at. Often these people feel propelled by alien forces, deprived of any feeling. In the case of patients . . . such pervasive valuelessness is a therapeutic liability" (italics mine).[36]

Thus, what must distinguish the un-conflicted *ba'al teshuvah* from the mental patient should be that certain superior religious sensitivity which seems to bring individuals closer in touch with a more profound sense of the generally-accepted reality rather than escape or withdrawal from that same reality. The hallowed acts, ceremonies and rituals of Judaism can become meaningless, fetishistic and trivial indulgences in the hands of an insecure, overanxious, depressed or otherwise disoriented individual. If it is the case that many *ba'alei teshuvah* harbor bothersome fears of backsliding of intensive guilt, this should be recognized and dealt with appropriately and halakhically so that these personal insecurities do not manifest themselves in some neurotic, clinging dependency, need for stringency and self-punishment. If not, then religion is indeed neurosis; i.e., the religion serves as a continuation of the neurosis or disorder which called this religious "penitence" into existence.

In this light, I return to the question of whether a clinician is ever justified in recommending the removal of a part of or a whole religious system so long as it also leaves a personality free of pathology. This question is difficult to answer halakhically for it involves individualized judgement before a competent halakhic authority, psychiatric *mumḥeh* (expert) and patient. One would need to consider the role of *sakanat nefashot* (danger to life), if it entered the picture, its extent and gravity. While there exists ample precedent in halakhic literature to waive specific religious requirements in the interests of preserving life and the quality of health,[37] it would be both halakhically problematical as well as psychiatrically rare to require the dissolution of an entire religious system in one personality in the 'interests' of mental health.

Suggesting another point of view, P. London writes that it would be ethically justifiable, from the psychiatric standpoint, for a therapist to offer psychotherapy to a religious client where such therapy might undermine the client's religious faith. "The problem presented to the therapist is one of disordered behavior, not of the attitudes that underlie it, and he must attack the disorder in whatever way he can. If he believes that the client's religious convictions help sustain the disorder, a confrontation with those convictions may be unavoidable. A conscientious therapist may have no choice but present his view."[38] Of course, "presenting his view" and actually advocating the practice of therapy which sets out to undermine religious belief are two different things, and calling for therapists to decide in favor of mental health over religious belief already seems to assume the role of moral arbiter. In the case of the Christian Scientist treated for compulsive disorders by Cohen and Smith,[39] Halleck[40] correctly notes that while knowing full-well that Christian Scientists reject medical and psychiatric intervention, Cohen and Smith's *very accepting* of the case implies a rejection of this aspect of the client's belief system.

Within certain ranges of emotional disorder, such as the psychoses or chronic affective disorders, disagreement with London's position is difficult to defend. However, one cannot generalize a London point of view across all milder forms of emotional imbalance. Second, the therapist in this case is certainly not *just* presented with "disordered behavior" — what I call the "particularistic fallacy;" i.e., the belief that in therapy one deals with only an isolated aspect of personality or only with 'bits' of disordered behavior — but rather with a *person* who has found meaning in life through a system, religion, which we know independently speaks to man through transcendent symbols and in meaningful terms and expectations. Third, while a professional may feel that a client is practicing religious ritual 'x' for rigid, anxiety-wrought reasons, the ritual *per se* may still be no less a religious obligation as long as the overall religious commitment is intact and there is no threat of harm to life through this ritual's observance. My opinion and practice is that therapy with such cases will usually need be done from within the religious belief system but, at the same time, around the defensive uses of that same religion; juggling for graduated levels of adjustment between quality (but not quantity) of religious observance and the elimination of psychopathology.

Summarizing to this point, it seems as if the past tendency of some psychoanalytic doctrines to explain away the value and legitimacy of religion and, in extension, their representing a threat to Halakhah in this regard, is a dated concern. The ability of psychotherapy to confine itself to the clinical arena and to hold back judgement on social entities, such as religion, which do not rightly fall into psychiatry's province, enhances Halakhah's ability to subsume psychotherapeutic technique and other compatible psychiatric philosophies under its purview.

III

Another potential value conflict between psychiatry and Judaism concerns their respective assumptions about sin and the value of guilt. The general psychoprophylactic view is that any intrapsychic variable is dysfunctional to the degree that it is neurotogenic; i.e., to the degree that its function is largely defensive, illusory or moves the individual away from health and reality toward neurosis. Again, there is no logical requirement that this principle include a corollary that "since religion is illusory and defensive, its preoccupation with the concept of sin is neurotogenic because it bids man make himself beholden to imaginary deities, mythical needs for perfection, etc." For, as made clear in the previous section, psychiatry can confine itself to the clinical realm which means that it can take a stance that a belief in sin is not necessarily a dysfunctional belief. On the other hand, even the religious therapist observes many situations where an already extant personality disorder uses the belief in sin and the potentially self-punishing effects of guilt to conform personality to pathological expectations or to fulfill pathological needs.[41] Certain concerned Orthodox Jewish scientists have written that psychiatry denies the worth of sin and the use of guilt trying to create a guiltless society.[42] While it may be true that some therapeutic schools have attempted to uphold such a world-view, it is clearly not the general psychotherapeutic view.

Indeed, the rational approach would be to distinguish between those schools which totally discount the benefits of the experience of guilt and the role of a belief in sin in meaningful, normal living, from those which accept their basic functionality.[43] Consider, for example, Albert Ellis' Rational Emotive Therapy. RET is a radical therapeutic approach which contends that it is not things-in-themselves which cause psychopathology but rather our *misconceptions* about and *inappropriate feelings* about such things; e.g., the death of a hated parent in childhood cannot 'cause' adult depression, but inappropriate guilt feelings about that event can cause unnecessary misery and depression. Cure? Re-educating oneself to no longer entertain such erroneous beliefs and feelings.[44] Similarly, RET would conceivably call for a patient's disavowal of the belief in sin if laboring under such a belief causes negativity, neurosis or depression, given RET's assumption that *thoughts about* sin rather than "sin", itself, cause unhappiness. Under such a therapeutic model, a client might be told that there is nothing implicitly wrong and, therefore, guilt-provoking about masturbation — but that wallowing in guilty thoughts about masturbation can be depressing. Such advice would obviously lead to a value conflict with an observant Jewish patient.

At the same time, using the same example, a halakhically-minded therapist would also initially try to hold guilt feelings of the client in abeyance in the therapeutic interests of allaying whatever deeper anxieties or psychosexual dynamics play a causative role in the development of this specific symptom. Later, this same therapist would accept and deal with the original masturbatory guilt and perhaps discuss the degree to which the halakhic category of *ones* (accidental, or completely unintended occurrence) might enter the specific situation. Yet, no attempt would ever be made by the halakhically-minded therapist to convince the client of a false view of the halakhic opinion in this or the other act (when considered not as a psychiatric symptom).

Despite possible complications, RET is but one of many therapeutic approaches which basically have as their common goal the alleviation of guilt when its proportions and pervasiveness seem destructive. Even Freud realized that without the integral role played by guilt, society as we know it could not continue.[45] Also wielding a growing influence in modern psychotherapy are the so-called existential psychiatric views of May, Boss and Frankl, to name a few, which accept the necessary worth of reality-based, *existential guilt* and *anxiety* as relevant for total, authentic psychic functioning or *being*.[46] These latter views are most in accord with the halakhic conception of guilt and anxiety *as danger signals of moral and spiritual weakness* or inauthentic living.

I have elsewhere argued in some detail that those religious practices in Judaism which assume the reality of sin, anxiety and guilt have been developed not to promote neurosis or continuous fear states but rather to affect a constant vigilance over existential weaknesses — weaknesses rooted in the very nature of human life, existence and worth vis-à-vis God and the Torah's expectations — inherent in the man-God encounter and human interrelations.[47] To be more specific, Maimonides makes it clear that one who is filled with anxiety and worry over past events, and with the fear which comes over the danger of backsliding, is comparable to one who laments the fact that he is a man and not an angel or a star — as one who is insane.[48] He makes it clear in his code that the *expectation* of forgiveness and the *experience* of consolation are to be construed as components of the *teshuvah*-process.[49] However, this view must also be made compatible with these Talmudic and Midrashic statements: "And my sin shall be before me always;" "Anxiety [*mardus* — pangs of conscience] in a man's heart is better than 100 lashes;" "He who is made anxious by his own conscience is greater than he who is shamed by others;" "All who sin and are made anxious [through shame] are forgiven for all their sins."[50] Recall also R. Eliezer's famous dictum: "Repent one day prior to your death . . . so that all your days shall be spent in repentance."[51] From these quotations, one would get the impression that Judaism advocates self-flagellation and encourages neurotic self-pity, to the contrary of Maimonides' halakhic view.

In truth, the contradiction blends into one view following this distinction suggested by the existential point of view, and apparently anticipated by the Sages, between *existential anxiety* and *fears* of imperfection versus the *elemental,* "psychiatric" versions of these emotions. Simple elemental fear is more the instinctual survival response — not differentiated from animal fear except in number of objects to which this basic fear is shown — and is the type of fear which easily becomes pathological and which is discouraged by Halakhah. Witness, "Do not appear guilt-ridden (evil) in your own eyes," "Fear breaks a man's strength."[52] This is why *teshuvah* motivated by fear of God, or fear of punishment, is less effective than *teshuvah* motivated by love of God.[53] On the other hand, *existential anxiety* or *guilt* — the intuitive experience of *being* meaningless, worthless; the fear of nothingness — are desirable affective responses in the Jewish world-view. This is why "anxiety is better than one hundred lashes," why for such anxiety "one is forgiven for all one's sins," etc. For this type of root-anxiety points to a healthy awareness of imperfections in one's God-centered living. It represents a *fear of loss of God's love* which, at the same time, presupposes *bonds* of love. Such anxiety, then, is really an *anxious longing* for God's return to man.[54] The awareness of this heightened psychological state of emotion in repentence as being the halakhic desideratum rather than elemental melancholia is apparent in the works of Rav Kook and is echoed in this aphorism attributed to Reb Shmelke of Nikolsburg, "And know you that all the weeping in this day (*Yom Kippur*) will be of no avail if there is sadness in it."[55]

Another useful perspective on this aspect of the relationship between psychiatric and halakhic views of sin can be along the lines of what Waldman calls the "sin-neurosis complex."[56] That is, sin and neuroses are actually two different perspectives on essentially similar types of human conduct insofar as both describe conduct which reflects fundamental contradictions in the human situation. Following Tillich's conceptualization of the human predicament as a constant dialectic between man's yearnings for freedom and limitlessness *versus* his inescapable human limitations and finitude, one can easily see a halakhic world-view reflected in a conception of sin as exaggeration of human freedom in the presence of the Infinite and man's conceited refusal to admit his limitations as he confronts the Eternal. Consider, "No man sins unless there enters in him a spirit of *madness,*" "Jealousy, appetite and glory remove a man from the world," etc., which, taken together, indicate that man's greatest folly, and hence his greatest sin, is his inability to recognize his limitations.[57]

Neurosis can be similarly conceptualized as the result of man's inability to tolerate estrangement, ambiguity and pretense in the face of our existing social structure. The result in both cases is a neurotic/sinful devotion to self-concern or narcissism to a point where ego boundaries, optimally oriented to include others and to seek out dialogical encounter with fellows and with God, constrict and entrap the afflicted individual in his or her autistic world. Thus, both Judaism and psychotherapy could agree that idolatry — worshipping the self rather than limiting it — accounts as man's most rebellious sin. This is perhaps why conceit is considered an offense as heinous as idol worship.[58] Freud and rabbinic Judaism can agree that man fights a constant battle against succumbing to the urge to destroy authority figures and surrendering to blind instinctual, appetitive gratification. "No one can be called holy until death has put an end to man's constant struggle with the ever-lurking tempter within and man lies in the earth with the victor's crown of peace on his head."[59]

Of course, not all sins are neurotic, in the psychiatric sense of the term, and not all neurosis is sinful, in the halakhic sense of the term — yet both concepts imply a lack of insight into one's self, both are symptomatic of regression or a relapse into infantile, socially/halakhically unacceptable behavior, both represent disordered personality.[60] It would therefore seem that a rapprochement between these two disciplines and their approaches to behavior disorder in certain circumstances should not be too difficult to imagine. A practical concern which exists in this regard is how many psychotherapists actually consult a religious expert when it is evident, somehow, that a client's own religious awarenesses and understandings are neurotically or otherwise limited? Nonetheless, it would appear that the appropriate reaction to this problem should not be one of blanket distrust of all therapies and therapists but rather one of thoughtful and cautious selectivity in choosing one's therapist.

I have presented several complex issues involving the working relationship between psychiatry and psychotherapy, as world-views and as practical techniques, and halakhah. This interface needs continuous monitoring both by halakhists as well as by religious psychiatric professionals in the interests of safeguarding the ultimate usefulness of psychiatry and psychotherapy and in the interests of preserving a fluid yet autonomous Halakhah that can confront and incorporate modern medical problems, advances and philosophical challenges.

Can psychiatry, by virtue of its own inherent ability to meet some of man's existential and uniquely human needs, ever successfully supplant religion as an ultimate *way of life*? That is, after having reached a point — when and if it does — where psychiatry can claim to "know" all the reasons why men promulgate religions, why man needs concepts like God, heaven, revelation, dialogue, etc., why man is made secure by certain symbolic systems, and after psychiatry feels certain that it has made man aware of these needs and of alternative ways in which to achieve satisfaction for them, will it then be capable of sustaining man in a manner qualitatively similar to the ways in which religion had earlier sustained mankind? This, as all the questions posed thus far, is no simple one to answer as it involves qualifying so many variables. Yet, some considerations can be suggested.

Earlier, I noted that on the clinical level, there is no halakhic doubt that Judaism can provide certain psychosocial benefits and that this latent function of religion has halakhic legitimacy. Equally, however, to rely on religion as a therapeutic crutch when true psychotherapy is what is really called for — as so many disheartened adolescents are doing today as they contemplate entrance into cult movements and other mystical pseudo-religions — is also to ask too much from religion.

On the other hand, to ask from modern therapeutics and their offshoots — Erhard Sensitivity Training, Transcendental Meditation (when used for more than specific therapeutic application), logotherapy, group therapy marathons, primal therapy, encounter groups, psychosynthesis, biofeedback, etc. — that they serve as all-inclusive responses to man's eternal quest for cosmic and Divine relatedness, religious transcendence, or that these be true symbolic expressions of man's deepest potentials, seems to ask the wrong thing from psychotherapy. For they reject *a priori* the fact that besides man's search for God, God is ever in search of man and has already revealed to man His definition of religious growth and what methods best achieve true God-consciousness. Indeed, man's pitiful persistence in accepting various finite, limited and fetishistic types of solutions — idolatries of sorts — through which to mediate his needs for transcendency suggests, perhaps, the patent inability of any of these ephemeral modes of salvation to measure up. Psychotherapy still speaks its own language even when addressing issues admittedly belonging to the religious domain. There is still a tendency toward psychological reductionism in these "therapeutic religions" and among their proponents in accepting the mistaken assumption that modern psychology will ever or has finally plumbed the depths of man's psychic needs and experiences. Authentic religious commitment is distinguished in that its *ultimate* concern is not in the providing of mere psychological support nor is it in fashioning sophisticated institutionalizations of man's neurotic needs to feel invincible and immortal.[61] Thus, the current worship of therapeutic religions and cult ways of life will eventually fail for though they may have achieved some fortuitous theory of man, they have still not secured any meaningful doctrine of belief in God.

Psychiatry seems to be a reasonable means by which to make occasional "midcourse corrections" in a religiously-oriented approach to God-centered living. The level of mental well-being so highly advocated by psychiatry is surely a prerequisite for success in securing a productive religious life. Because the development of psychiatric philosophies and techniques cannot be constant in the same sense as is the halakhic understanding of man, the former will appear to be at odds with Halakhah at various stages in psychiatry's unfolding maturation. Whereas Halakhah is non-relativistic, psychiatry often must be. Psychotherapy, more importantly, does not have among its goals *sanctification or redemption* of man — elements so critical to the halakhic mode. Though both psychotherapy and Halakhah recognize that man must exercise his freedom, only Halakhah directly demands *via* its ethico-moral imperatives what man *must* do *with* his freedom. However, this alone cannot prevent Halakhah from benefiting from those psychiatric models and related techniques that are otherwise compatible and occasionally shed unique light on the Jewish approach to man, his strengths and weaknesses. Psychiatry does offer many such legitimate responses to disturbed, unhappy, confused and unfulfilled individuals which transcend the limitations of its relativistic world-view. The observant Jewish individual would appear to be duty-bound to incorporate such practices where halakhically appropriate and where such intervention enhances religious commitment.

NOTES

1. Examples of the heuristic approach in psychology and Judaism might be "Dream Psychology in the Talmud," p. 123-132 and P. Bindler's "A Psychological Analysis of *Kavvanah* in Prayer," p. 133-144 both in the *Proceedings of the Association of Orthodox Jewish Scientists,* 1976, vol. 3-4. A useful source which collects and annotates articles dealing with this subject is the *Critical Review in Psychology and Judaism* of the *Journal of Psychology and Judaism* (1976).

2. See Arieti, S., *American Handbook of Psychiatry,* New York: Basic, 1964 ed., vol. I, p. 2-58.

3. Brown, F., "Clinical Psychology," p. 1616-1621. In A. Freedman and H. Kaplan (eds.), *Comprehensive Textbook of Psychiatry,* Baltimore: Williams & Wilkins, Co., 1967 ed.

4. Wittman, M. "Social Work Manpower in the Health Sciences," *Am. J. Pub. Heal.,* 1965, 55, p. 393-399.

5. See Wolberg's "The Medical: Non-Medical Controversy," p. 331-341 in L. Wolberg, *The Techniques of Psychotherapy,* New York: Grune & Stratton, 1967 ed.

6. Freud, S., "The Question of Lay Analysis," p. 138-258, in *Standard Edition of the Complete Works of Sigmund Freud,* London: Hogarth, Vol. 20, (1926) 1958.

7. Weiner, I., *The Principles of Psychotherapy,* New York: Wiley & Sons, 1975 and L. Wolberg "The Scope, Types and General Principles of Psychotherapy," p. 1-440 in Wolberg, *The Techniques of Psychotherapy, op. cit.* see also T. Wen-Shing & J. McDermott, "Psychotherapy: Historical Roots, Universal Elements and

Cultural Variations," *Am. J. Psych.* 1975, 132(4), p. 378–384.

8. These medical techniques are discussed in detail elsewhere.

9. See my discussion in "On the Relationship Between Psychotherapy and Judaism," *Journal of Psychology and Judaism,* 1976, 1(1), p. 15–36 and see P. Kahn, "Judaism and the Challenge of Modern Psychology," *Intercom,* 1976, 16(1), p. 3–6. Notorious in this regard are the sweeping generalizations of A. Amsel in his *Judaism and Psychology* (1969) and *Rational Irrational Man* (1976), New York: Feldheim.

10. Mermelstein, J., "Halachik values and the Clinical Practice of Psychotherapy," *Intercom,* 1976, 16(2), p. 4–9.

11. Under the editorship of Dr. Reuven P. Bulka, 1747 Featherston Drive, Ottawa, Ontario, Canada, K1H 6P4.

12. Assoc. of Orthodox Jewish Scientists, *Intercom,* 1976, 16(2).

13. Jakobovits, I., *Journal of a Rabbi,* London, 1967, p. 172.

14. Some of which have been reviewed in the *Critical Review* of the *JPJ* (see note 11).

15. E. G., Amsel's two works (note 9).

16. In Wolf, Y. A., *Torat ha-Nefesh,* B'nai B'rak, 1969, p. 12.

17. Tillich, P., "Existentialism, Psychotherapy and the Nature of Man," In S. Doniger (ed.) *The Nature of Man in Theology and Psychotherapy,* New York: Harper, 1962.

18. Spero, *op. cit.,* 1976.

19. See J. Masserman, "The Timeless Therapeutic Trinity," p. 611–623 In J. Masserman (ed), *Current Psychiatric Technique,* New York: Grune & Stratton, 1963.

20. Skinner, B. F., *About Behaviorism,* New York: Knopf, 1974.

21. Proverbs 3:17; cf. *Yoma* 85b. Rambam, *Moreh* 3:27 states that Deuteronomy 6:24 teaches that the commandments enable man to live in peace in an ordered society. see *Genesis Rabbah* 44:1; *Perush ha-Mishnayot, Pe'ah* 1:1; Ramban on Deut 22:7 — the commandment of *shiluah ha-kan; Hinukh* 239.

22. Izenberg, G. *The Existential Critique of Freud: The Crisis in Autonomy,* Princeton: Princeton University Press, 1976; Schultz, D., *A History of Modern Psychology,* New York: Academic Press, 1969, p. 182–211; Chaplin, J. and Krawiec, T., *Systems and Theories of Psychology,* New York: Holt, 1960; Hall, C. and Lindzay, G., *Theories of Personality,* New York: Wiley & Sons, 1970 ed., p. 476.

23. The debate about dropping homosexuality from the Diagnostic Statistical Manual-II and the WHO's own DSM continues with much heat and has obvious implications for the halakhic therapist.

24. Arieti, S., "Psychiatry Controlling Man's Ethical Dimension," *Am. J. Psychiatr.,* 1975, 132(1), p. 39–42 and Greben, S. & Lesset, S., "The Question of Neutrality in Psychotherapy," *Am. J. Psychother.,* 1976, 30(4), p. 623–630.

25. See Weiner, *op. cit.,* 1975. This has been especially stressed by the phenomenological-perceptual schools such as Carl Rogers' Client-Centered Therapy.

26. A. Amsel, *Rational Irrational Man,* New York: Feldheim, 1976, p. 247–253; 9–11.

27. Chessick, R., *The Technique and Practice of Psychotherapy,* New York: J. Aronson, 1974, p. 311–327.

28. Freud, S., *Moses and Monotheism* (1939) and *The Future of an Illusion* (1927).

29. See Shakow, D., "Ethics for a Scientific Age: Some Moral Aspects of Psychoanalysis," *Psychoanal. Rev.*, 1965, 52(3), p. 5-18. Other authors have argued that psychoanalysis has positive values to contribute to the development of morality, such as J. C. Flugel, *Man, Morals and Society*, London, 1955; E. Erikson, *Insight and Responsibility;* New York: Norton, 1964; E. Frenkel-Brunswick, "Contributions to the Analysis and Synthesis of Knowledge," *Proc. Acad. Arts. & Sci.*, 1964, no. 80; H. Hartmann, *Psychoanalysis and Moral Values*, New York: Int. Univ. Press, 1960. On the other hand, a vocal detractor has been O. H. Mowrer, *The Crisis in Psychiatry and Religion*, Princeton: Van Nostrand, 1961.

30. *Avot* 2:6; 2:18; Isaiah 29:13, *Emunot Ve-De'ot* and in the introduction of the *Sefat Emet* quoted in D. Katz, *Tenu'at ha-Mussar*, 1950, I, p. 364.

31. In A. J. Heschel, *A Passion for Truth*, New York: Farrar, Straus & Giroux, 1973, p. 18.

32. Novey, S., "Considerations on Religion in Relation to Psychoanalysis and Psychotherapy," *J. Nerv. Ment. Dis.*, 1960, 130(4), p. 315-324.

33. Novey, S., "Utilization of Social Institutions as a Defense Technique in Neuroses," *Int. J. Psychoanal.*, 1957, 38(1), p. 82-91, p. 90. Cf. comments of P. London in A. Apolito, "Psychoanalysis and Religion," *Am. J. Psychoanal.*, 1970, 30(2), p. 115-123: "As long as the therapist is concerned with happiness, death, security, and the 'meaning of life', he is primarily a moralist and not a scientist; he is replacing the religious ministry more than he is being a physician" (p. 119). See also the discussion following Apolito's essay by A. Franzblau (p. 123-126). Other articles dealing with the positive relationship between religion, psychoanalysis and psychotherapy are: M. H. Spero, "Neurotic Aspects of the Religious Personality: Treatment Considerations, *J. App. Soc. Sci.*, 1976, 1(1), p. 1-18; A. Kaplan, "Maturity in Religion," *Bull. Phila. Assn. Psychoanal.*, 1963, 13, p. 101-119; H. Guntrip, "Religion in Relation to Personal Interaction," *Brit. J. Med. Psychol.*, 1969, 42, p. 323-333; P. Homans, *Theology after Freud: An Interpretive Inquiry*, Indiana: Bobbs-Merrill, 1970 and P. Homans, "Toward a Psychology of Religion by way of Freud and Tillich," *Zygon*, 1967, 2, p. 97-119; H. Meng & E. L. Freud (eds.), *Psychoanalysis and Faith: The Letters of S. Freud and Oskar Pfister*, New York: Basic, 1964.

34. Spero, M. H., "Neurotic Conflict in the Religious Personality: Treatment Consideration," *J. App. Soc. Sci.*, 1976, 1(1), p. 1-18 and see J. Rubins, "Neurotic Attitudes Towards Religion," *Am. J. Psychoanal.*, 1955, 5(1), p. 56-67.

35. See my conclusion in "Man's Evil Nature: A Reinterpretation of the *Yezer ha-Ra*," *Proceedings of the AOJS*, vol. 5.

36. Menninger, K. and Pruyser, P., "Morals, Values and Mental Health," p. 1254 in A. Deutsch and H. Fishman (eds.), *Encyclopedia of Mental Health*, 1963, vol. 4.

37. *Hullin* 10a; *Sukkah* 14b. re: *safek sakanah* see *Berakhot* 3a; *Pesaḥim* 112a; *Hullin* 10a; *Ecclesiastes Rabbah* 3:2; Jerusalem *Berakhot* 4:4; *Shulḥan Arukh Oraḥ Hayyim* 328:10,4; 327:2; *Yoreh De'ah* 116 and see Resp. *Paḥad Yiẓḥak* (I. Lampronti), no. 71.

38. London, P. "Psychotherapy for Religious Neuroses? Comments on Cohen and Smith," *J. Consult. Clin. Psychol.*, 1976, 44(1), p. 146.

39. Cohen, R. and Smith, F., "Socially Reinforced Obsessing: Etiology of a Disorder in a Christian Scientist," *J. Consult. Clin. Psychol.*, 1976, 44(1), p. 142-144.

40. Halleck, S., "Discussion," *ibid.*, p. 147.

41. See Spero, *op. cit.*, 1976 and Menninger and Pruyser, *op. cit.*, 1963.

42. Amsel, *op. cit.*, 1976.

43. E.g., H. B. Lewis, *Shame and Guilt in Neurosis,* New York: Int. Univ. Press, 1971 and Menninger and Pruyser, *op. cit.*, 1963.

44. Ellis, A., *Humanistic Psychology,* New York: McGraw-Hill, 1973, p. 1–18 and see also Ellis' "The Case Against Religion: A Psychotherapist's View," *Mensa Bulletin,* 1970, 28, p. 5–6. see also "Rational Emotive Therapy," p. 49–76 in C. Patterson, *Theories of Counseling and Psychotherapy,* New York: Harper & Row, 1973.

45. S. Freud, *Civilization and its Discontents,* London: Hogarth, 1930.

46. R. May, *Existence,* New York: Clarion, 1958, p. 50–55; G. Condrau and M. Boss, "Existential Analysis," p. 488–519 in J. Howells (ed.), *Modern Perspectives in World Psychiatry,* New York: Bruner/Mazel, 1871 — see their discussion of guilt and their concept of the experience of "debt to existence" — also, "Frankl's Logotherapy," p. 428–456 in Patterson, *op. cit.*, 1973.

47. Spero, M. H., "Anxiety and Religious Growth: A Talmudic Perspective," *J. Relig. Heal.,* 1977, 16(1), p. 52–57.

48. Rambam, *The Preservation of Youth: Essays on Health,* H. L. Gordon (Trans.), New York: Philosophical Library, 1958, p. 66–67.

49. *Hilkhot Teshuvah* 1:2.

50. Psalms 51:5; *Berakhot* 7a (see Rashi *loc. cit*); *Ta'anit* 15a; *Berakhot* 12b; see also the Maharal, *Netiv Teshuvah,* intro. to Chapter 5.

51. *Shabbat* 153a.

52. *Avot* 2:18; *Zohar* 202a (Goldman, Warshaw 1878); *Gittin* 70b.

53. *Yoma* 86b; *Eruvin* 19a.

54. See my discussion of the philosophical relevance of this existential emotion in "Religious Anxiety, the Experience of God and the Ontological Argument", *Judaism,* 1977, 26 (2). See also Hiltner, S. and Menninger, K., *Constructive Aspects of Anxiety,* New York: Abingdon, 1963.

55. (S. Y. Agnon, *Days of Awe,* New York: Schocken, 1948, p. 207). Cf. *Orot ha-Teshuvah,* 3, where Rav Kook refers to a general repentence — a kind of deep shame, a sense of God's absence, a vague apprehension of threat to one's being — which should be compared with Rollo May's definition of existential anxiety (*The Meaning of Anxiety,* New York: Roland, 1950, p. 51, 191).

56. Waldman, R., "The Sin-Neurosis Complex: Perspectives in Religion and Psychiatry", *Psychoanal. Rev.,* 1970, 57(1), p. 143–152. see also Rabbi J. B. Soloveichik's discussion of similarities between sin and (mental) illness in *Al Ha-Teshuvah,* P. Peli (ed.), Israel: Torah Education Department of the WZO, 1975, p. 108–110.

57. *Sotah* 3a; (sin confuses, *metamtemet,* the heart of man — *Yoma* 39a); *Avot* 4:28; Proverbs 16:5.

58. *Sotah* 4b, 5a; *Ecclesiastes Rabbah* 4:18; in the *Kunteres Aharon* of the *Hazon Ish* (no. 94–95) we find, "There is no difference between the sinful and the mentally ill in our reacting towards them with understanding" (i.e., with the therapeutic goal of imparting insight). see also E. Fromm, *Psychoanalysis and Religion,* New Haven, 1958, last chapter. Other allusions to sin: illness are Psalms 103:1–4 and Isaiah 6:10; 57:19.

59. Midrash on Psalms 16:2.

60. See notes 57 and 58 and my essay "The Aveirah Syndrome", *Jewish Observer,* 1973, 9(1), p. 18–21.

61. For further discussion of this important issue, see E. Becker, *The Denial of Death,* New York: Free Press, 1974 (last chapters deal with the possibility of psychotherapy as a way of life); J. McFadden, "Psychology and Unbelief,"

Religious Education, 1969, 6, p. 491–498 (talks of man's increasing incapacity to sustain the tension of religious belief); O. Rank, *Psychology and the Soul,* New York: Barnes, 1950 (Rank's landmark exposition on man's spiritual strivings and psychology's role in accepting same); J. Masserman, "The Biodynamic Approaches" in S. Arieti, *Am. Hand. Psychiatr.* 1964: vol. 2. (Masserman's notion of the three, universal "Ur-defenses" by which man defends himself against reality, one of which is man's belief in his immortality and in the omnipotence of various authority figures, supported by the institution of religion); compare the foregoing with an excellent essay by R. Hoehn-Saric, "Transcendence and Psychotherapy," *Am. J. Psychother.* 1974, 28(2), p. 252–264 (notes the differences between psychotherapy's domain and man's transcendental goals, yet advocates that for those individuals who have no foundation with which to meet the current psychic requirements for living, psychotherapy can aid religion or work in its place).

14
Drugs:
A Jewish View

MENACHEM M. BRAYER

The use of mind-affecting drugs is not a new phenomenon. Throughout history, men have taken drugs to evade reality or to stimulate religious experience. American Indians used peyote as part of their worship, and the Mexicans ate mushrooms. The Moslems — hashish, the Zoroastrians — haoma; the list is endless. The opium of the Orientals is already mentioned in the Jerusalem Talmud and by Maimonides.

These drugs are not narcotics, tranquilizers or energizers. They are known as consciousness-expanding, altering perspective and perception in new dimensions of experience. By far, the most controversial among them in terms of its effect on the individual's psyche and personality is LSD, on which this paper will focus.

Lysergic Acid Diethalamide was first discovered by Dr. Albert Hoffman in 1938. Publicized by Timothy Leary as the utopian hope by which he wants "to turn on the whole world," its use has spread from the breeding grounds of the avant-garde to college campuses all over the country. Approximately 5 percent of the nation's college youth have taken LSD at least once; evidence shows that the age of its users is dropping.

Dr. Donald B. Louria, a Cornell medical professor and head of the infectious disease laboratory at Bellevue, reports that 130 persons with LSD-induced psychoses have been admitted in the last eighteen months.

He has attested to the fact that effects of the drug hallucinations may reappear weeks later under stress, and that a single dose is sufficient to cause permanent personality changes.[1] Many of those hospitalized suffered from strong terror and others exhibited homicidal or suicidal tendencies. Its potency and the dangers of taking an overdose are dramatic: a single ounce is enough of a dosage for 300,000 people. The average dosage of 200 micrograms, synthesized easily by any chemistry student, is available in the

Reprinted from *Tradition* (Summer, 1968). Copyright © 1968 by the Rabbinical Council of America.

Greenwich Village area for a few dollars. Dr. Louria is perhaps the most outspoken advocate of strict curbs and severe penalties for LSD users.[2] The question is not alcohol or marijuana, but "whether we should add to our alcohol burden another intoxicant."

On the other hand, its adherents claim for LSD the ability to expand consciousness, transport the user to primal dream-like conditions, increase depth-introspection and allow the experience of one's inner world.[3] There is a sense of transcending time and space. In short, its effects seem to reproduce the experience of mystics. Thus, even attainment of genuine religious experience has been ascribed to it.[4]

This paper will attempt to evaluate the personality changes claimed for the drug from a psychological viewpoint, and the validity of religious claims from the *weltanshauung* of Halakhah and Jewish thought. Finally, perhaps an insight will be gained as to what the contemporary generation of youth is seeking from these drugs, and why they are being driven in this direction.

The Adolescent Personality

Sociologists claim that there are three socially-developed guides for the individual's behavior: Tradition-directed, inner-directed, and other-directed. In the American setting, other-orientation seems to be the dominant pattern. One is judged by the group in terms of how well he conforms to the group norms. The group most dominant in determining our behavior is called the reference group, and our self-image is developed in terms of its values.[5]

Other-directedness is in consonance with Jewish teaching, at least as a partial determinant of one's behavior. *Ru'ah ha-beriyot* is equated with *ru'ah ha-makom;* social acceptance is a correlative to Divine approval.[6] In Hasidism,[7] the precept of *ahavat Yisra'el* (Love of Israel) is equivalent to the command of *ahavat ha-shem* (Love of God).

Most personality characteristics of adolescents show substantial relationships to social acceptability. Since they are striving to find their place in society, there are great fluctuations in their values. Eventually, the adolescent will be freed from the strictures of parental control and will stabilize his other-directedness, but such processes of growth should be consummated gradually.

Adolescence is also a period of great emotional hunger. Not always is this hunger for familial approval, peer acceptance, and heterosexual popularity based on a real lack of gratification in life. In addition to the psychological suffering of the youth in his autoplastic adjustment, or changing of the self, he must contend with the change of his environment simultaneously.

In the words of Anna Freud, "Adolescence is by definition an interruption of peaceful growth. The adolescent manifestations come close to symptom formation of the neurotic, the psychotic, or dissocial order and verge almost imperceptibly into borderline states and initial, frustrated or fully fledged forms of almost all the mental illnesses. . . . Such fluctuations between extreme opposites would be deemed highly abnormal at any other time of life. At this time they may signify no more than that an adult structure of personality takes a long time to emerge, that the ego of the individual in question does not cease to experiment and is in no hurry to close down on possibilities."[8] It is for this reason that psychoanalysts dubbed adolescence "the schizophrenic age."[9] Thus, the normal adolescent who takes these drugs as a false anaesthesia from fear or doubt in a perennial search for himself is also liable to the effects the drug has on the mentally deranged.

In a study entitled "Motivational Patterns in LSD Usage," the types of users are differentiated.[10] So far as it is used by neurotics, LSD was found to have a cathartic effect similar to that achieved in conventional psychotherapy, albeit in a fraction of the time.

Psychotics, on the other hand, who self-treated themselves in a desperate attempt to "break through," were usually left in a more chaotic mental state than before. "Such 'cases' would never be given LSD . . . [by doctors] . . . [but] would be provided with close therapeutic support of a *realistic* sort. . . ."[11]

We should not categorically oppose supervised experimentation with this drug. The American Psychiatric Association's report of August 1966 states that "there is sufficient information to justify continuing research of its possible values." Masters and Houston write that "LSD is exactly like atomic energy. It has enormous potential for good or evil. Right now we are just seeing the mental Hiroshimas . . . the value of the drug is not the drug itself but how the insights are implemented in one's daily life."[12]

Granted, then, that LSD has potential in certain areas of psychological imbalance. However, the adolescent who takes it does so from a different motivation, for the "neurotic" in him is unrecognized by the subject. In actuality, the adolescent user often develops into a Dostoevskian "underground man," whose vision of the future contains radically new relationships between the individual and society.[13]

In a society as impersonal and tension-charged as ours, where the sense of identity is lacking, and belonging is replaced by emotional insecurity, man finds himself tragically lonely. The adolescent student, more than others, is beset by a deep sense of unbearable isolation.[13a] Escape mechanisms of all sorts are therefore employed to defend one's ego from the devastating dangers to which he is so critically exposed. Instead of seeking his Ego-ideal in the real world, the *olam ha-asiyah,* the search is carried on in distortion. The colorama viewer who claims he is undergoing a voluntary psychoanalysis is deluding himself. His claim that he has "found himself" is true only to the extent that he has seen but a minute part of his potential, in unreal circumstances. Says Dr. Louria, "Those who frequently use the drug almost inevitably withdraw from society and enter into a solipsistic, negativistic existence, in which LSD is not merely an experience in the totality of living, but rather becomes synonomous with life itself."[14]

The "Real" in Judaism

An offense, even when committed without conscious knowledge, is considered by the rabbis to be a "bad symptom."[15] It is an indication of mental weakness and moral disequilibrium. Thus, the rabbis said, "Sinful thoughts are more severe than the sinful act itself,"[16] for the thoughts are indicative of a blemished personality. This, too, is the impact of the Talmudic comment that man sins only when possessed by a *ru'aḥ shtut* (spirit of folly).

We know from clinical practice that neurotic demands are usually selfish desires. These cravings, outcroppings of the neurosis, are unconscious reactions. Our rabbis envisioned sin much as the psychoanalyst views the neurotic; both the sin and the neurotic act are evidence of internal conflict.

The hallucinatory state of mind, where one's actions lack control and conscious awareness, may be the same as the lapse into neurotic or sinful behavior. Not only are the acts committed under drug influence mirrors of the user's subconscious, but taking the drugs itself is a lapse into infantile, socially-unacceptable behavior. The attempt to escape reality is in itself neurotic.

We thus can see that, discounting the possible neurotic and psychotic effects on the student user, the normal youthful motivation is in itself contrary to Jewish thought. For Judaism the real is the world of creation in all its diversity, and man's role in it is to act as a partner in hallowing all of its aspects. If the state of the world is depressing, "neither are you free to set yourself apart from it." If social institutions such as marriage and family have disintegrated, the Jewish answer is not their abandonment. The salvation of man is dependent on his capability to raise up *his* world, not on his ability to raise himself out of it.

Some claim that the drug experience gives the user character traits that will be useful upon his return to normal consciousness. The fact that one has increased sensitivity while under drug influence would not justify their use unless this sensitivity extended into the *olam ha-asiyah*. (This eliminates from our consideration all those who use LSD for aesthetic or hedonistic reasons alone. Regarding this claim, there is no evidence available in current research.)

On the contrary, it has been pointed out that the Indians of the Southwest and Mexico who make extensive use of hallucinogens have passive, stagnant cultures. In an important series of experiments, the authors report that "These drugs attack some of the deepest values of our culture — competition, material achievement, striving, . . . social responsibility. . . ."[17]

As mentioned above, the only recurrent traits in the drug seem to be their negative effects, as pointed out by Dr. Louria. His evidence of an adverse "pleasure-to-risk ratio" should be considered halakhically. Self-injury — ha-hovel be-azmo — is clearly prohibited. This principle was codified by Maimonides who states that "man is forbidden to inflict injury upon himself or upon others . . ."[18] in addition to the halakhic consideration of hamira sekanta me'issura, involving not only individual but collective injury.[19]

In fact, causing fright and emotional stress to others even without concrete damage is an offense which, though exempt from the judgments of man, makes one liable be-dinei shamayim (judgment of God).[20]

It may also be stated that enticing one into the use of psychedelics entails also the issur of ve-lifne iver lo titen mikhshol[21] — placing a stumbling block before the inexperienced and naive. Violation of such an ethical precept involves a large variety of moral principles bordering on wrong counsel and ill advice, which are an expression of human callousness and disrespect for our fellowmen. Maimonides in his Regimen Sanitatis reiterates "the deep concern of the Torah for the mental welfare of the Israelites, whether they be sinful or righteous." In many of his medical works, he stresses "the importance of mental health, the improvement of behavior which is the cure of the mind and its faculties," stating repeatedly "how dangerous it is to indulge in medicine, tranquilizers, sedatives or stimulants and becoming habituated to them."[22]

Many of the rabbinic regulations concerning the "better adjustment of society" point to the fact that damage or injury perpetrated on a rabbim, involving a group, is considered a more serious offense, hezeika de-rabbim, than any other injury concerning the individual. In this sense we can consider the hallucinogenic craze as an hezeika de-rabbim, a hazard for the entire community, and a direct threat to organized society.[23] New bio-medical evidence points to the genetic damage caused by LSD to the chromosomes, which according to Dr. Maimon Cohen of the State University School of Medicine, could lead to mental retardation and physical abnormalities in the offsprings of LSD users as shown in a number of maternity cases.

Traditionally viewed, then, taking psychedelic drugs and exposing oneself to a "bad trip" with all the possible psychotic repercussions would be considered a transgression of the positive commandment for man's welfare in the Torah, ve-nishmartem me'od le-nafshoteikhem (taking protective measures to guard one's health), committing an act of *ḥavallah be-aẓmo* (self-damage) and hampering his homeostasis and mental balance from performing the Divine way of life properly.

Religious Experiences

Not a few "trippies" have reported on the similarity of their experiences to the reports of religious mystics and quite a few papers have discussed the drug's religious implications.

From our point of view we must address ourselves to several questions. Is the mystical experience in general a religious experience, synonomous with Jewish religious experience, or is it even a legitimate part of Jewish living?

On the first question, opinion seems to be divided. Walter Pahnke, a psychologist and theologian, writes, ". . . all mystical experience is not necessarily religious. If one makes the concept of a 'personal God' central to the definition of religion, many forms of mystical experience could not be considered religious. The phenomena of mystical experience may occur outside the framework of any formal religion. . . . Whether or not mystical experience is religious depends upon one's definition of religion. . . ."[24]

Gershom Scholem is of another opinion: ". . . there is no such thing as mysticism in the abstract . . . which has no particular religious system. . . . But only in our days has the belief gained ground that there is such a thing as an abstract mystical religion."[25]

If one keeps in mind that Scholem's analysis is chiefly historical, while Pahnke speaks from the results of experimental data, the contradiction may resolve itself. Historically, mystics were people deeply concerned with their particular religions who integrated the experience into their philosophy or theosophy of religion. Nonetheless, one can readily see certain psychological phenomena which are common to all religious mystics, which Scholem readily affirms. From Dr. Pahnke's evidence, it would seem that LSD has the ability to duplicate the psychological phenomena of unity, ego-transcendence and the noetic feeling described by James, in a person who has no conscious religious life. Hence, the severing of the mystical from the religious. From the point of view of religion, it is a counterfeit experience.

In Buber's criticism of Aldous Huxley's counsel to the use of mescaline as a means to acquire mystical insight, he states: "Man may master as he will his situation . . . he may alter it, exchange it for another, but the fugitive flight out of the claim of the situation into situationless-ness is no legitimate affair of man. And the true name of all paradises which man creates for himself by chemical or other means is situationlessness . . . It is a flight from the authentic spokenness of speech in whose realm a response is demanded, and response is responsibility."[26]

We spoke before of man's place in the world of reality. Mystical experience is no doubt a part of Judaism, and it may be the *summum bonum* of religious experience, but it must arise from the involvement of man in the *real* world and it must enable him to return to it. It is the final rung on a ladder whose legs are resting on the ground. One doesn't fly to the top; one climbs.

Religious experience in its true sense is from within. It is the fervor of the soul — the divine spark — to unite itself with the eternal flame. Such mystic fervor which one sees in the ḥasidic ecstasy aroused by *tefillah* (prayer) — a sound, healthy revelation is the encounter of the purified soul with the Holy — can hardly be compared to a drug experience. On the one hand, the experience is the climax of *hirhur teshuvah* (thinking of repentance) and *ḥeshbon ha-nefesh* (self-analysis). In the latter case, it is the experience of a person lacking discipline. In the former, it is the result of a total orientation of the self toward accepting a certain mode of life. In the hippie, it is the result of a haphazard attempt to escape the reality of a purposeless existence. Into what frame of reference can the hippie channel this ambiguous feeling?

Contemporary youth is lacking in stability and orientation towards an ethico-religious code of values. They must be taught that religion wants man to play a role in society — *hamakir et mekomo* (knowing one's place). If there is a self-accepted discipline of a *torat ḥayyim,* repression is never necessary. They must also learn that healthy, interpersonal behavior, which senses affection and acceptance, is another genuine expression of one's real self.

A key word among the hippies is "love" — a deficiency they severely feel. Ḥasidim tell of a father who complained to the Ba'al Shem that his son had forsaken God. "What, Rebbe, shall I do?" "Love him more than ever" was the Ba'al Shem's reply.[27] Aside from showing then that love in all its forms is a cornerstone of Judaism, parents must actively provide love and security to their children in this age-period of upheaval and adjustment.

We must not evade responsibility and mature growth, nor fear reality and escape into a chemically-induced transcendentalism, but we must accept and master our *olam ha-zeh* — this world. In his anguished cry for identity, purposefulness, and self-discovery from the refrigerating alienation and depersonalization, man must "turn on" his inner resources and redirect from subliminally towards a more affiliative, symbiotic and sociable personality. By rechanneling his psychic "economy" towards self-improvement, better inter-personal relations, and a sincere human understanding, man can rediscover his true Self.

Experiences in self-discipline, which correct the baseness of orgiastic passions and represent impulses, fortify the mind with enlightened and useful knowledge and bring in their wake inner serenity and hopeful existence. Knowing that fellow men will comprehend affliction because an omniscient God understands human frailties and suffering, moves man to heights of spiritual elevation and closer encounter with his Maker. In this way, man can become a co-worker with God, and achieve integration and spiritual redemption.

NOTES

1. Donald B. Louria, in "Therapeutic Notes," Parke, Davis & Co.

2. Donald B. Louria, "The Abuse of LSD," *LSD, Man & Society,* ed. De Bold and Leaf (Wesleyan U. Press: 1967), p. 3ff.

3. R. E. L. Masters and Jean Houston, *The Varieties of Psychedelic Experience* (New York: Holt, Rinehart and Winston, 1966).

4. Walter N. Pahnke and W. A. Richards, "Implications of LSD and Experimental Mysticism," *Journal of Religion and Health,* V, no. 3 (1966). Also R. C. Zaehner, *Mysticism: Sacred and Profane* (New York: Galaxie Books, 1961).

5. Earl H. Bell and Sir John Sirjamaki, *Social Foundations of Human Behavior* (New York: Harper and Row, 1965), p. 272.

6. *Avot* 3:13. Compare Malachi 3:16 and *Sukkah* 49b, Numbers *Rabbah II, Sifrei Zuta Naso* 22; in Latin, *Vox populi vox Dei. Yalkut Shimoni Naso* 711.

7. "By Reb A. J. Heschel of Apt," from *Ms. on Rijn and Sadagora,* in the family archives of the Boyaner Rebbe, (M. S. Friedman).

8. Freud, Anna, "Adolescence," *Psychoanalytic Study of the Child,* Vol. XIII, New York, International University Press, (1958).

9. Sandor Lorand and Henry Schneer, *eds., Adolescents, Psychoanalytic Approach to Problems and Therapy,* (New York, P. B. Hoeber, Inc. 1961).

10. Frank Barron, in LSD, *Man and Society,* p. 12.

11. *Ibid.*

12. *Varieties.*

13. Barron, p. 14.

13a. Kurt-Lewin, *A Dynamic Theory of Personality,* 1935, also Bringing Up the Jewish Child, *The Menorah Journal,* vol. 28 (1940).

14. "The Abuse of LSD," p. 41.

15. *Ḥagigah,* 5a. Compare *Bava Meẓia* 33b, *Ḥullin* 15a (*kansinan shogeg atu mezid*), *Bava Kamma* 32b.

16. *Sotah* 3a.

17. John C. Pollard, L. Uhr, and B. Stern, *Drugs and Fantasy* (Boston: Little, Brown and Co., 1965), p. 203.

18. *Mishnah, Bava Kamma,* VII, 8, Maimonides, Code, *Hilkhot Ḥovel u-Mazik,* 5:1; *Ibid. Hilkhot Shavuot,* 5:17; *Semag, Lavin* 70, 238.

19. *Ḥullin* 10a, *Sukkah* 14b. Maimonides warns sternly against experimenting with drugs, see *Pirkei Moshe,* Chapters 17 and 21. Compare *Ecclesiastes Rabbah* 3 and *Shulḥan Arukh, Oraḥ Ḥayyim,* 328:10.

20. See *Bava Kamma* 56a, Maimonides, Code, *Hilkhot Ḥovel u-Mazik* 5:9 and infer *a fortiori* for *nizkei nefesh.*

21. Leviticus 10:13, See *Semag, Lavin* 168 based on *Sifra, ad loc., Pesaḥim* 22b. and *Zohar Kedoshim* 85a. Compare Deuteronomy 27:18 Rashi *ad loc.*

22. Maimonides, *Pirkei Moshe,* 8; see also *Eight Chapters,* 1.

23. *Bava Batra* 2b and 59b, *Kiddushin* 39b. Compare *Mo'ed Katan* 13a, *Sanhedrin* 72a, *Hullin* 142a, where man is always considered *mu'ad* even *be-shogeg*. See also *Zohar Bereshit* 111a.

24. Walter N. Pahnke, "LSD and Religious Experience," *LSD, Man and Society*, p. 68.

25. Gershom G. Scholem, *Major Trends in Jewish Mysticism* (New York: Schocken Books, 1946), pp. 5–6.

26. Martin Buber, *The Knowledge of Man* (New York: Harper and Row, 1966).

27. *Siyah Sarfei Kodesh* (Lodz: 1929), III. p. 147.

Death and Dying

15

The Jewish Attitude Toward Euthanasia

FRED ROSNER

The word euthanasia is derived from the Greek "eu" meaning well, good, or pleasant and "thanatos" meaning death. Webster's dictionary defines euthanasia as the mode or act of inducing death painlessly or as a relief from pain. The popular expression for euthanasia is mercy killing. Perusal of the medical literature of the last two decades reveals a host of books,[1-3] articles,[4-33] editorials,[34-38] and letters to editors of journals[39-41] dealing with this subject. This is exclusive of the legal, theologic, psychologic, and social literatures. Even the lay press is replete with writings on euthanasia[42] dating back to February, 1873, when both the *Fortnightly Review* and the *Spectator* carried feature articles on the subject.[8] A recent lead article in the *Times* of London on the acquittals of parents, relatives, and a physician charged with murdering a thalidomide-damaged child raised such interest from readers that 42 of the numerous letters written to the *Times* in response to the article were published in a subsequent issue.[40]

There is thus little doubt as to the tremendous interest in euthanasia today. The present report is an attempt to review briefly the subject of euthanasia by providing classification and terminology, citing selected examples, describing the legal attitude toward euthanasia in various countries, discussing the arguments put forth for and against euthanasia, briefly mentioning the Catholic and Protestant viewpoints on euthanasia, and finally presenting in detail the Jewish attitude toward euthanasia.

Classification and terminology

As already stated, euthanasia is popularly spoken of as "mercy killing." A less painful term used by euthanasia societies is "merciful release"[32] or "liberating euthanasia."[24] Some people classify euthanasia into three types: eugenic, medical, and preventive.[24, 28] A more meaningful

Reprinted from the *New York State Journal of Medicine* (vol. 67, September 1967). Copyright © 1967 by the Medical Society of the State of New York.

classification speaks of eugenic, active medical, and passive medical euthanasia.[32] Eugenic euthanasia would encompass the "merciful release" of birth monsters and socially undesirable individuals such as the mentally retarded and psychiatrically disturbed. Perhaps an extreme example of this method of extermination was the Nazi killing of all the socially unacceptable or socially unfit. To many, this German practice as well as all eugenic euthanasia is considered nothing less than murder, and thus there are very few proponents of this type of euthanasia.

Active medical euthanasia is exemplified by the case where a drug or other treatment is administered, and death is thereby hastened. This type of euthanasia may be voluntary or involuntary, that is, with or without the patient's consent.

Passive medical euthanasia is defined as the situation in which therapy is withheld so that death is hastened by omission of treatment. This type of euthanasia has also been called automathanasia[30] meaning automatic death, such as without therapeutic heroics. This passive form of euthanasia can also be voluntary or involuntary.

A new term, antidysthanasia, has been put forth by one of the most outspoken proponents of euthanasia in this country, the Anglican minister Joseph Fletcher.[43] This new word seems only to add to the confusion.

Exemplification of the problem

Many a physician has had to wrestle with the problem of an incurably ill, suffering patient. Such physicians fully realize that "whereas life is lengthened, man's period of usefulness is not always lengthened."[25] Some are of the opinion that advanced medicine should "serve only to improve the condition of human life as it increases the life span and not the useless prolongation of human suffering."[25] Thus, on December 4, 1949, H. N. Sander, M.D., a general practitioner in Manchester, New Hampshire, ended a cancer patient's suffering by injecting into the patient a substantial quantity of air intravenously. He was acquitted.[24] On March 9, 1950, Miss C. A. Paight of Stamford, Connecticut, shot and killed her father who was dying of incurable cancer. She was acquitted.[24]

The problem is far from localized to the shores of the United States. In December, 1961, Giuseppe Faita, having settled in France, was struck with an incurable disease. He summoned his brother Luigi and convinced the latter to kill him, which Luigi did. The jury acquitted Luigi.[27]

One of the most famous instances exemplifying many of the problems surrounding euthanasia is the case of Maurice Millard, M.D., son of the founder of the British Euthanasia Society. Dr. Millard told a Rotary meeting: "To keep her from pain . . . I gave her an injection to make her sleep."[25] His objective as specifically stated was to relieve pain, not to put an end to the patient's life. An outcry in the British press followed, labeling the incident "a mercy killing." Even the British Euthanasia Society admitted that from a strictly legal sense mercy killing is murder, but it backed Dr. Millard by insisting that "every doctor must be guided by his own conscience." Many physicians disagreed, saying euthanasia is only legalized murder. Others cited the Hippocratic oath which states: "I will give no deadly medicine to anyone if asked, nor suggest any such counsel." Still others were of the opinion that the Hippocratic oath refers only to premeditated murder. The medical council refused to act against Dr. Millard unless the family of the deceased lodged a formal complaint. However, the family consented to Dr. Millard's actions. Thus, all the ingredients to emphasize the problem of euthanasia are present in this case: the incurable patient in great pain, the request for euthanasia by patient and family, and the physician's acquiescence and participation.

The list of examples one could cite is endless. The aforementioned illustrative cases serve as background for the ensuing discussion.

Legal attitude

Although suicide is not legally a crime in most American jurisdictions, aiding and abetting suicide is a felony.[16] Euthanasia in the United States, even at the patient's request, is legally murder. In England the Suicide Act enacted into law in 1961 states that it is no longer a criminal offense for a person, whether in sickness or in health, to take his own life or to attempt to do so. However, any individual who helps him to do so becomes liable to a charge of manslaughter.[44] Euthanasia per se does not exist in the law books of France and Belgium, and in both countries it is considered premeditated homicide.[27,28,30] However, a bill to legalize euthanasia for some "damaged" children came before the Belgian government on November 26, 1962, following the famous *Liège* trial involving parents, relatives, and a physician charged with murdering a thalidomide-damaged child.[40]

In Italy, euthanasia is only a crime if the victim is under eighteen years of age, mentally retarded, or menaced or under the effect of fear.[28] More tolerant attitudes also exist in Denmark, Holland, Yugoslavia, and even Catholic Spain.[28] In Russia, euthanasia is considered "murder under extenuating circumstances" and punishable with three to eight years in prison.[24] Switzerland seems to have the most lenient legislation.[28] The Swiss penal code was revamped in 1951 and distinguishes between killing with bad intentions, that is, murder, and killing with good intentions, that is, euthanasia.[24] In addition, in 1964 in Sweden, passive euthanasia was legalized.[45]

Even in the countries where euthanasia is legally murder, "the sympathies of juries towards mercy killings often cause the law to be circumvented by various methods, making for great inequities of the legal system.''[16] In the several sample cases cited here, the defendants were all acquitted. Although judges and juries are usually very lenient, a recent case of euthanasia is described from Perth, Australia, in which the death penalty was imposed.[30]

In 1935 the first Euthanasia Society was founded in England by C. Killick Millard, M.D., for the purpose of promoting legislation which would seek to ''make the act of dying more gentle.''[44] In 1936, one year after the founding of the Society, a bill was introduced into the House of Lords which sought to permit voluntary euthanasia in certain circumstances and with certain safeguards. Following a rather heated debate, it was decided that ''in view of the emergence of so many controversial issues, it would be best to leave the matter for the time being to the discretion of individual medical men . . . the bill was rejected by 35 votes to 14.''[44] The Euthanasia Society of England is quite active today under the presidency of the Earl of Listowel and the chairmanship of Leonard Colebrook, M.D., and its goal is to see implemented a ''Plan for Voluntary Euthanasia which would permit an adult person of sound mind, whose life is ending with much suffering to choose between an easy death and a hard one; and to obtain medical aid in implementing that choice.''[44]

In 1938, three years after the inception of the British group, the Euthanasia Society of America, Inc., was founded by Charles Frances Potter. This nonsectarian, voluntary organization currently presided over by Rev. Donald W. McKinney, rather than seeking to have legislation enacted to legalize euthanasia, is attempting to achieve a more enlightened public understanding of euthanasia through dissemination of information. This goal is being strived for through discussions of euthanasia in medical societies and other professional groups, research studies and opinion polls, dissemination of literature, a speaker's bureau, and other responsible media of communication.[46]

Other euthanasia societies have cropped up in Sweden and Japan. Support for these societies and their work comes from various other groups such as the American Humanist Association and the Ethical Culture Society.[45] Opposition to euthanasia is also strong, however. Thus, the Academy of Moral and Political Sciences of Paris voted on a motion completely outlawing, forbidding, and rejecting euthanasia in all its forms.[24] In addition, the Council of the World Medical Association, meeting in Copenhagen in April, 1950, recommended that the practice of euthanasia be condemned.[1] The debate continues, and some of the arguments presented by proponents and opponents of euthanasia will be presented here.

The problem has been well stated by Filbey[32]: ''When a tortured man asks: 'For God's sake, doctor, let me die, just put me to sleep,' we have yet to find the answer as to whether to comply is for God's sake, the patient's sake, our own, or possibly all three." Even if the moral issue of euthanasia could be circumvented, other questions of logistics would immediately arise: Who is to initiate euthanasia proceedings? The patient? The family? The physician? Who is to make the final decision? The physician? A group of physicians? The courts? Who is to carry out the decision if it is affirmative? The physician? Others?[26]

Pros and cons

Arguments in favor and against euthanasia are numerous, have and continue to be heatedly debated in many circles, and will be only briefly summarized here.

Opponents of euthanasia say that if voluntary, it is suicide. Although by British law suicide is no longer a crime,[44] Christian and Jewish religious teachings certainly outlaw suicide. The answer offered to this argument is that martyrdom, a form of suicide, is condoned under certain conditions. However, the martyr seeks not to end his life primarily but to accomplish a goal, death being an undesired side product. Thus, martyrdom and suicide do not seem comparable.

It is also said that euthanasia, if voluntary, is murder. As one writer so aptly put it: "Euthanasia must be defined within the knife's edge area between suicide and murder."[29] Murder, however, usually connotes premeditated evil. The motives of the person administering euthanasia are far from evil. On the contrary, such motives are commendable and praiseworthy, although the methods may be unacceptable.

A closely related objection to euthanasia says that it transgresses the Biblical injunction "Thou shalt not kill." To overcome this argument, some modern Biblical translators substitute "Thou shalt not commit murder" and, as just mentioned, murder usually represents "violent killing for purposes of gain, or treachery or vendetta"[44] and is totally dissimilar to the "merciful release" of euthanasia.

That God alone gives and takes life as it is written in Deuteronomy 32:39: "I kill and I make alive" and Ezekiel 18:4: "Behold, all souls are Mine" and that one's life span is divinely predetermined, is not denied by the proponents of euthanasia. The difficulty with this point, however, seems to be the question of definition as to whether euthanasia represents shortening of life or shortening of the act of dying.

To complete the religious argumentation, it is said that suffering is part of the divine plan with which man has no right to tamper. This phase of faith remains a mystery and is best exemplified by the story of Job.

It is further argued by opponents to euthanasia that since physicians are only human beings, they are liable to error. There is no infallibility in a physician's diagnosis of an incurably ill patient, and mistakes have been made. Rabinowitch and MacDermot,[7] in an address on the subject of euthanasia delivered before the Medical Undergraduates Society of McGill University on March 21, 1950, quote Rabinowitch's own case. Eighteen years earlier a diagnosis of carcinoma of the esophagus had been made, yet Dr. Rabinowitch was very much alive when he spoke at McGill University eighteen years later. Such mistaken diagnoses are exceedingly rare, but they do occur. The same is true of spontaneous remission of cancer: It has been reported, but only in very rare instances.

The need for euthanasia today is minimized by some because the availability of hypnotics, narcotics, anesthetics, and other analgesic means is sufficient to keep any patient's pain and distress at a tolerable level. This fact, in general, may be true, but occassional patients develop severe pain which is refractory to all drugs and requires surgical interruption of the nerve pathways for relief.

The Hippocratic oath or a similar vow which all physicians swear to on graduation from medical school is conflicting. On the one hand, it states that a physician's duty is to relieve suffering yet, on the other hand, it also states that the physician must preserve and protect life. This oath is used as an argument by both proponents and opponents of euthanasia.

A very valid point of debate is the suggestion that if euthanasia for incurably ill, suffering cancer patients were legalized, then extension of such legislation to the grossly deformed, psychotic, or senile patients might follow. A recent editorial stated: "If euthanasia is granted to the first class, can it long be denied to the second? . . . Each step is so short; the slope so slippery; our values in this age, so uncertain and unstable . . ."[35]

Further debatable questions are the sincerity of patient and/or family in requesting euthanasia. A patient racked with pain may make an impulsive but ill-considered request for merciful release which he will not be able to retract or regret after the fait accompli. The patient's family may not be completely sincere in its desire to relieve the patient's suffering. The family also wishes to relieve its own suffering.[30] Enemies or heirs of the patient may request hastening of the patient's death for ulterior motives.[1] These and further arguments both for and against euthanasia are discussed at greater length by Fletcher,[1] Sperry,[2] and others.[22, 24]

Ideally, euthanasia should not be necessary if medicine had all the answers to the problems of presently incurable disease. This thesis was well enunciated by a recent writer who stated: "Let us hope that with the advances of medical science, the requests for euthanasia would be few and far between, for each request represents a failure in our present methods of providing adequate relief . . ."[41]

Catholic attitude

The New Testament in at least five places (*Matthew* 5:21, *Matthew* 19:18, *Mark* 10:19, *Luke* 18:20, *Romans* 13:9) contains the Biblical admonition "Thou shalt not kill." Based on this, the attitude of the Catholic Church in this matter is cited as follows:

> . . . The teaching of the Church is unequivocal that God is the supreme master of life and death and that no human being is allowed to usurp His dominion so as deliberately to put an end to life, either his own or any one else's without authorization . . . and the only authorizations the Church recognizes are a nation engaged in war, execution of criminals by a Government, killing in self defense . . . The Church has never allowed and never will allow the killing of individuals on grounds of private expediency; for instance . . . putting an end to prolonged suffering or hopeless sickness . . .[7]

Thus we see a blanket condemnation of active euthanasia by the Catholic Church as murder and, therefore, a mortal sin. The reasons behind this teaching include the inviolability of human life or the supreme dominion of God over His creatures and the purposefulness of human suffering.[22] Man suffers as penance for his sins, perhaps an earthly purgatory; man endures pain for the spiritual good of his fellow man; suffering teaches humility and helps the Catholic identify with his crucified Lord.

Passive medical euthanasia is treated quite differently. The Church distinguishes between "ordinary" and "extraordinary" measures employed by physicians when certain death and suffering lie ahead. In this day of auxiliary hearts, artificial kidneys, respirators, pacemakers, defibrillators, and similar instruments, the definition of "extraordinary" is unclear and nebulous. Pope Pius XII, in the last year of his life, issued an encyclical not requiring physicians to use heroic measures in such circumstances.[27, 29, 33] Thus, passive euthanasia is sanctioned by the Catholic Church. In an address to the congress of Italian anesthetists on February 24, 1957, the Pope further stated: "Even if narcotics may shorten life while they relieve pain, it is permissible."[27]

Protestant attitude

In the Protestant Church there are "all possible colors in the spectrum of attitudes toward euthanasia."[22] Some condemn it, some favor it, and many are in between, advocating judgment of each case individually. Perhaps the greatest Protestant advocate of legalized euthanasia is the Anglican minister Joseph Fletcher. His three main reasons are the following: (1) Suffering is purposeless, demoralizing, and degrading; (2) human personality is of greater worth than life per se; and (3) the phrase "Blessed are the merciful, for they shall obtain mercy" is as important as "Thou shalt not kill."

Jewish attitude

Before tracing the Jewish attitude toward euthanasia through rabbinic sources, it would seem appropriate to cite Biblical references to this matter. In the book of Genesis, 9:6, we find: "Whoso sheddeth man's blood, by man shall his blood be shed . . ." In the second book of the Pentateuch, Exodus 20:13, it is stated: "Thou shalt not murder" and further in the next chapter, Exodus 21:14, is the following sentence: "And if a man come presumptuously upon his neighbor, to slay him with guile: thou shalt take him from Mine altar, that he may die." In Leviticus 24:17, is the phrase "And he that smiteth any man mortally shall surely be put to death" and four sentences later we find again ". . . And he that killeth a man shall be put to death." In the book of Numbers it is stated (35:30): "Whoso killeth any person, the murderer shall be slain at the mouth of witnesses . . ." Finally in Deuteronomy, the sixth commandment of the decalogue is repeated (5:17): "Thou shalt not murder." Thus, in every book of the Pentateuch, we find at least one reference to murder or killing. Accidental death or homicide is dealt with separately in the Bible and represents another subject entirely.

Probably the first recorded instance of euthanasia concerns the death of King Saul in the year 1013 B.C.E. Thus at the end of the first book of Samuel, chapter 31:1-6, we find the following:

> Now the Philistines fought against Israel, and the men of Israel fled from before the Philistines and fell down slain in Mount Gilboa. And the Philistines pursued hard upon Saul and upon his sons; and the Philistines slew Jonathan and Abinadab and Malchishua, the sons of Saul. And the battle went sore against Saul and the archers overtook him and he was greatly afraid by reason of the archers. Then said Saul to his armorbearer: "Draw thy sword, and thrust me through therewith, lest these uncircumcised come and thrust me through and make a mock of me." But his armor-bearer would not; for he was sore afraid. Therefore, Saul took his sword and fell upon it. And when the armor-bearer saw that Saul was dead, he likewise fell upon his sword and died with him. So Saul died and his three sons, and his armorbearer, and all his men, that same day together.

From this passage it would appear as if Saul committed suicide. However, at the beginning of the second book of Samuel when David is informed of Saul's death, we find the following (chapter 1:5-10):

And David said unto the young man that told him: "How knowest thou that Saul and Jonathan his son are dead?" And the young man that told him said: "As I happened by chance upon Mount Gilboa, behold Saul leaned upon his spear; and lo, the chariots and the horsemen pressed hard upon him. And when he looked behind him, he saw me, and called unto me. And I answered: Here am I. And he said unto me: Who art thou? And I answered him: I am an Amalekite. And he said unto me: Stand, I pray thee, beside me, and slay me, for the agony hath taken hold of me; because my life is just yet in me. So I stood beside him, and slew him, because I was sure that he would not live after that he was fallen. . . ."

Many commentators consider this a case of euthanasia. Radak specifically states that Saul did not die immediately on falling on his sword but was mortally wounded and in his death throes asked the Amalekite to hasten his death. Ralbag and Rashi also support this viewpoint, as does *Meẓudat David*. Some modern scholars think that the story of the Amalekite was a complete fabrication.

The Mishnah states as follows (*Semaḥot* 1:1): "One who is in a dying condition (*goses*) is regarded as a living person in all respects." This rule is reiterated by later codifiers of Jewish law including Maimonides and Caro as described below. The Mishnah continues (*Semaḥot* 1:2 to 4):

One may not bind his jaws, nor stop up his openings, nor place a metallic vessel or any cooling object on his navel until such time that he dies as it is written (Ecclesiastes 12:6): "Before the silver cord (Midrash interprets this as the spinal cord) is snapped asunder."

One may not move him nor may one place him on sand nor on salt until he dies.

One may not close the eyes of the dying person. He who touches them or moves them is shedding blood because Rabbi Meir used to say: this can be compared to a flickering flame. As soon as a person touches it, it becomes extinguished. So too, whosoever closes the eyes of the dying is considered to have taken his soul.

Other laws pertaining to a *goses* or dying person, such as the preparation of a coffin, inheritance, marriage, and so forth, are then cited. These latter laws are not pertinent to our discussion of euthanasia and will not be further commented on here.

The Babylonian Talmud (*Shabbat* 151b) mentions as follows: "He who closes the eyes of a dying person while the soul is departing is a murderer (literally, he sheds blood). This may be compared to a lamp that is going out. If a man places his finger upon it, it is immediately extinguished." Rashi explains that this small effort of closing the eyes may slightly hasten death.

The code of Maimonides (Judges, Laws of Mourning 4:5) treats our subject matter as follows:

> One who is in a dying condition is regarded as a living person in all respects. It is not permitted to bind his jaws, to stop up the organs of the lower extremities, or to place metallic or cooling vessels upon his navel in order to prevent swelling. He is not to be rubbed or washed, nor is sand or salt to be put upon him until he expires. He who touches him is guilty of shedding blood. To what may he be compared? To a flickering flame, which is extinguished as soon as one touches it. Whoever closes the eyes of the dying while the soul is about to depart is shedding blood. One should wait a while; perhaps he is only in a swoon . . .

Thus, we again note the prohibition of doing anything that might hasten death. Maimonides does not specifically forbid moving such a patient as does the Mishnah, but such a prohibition is implied in Maimonides' text. Maimonides also forbids rubbing and washing a dying person, acts which are not mentioned in the Mishnah. Finally, Maimonides raises the problem of the recognition of death. This problem is becoming more pronounced as scientific medicine improves the methods for supporting respiration and heart function.

The sixteenth century code of Jewish law, the *Shulḥan Arukh,* by Rabbi Joseph Caro, devotes an entire chapter (*Yoreh De'ah,* 339) to the laws of the dying patient. The individual in whom death is imminent is referred to as a *goses.* Caro's code begins as do Maimonides and the Mishnah, with the phrase: "A *goses* is considered as a living person in all respects," and then Caro enumerates various acts that are prohibited. All the commentaries explain these prohibitions "lest they hasten the patient's death." One of the forbidden acts not mentioned by Maimonides or the Mishnah is the removal of the pillow from beneath the patient's head. This act had already been prohibited two centuries earlier by the *Tur (Yoreh De'ah,* 339). Caro's text is nearly identical to that of the *Tur.* The *Tur,* however, has the additional general explanation: "the rule in this matter is that any act performed in relation to death should not be carried out until the soul has departed." Thus, not only are physical acts on the patient such as described forbidden, but one should also not provide a coffin or prepare a grave or make other funeral or related arrangements lest the patient hear of this and his death be hastened. Even psychological stress is prohibited.

On the other hand, Rabbi Judah ben Samuel, the Pious, author of the thirteenth century work *Sefer Ḥasidim,* states in number 723, page 173: ". . . if a person is dying and someone near his house is chopping wood so that the soul cannot depart then one should remove the (wood) chopper from there . . ."

Based on the *Sefer Ḥasidim,* the Rema states (*Shulḥan Arukh, Yoreh De'ah,* 339:1) that

> if there is anything which causes a hindrance to the departure of the soul such as the presence near the patient's house of a knocking noise such as wood chopping or if there is salt on the patient's tongue; and these hinder the soul's departure, then it is permissible to remove them from there because there is no act involved in this at all but only the removal of the impediment.

Furthermore, Rabbi Solomon Eger, in his commentary on Caro's code (*Yoreh De'ah,* 339:1) quotes another rabbinic authority (*Beit Ya'akov,* 59) who states "it is forbidden to hinder the departure of the soul by the use of medicines." Other rabbinic authorities, however, (*Shevut Ya'akov,* 3: 13) disagree with this latter view. The *Shiltei ha-Gibborim* pleads at the end of chapter 3 of tractate *Mo'ed Katan* for the abolition of the custom of those who removed the pillow from below the dying person's head following the popular belief that bird feathers contained in the pillow prevent the soul from departing. He further states that Rabbi Nathan of Igra specifically permitted this act. The *Shiltei ha-Gibborim* continues: "After many years I found in the *Sefer Ḥasidim* (723) support for my contentions, as it is written there that if a person is dying but cannot die until he is put in a different place, he should not be moved." This law is not contradictory to the earlier statement of the *Sefer Ḥasidim* as both the *Shiltei ha-Gibborim* and Rema (in his commentary on the *Tur Yoreh De'ah* 339) explain: To do an act which prevents easy death such as chopping wood is forbidden and on the contrary, such impediments to death should be removed. On the other hand, it is definitely forbidden to perform any act which hastens death such as moving the dying person from one place to another.

A more extensive discussion and bibliography of sources dealing with these and other aspects of a dying person according to Jewish law is found in the fifth volume of the monumental *Talmudic Encyclopedia.*[47]

The sum total of this discussion of the Jewish attitude toward euthanasia seems to indicate, as expressed by Jakobovits[3,23] that ". . . any form of active euthanasia is strictly prohibited and condemned as plain murder . . . anyone who kills a dying person is liable to the death penalty as a common murderer. At the same time, Jewish law sanctions the withdrawal of any factor — whether extraneous to the patient himself or not — which may artificially delay his demise in the final phase." Jakobovits is quick to point out, however, that all the Jewish sources refer to an individual in whom death is expected to be imminent, three days or less in rabbinic references. Thus, passive euthanasia in a patient who may yet live for weeks or months may not necessarily be condoned. Furthermore, in the case of an incurably ill person in severe pain, agony, or distress, the removal of an impediment which hinders his soul's departure, although permitted by Jewish law (as described by Rema), may not be analogous to the withholding of medical therapy that is perhaps sustaining the patient's life unnaturally. The impediments spoken of in the code of Jewish law, whether far removed from the patient as exemplified by the noise of wood chopping, or in physical contact with him such as the case of salt on the patient's tongue, do not constitute any part of the therapeutic armamentarium employed in the medical management of this patient. For this reason, these impediments may be removed. However, the discontinuation of instrumentation and machinery which is specifically designed and utilized in the treatment of incurably ill patients might only be permissible if one is certain that in doing so one is shortening the act of dying and not interrupting life. Yet who can make the fine distinction between prolonging life and prolonging the act of dying? The former comes within the physician's reference, the latter does not.

NOTES

1. Fletcher, J.: Euthanasia: our right to die, in *Morals and Medicine,* Princeton, New Jersey, Princeton University Press, 1954, chap. 6, p. 172.

2. Sperry, W. L.: The prolongation of life, euthanasia-pro and euthanasia-con, in *The Ethical Basis of Medical Practice,* New York, Medical Dept., Paul B. Hoeber, Inc., 1950, chaps. 10 to 12, p. 124.

3. Jakobovits, I.: The dying and their treatment. Preparation for death and euthanasia, in *Jewish Medical Ethics,* New York, Bloch Publishers, 1959, chap. 11, p. 119.

4. Horder, T. J.: Signs and symptoms of impending death, *Practitioner* 161: 73 (1948).

5. Barber, H.: The act of dying, *ibid.* 161: 76 (1948).

6. Leak, W. N.: The care of the dying, *ibid.* 161: 80 (1948).

7. Rabinowitch, I. M., and MacDermot, H. E.: *Euthanasia,* McGill M. J. 19: 160 (1950).

8. Banks, A. L.: Euthanasia, *Bull. New York Acad. Med.* 26: 297 (1950).

9. Davis, E.: Should we prolong suffering?, *Nebraska M. J.* 35: 310 (1950).

10. Hebb, F.: The care of the dying *Canad. M. A. J.* 65: 261 (1951).

11. Alvarez, W. C.: Care of the dying, *J.A.M.A.* 150: 86 (1952).

12. Rud, F.: Euthanasia, *J. Clin. & Exper. Psychopath.* 14:1 (1953).

13. Symposium on euthanasia, *Maryland M. J.* 2: 120 (1953).

14. Rudd, T. N.: Family doctor at the deathbed; medical classics reconsidered, *Med. World* 85: 50 (1956).

15. Mitchison, N.: The right to die, *ibid.* 85: 159 (1956).

16. Friedman, G. A.: Suicide, euthanasia and the law, *M. Times* 85: 681 (1957).

17. Ogilvie, H.: Journey's end, *Practitioner* 179: 584 (1957).

18. Farrell, J. J.: The right of a patient to die, *J. South Carolina M. A.* 54: 221 (1958).

19. Rynearson, E. H.: You are standing at the bedside of a patient dying of untreatable cancer, *CA.* 9: 85 (1959).

20. Karnofsky, D. A.: "Why prolong the life of a patient with advanced cancer?", *ibid.* 10:9 (1960).

21. Betowski, E. P. S. J.: Prolongation of life in terminal illness, *ibid.* 10:25 (1960).

22. Torrey, E. F.: Euthanasia: a problem in medical ethics, *McGill M. J.* 30: 127 (1961).

23. Jakobovits, I.: The dying and their treatment in Jewish law. Preparation for death and euthanasia, *Hebrew M. J.* 2: 251 (1961).

24. Delhaye, C. P.: [Euthanasia or death by pity], *Union méd. Canada* 90: 613 (1961) (Fr.).

25. Levisohn, A. A.: Voluntary mercy deaths. Sociolegal aspects of euthanasia, *J. Forensic Med.* 8: 57 (1961).

26. Jones, K.S.: Death and doctors, *M. J. Australia* 49: 329 (1962).

27. Archambault, P. R.: [The problem of euthanasia considered by a Catholic physician], *Union méd. Canada* 91: 543 (1962) (Fr.)

28. Crinquette, J.: L'euthanasie, *J. sc. méd. Lillie* 81: 522 (1963).

29. McClanahan, J. H.: The patient's right to die. Moral and spiritual aspects of euthanasia, *Memphis M. J.* 38: 303 (1963).

30. Monnerot-Dumaine: Les notions d'euthanasie et d'automathasie, *Presse méd.* 72: 1458 (1964).

31. Picha, E.: Gedanken über die Euthanasie missgebildeter Neugeborener, *Wien. Med. Wchschr.* 114: 779 (1964).

32. Fibey, E. E.: Some overtones of euthanasia, *Hosp. Topics* 43: 55 (Sept.) 1965.

33. Hofling, C. K.: Terminal decisions, *Med. Opinion & Review* 2: 40 (Oct.) 1966.

34. Long, P. H.: On the quantity and quality of life, *M. Times* 88: 613 (1960).

35. Euthanasia, editorial, *Lancet* 2: 351 (1961).

36. Prolongation of dying, editorial, *ibid.* 2: 1205 (1962).

37. Bordet, F.: [Euthanasia], *Presse méd.* 70: 2022 (1962) (Fr.).

38. Farrar, C. B.: Euthanasia, *Am. J. Psychiat.* 119: 1104 (1963).

39. Symposium on terminal care (thirty-nine letters to the editor in regard to allowing the suffering, incurable, moribund patient to die quietly without the annoyance of radical procedures for short-period extension of life), *CA.* 10: 12 (1960).

40. Colebrook, L.: The Liège trial and the problem of voluntary euthanasia, *Lancet* 2: 1225 (1962).

41. Gillison, T. H.: Prolongation of dying, *ibid.* 2: 1327 (1962).

42. *Readers Digest,* December, 1960; *Harpers Magazine,* October, 1960; *Saturday Evening Post,* May 26, 1962, and September 10, 1966.

43. Fletcher, J. F.: *Anti-dysthanasia: The problem of prolonging death.* Address read at the annual meeting of the Euthanasia Society of America, New York, February 26, 1962.

44. *A Plan for Voluntary Euthanasia,* London, The Euthanasia Society, 1962, p. 28.

45. Mamis, J. F., executive secretary of the Euthanasia Society of America, Inc.: *Personal communication,* October 20, 1966.

46. *The Right to Die?,* New York, The Euthanasia Society of America, Inc.

47. Zevin, S. J., Ed.: *Talmudic Encyclopedia,* Jerusalem, 1963, vol. 5, p. 393.

16

The Quinlan Case:
A Jewish Perspective

J. DAVID BLEICH

Karen Ann Quinlan's tragic life — and protracted death — have not been in vain. Unconscious though she may be, she has served as the fulcrum of a recurring moral dilemma. Euthanasia, usually passive, but at times active, has been and continues to be practiced with a high degree of frequency, albeit clandestinely. The physicians at St. Claire's Hospital are to be commended for not opting for the path of least resistance and for their tenacity in scrupulously discharging the moral and professional duties with which they are charged. The controversy surrounding the care of Karen Quinlan has called attention to and sharpened the question which will be posed over and over again: Who is the arbiter of life and death, man or God?

The Quinlan case, particularly as tried in the press, presented three critical issues. The first: whether or not Karen should be pronounced dead, was a specious question from the start. It quickly became evident that Karen Quinlan is alive even according to the most liberal definitions of death. The second question was that of vicarious consent; may parents authorize withdrawal of treatment? From the legal perspective, proxy consent remains a clouded area; from the perspective of Jewish law parents have no standing whatsoever in this matter. The obligations which exist with regard to treatment of the sick are autonomous in nature and are not at all contingent upon the desire of parents, or for that matter, of the patient. Judge Muir's statement, ". . . the only cases where a parent has standing to pursue a constitutional right on behalf of an infant are those involving continuing life styles," is quite consistent with Jewish ethics. The third question is by far the most crucial: Does anyone have the right to choose death over life? Since the New Jersey Supreme Court had already ruled in a unanimous opinion that no one has a "right" to die, Judge Muir's decision

Reprinted from *Jewish Life* (Winter, 1976). Copyright © 1976 by the Union of Orthodox Jewish Congregations of America.

was a foregone conclusion. His decision was but a procedural prologue to a re-examination of this fundamental question by the New Jersey appeals court[1] and perhaps ultimately by the federal courts as well. It is this issue which will be debated in the months — and perhaps years — to come.

There was a time, not too long ago, when man could do but little when afflicted by serious illness and found himself powerless before the ravages of nature. Man could only proclaim with resignation: "The Lord hath given; the Lord hath taken; let the name of the Lord be blessed." In our day, many feel that since scientists and physicians have succeeded in prolonging life through the application of human intellect and technology it is therefore fitting and proper that members of the scientific community be the arbiters of whether the quality of such life is worth preserving. The argument acquires a measure of cogency when the decision to terminate life is reached for a purportedly higher purpose, such as transplantation of an organ from a moribund individual to a patient with greater chances for recovery. The new dictum appears to be: "Science hath given; science hath taken; let the cause of science be blessed."

The same argument is also heard in instances in which there is simply scant hope that the patient will recover. Man, it is argued, should not become the victim of his own technology. Man should not be forced to cling to life simply because he has the technical ability to do so. Nature should be permitted to take its course.

Man is instinctively repulsed by the prospect of becoming the agent responsible for the death of his fellow. This repugnance is keenly felt regardless of the patient's condition and of whether the contemplated act of euthanasia is active or passive. The reconciliation of termination of the life of a fellow human being with one's instinctive moral feelings is indeed a formidable challenge.

The widespread press coverage of the Quinlan case highlighted a most curious aspect of contemporary thought processes. Now that a decision has been handed down and the case is being appealed before the Supreme Court of the State of New Jersey, every informed person recognizes that the issue being adjudicated is that of "refusal of treatment", that is, does a person— or his proxy—have a right to demand that he be permitted to die or does the state have an overriding, compelling interest in the preservation of the life of each of its citizens. Yet, when the case first received publicity in the media it was presented in an entirely different guise. It was then presented as a "definition of death" case. We were urged, both on editorial pages and in what passed for straightforward news reports, to accept "brain death" as the scientifically precise criterion of cessation of life. This tactic was abandoned only when it became patently obvious that Karen Quinlan must be considered to be alive even if the newly-advocated definitions of death were to be accepted.

Why the confusion? Psychologically, it is not at all difficult to understand what has transpired. No one really wants to sanction murder. Homicide is abhorrent; man is endowed with a moral consciousness which recoils with shock at the very idea of taking the life of a fellow human being. No one wants to let another human being die. Man has a deeply-ingrained sense of responsibility for his fellow; man *does* perceive himself as his brother's keeper. Confronted with the tremendous emotional and financial toll exacted by the protracted care of a comatose patient, man finds himself impaled upon the horns of a dilemma. Moral sanction for abandoning the patient eludes him, yet the burden of sustaining life seems intolerable. The resolution of the problem is to pass between the horns of the dilemma by means of a lexicographical sleight-of-hand. If the patient may somehow be pronounced "dead" the problem is dispelled. Treatment may then be suspended without doing violence to ethical sensitivities.

This exercise in semantics can be, and has been, extended to resolve other bioethical problems. If one wishes to avoid the moral onus of snuffing out a human life when performing an abortion it is logically imperative that the fetus be denied status as a person. The transition from one position to the next is clearly delineated in a letter to the editor which appeared in *The New York Times* on March 6, 1972. The author, Cyril C. Means Jr., Professor of Constitutional Law at New York Law School, writes: "An adult heart donor, suffering from irreversible brain damage, is also a living human 'being,' but he is no longer a human 'person.' That is why his life may be ended by the excision of his heart for the benefit of another, the donee, who is still a human person. If there can be human 'beings' who are nonpersons at one end of the life span, why not also at the other end?" Once one moral concept is abrogated by the process of "redefinition" does any norm remain sacrosanct?

Another case in point is the problem of defective newborns. Babies born with severe congenital abnormalities or suffering from serious mental retardation are bound to be a burden to their parents, their siblings, and society. What can be done? Killing them is unthinkable. Abandoning the baby to custodial care in public institutions merely shifts the financial burden from parents to society at large and carries in its wake feelings of guilt to boot. Moreover, the extensive care and treatment which such infants require does create a genuine strain upon already limited and inadequate health care resources. Resolution: Let us redefine birth. Birth shall no longer be regarded as taking place at the moment of parturition but as occurring seventy-two hours after emergence of the infant from the birth canal. Since the baby is not yet born, in the event that it is found to be physically or mentally defective it could be destroyed with impunity up to the moment of "birth." This proposal was made, in all earnestness, by Dr. James Watson, codiscoverer of the double-helix in DNA. Situation ethicist Joseph Fletcher counsels that such infants should not be considered human children but should rather be viewed as "reproductive failures." And so the game continues.

Quite apart from theological considerations, definitions of death which, in reality, are value judgments in disguise are fraught with danger. Who is to decide at which stage of physical or mental deterioration life is no longer worthwhile? It is but a short step from the notion of "brain death" to the formulation of a definition of death centering around "social death," that is, an individual's capacity to serve as a useful member of society. It is entirely conceivable that eventually the concept of death will be broadened to include a person who consumes more of society's resources than he produces. Such a person is not productive and, from a *societal* perspective, his life appears to be hardly worth preserving. Fears such as these should not be dismissed as absurd. England's eminent biologist and Nobel Prize laureate, Dr. Francis Crick, has already advanced beyond this point in advocating compulsory death for all at the age of eighty as part of a "new ethical system based on modern science."

Human civilization has in the past witnessed attempts to make the right to life subservient to other values. Exposure of the aged to the elements was practiced by primitive societies; infanticide was not at all uncommon in 18th-century England; the Nazis broadened their infamous "final solution" to encompass the mentally ill and feebleminded. Each policy was undertaken in the name of enhancing the quality and dignity of human life. This is a road which men have trodden in the past. The achievement was never dignity, but ignominy.

It is quite true that man has the power to prolong life far beyond the point at which it ceases to be either productive or pleasurable. Not infrequently, the patient, if capable of expressing his desires and allowed to follow his own inclinations, would opt for termination of a life which has become a burden both to others and to himself. Judaism, however, teaches that man does not enjoy the right of self-determination with regard to questions of life and death. Generations ago our Sages wrote, "Against your will you live; against your will you die." While conventionally understood as underscoring the irony that a baby wishes to be born no more than an adult wishes to die, these words today take on new meaning. They may be taken quite literally as an eloquent summary of the Jewish view with regard to both euthanasia and the withholding of life-sustaining treatment. Judaism has always taught that life, no less than death, is involuntary. Only the Creator who bestows the gift of life may relieve man of that life even when it has become a burden rather than a blessing.

In the Jewish tradition the value with which human life is regarded is maximized far beyond the value placed upon human life either in the Christian tradition or in Anglo-Saxon common law. In Jewish law and moral teaching life is a supreme value and its preservation takes precedence over virtually all other considerations. Human life is not regarded as a good to be preserved as a condition of other values, but as an absolute basic and precious good in its own stead. Even life accompanied by suffering is regarded as being preferable to death. (See *Sotah* 20a).

Man does not possess absolute title to his life or his body. He is charged with preserving, dignifying, and hallowing that life. He is obliged to seek food and sustenance in order to safeguard the life he has been granted; when falling victim to illness or disease he is obliged to seek a cure in order to sustain life. The category of *pikku'ah nefesh* (preservation of life) extends to human life of every description and classification including the feeble-minded, the mentally deranged and yes, even a person in a so-called vegetative state. *Shabbat* laws and the like are suspended on behalf of such persons even though there may be no chance for them ever to serve either God or fellow man. The *mitzvah* of saving a life is neither enhanced nor diminished by virtue of the quality of the life preserved.

Distinctions between natural and artificial means, between ordinary and extraordinary procedures, and between non-heroic and heroic measures recur within the Catholic tradition, but no precisely parallel categories exist within Jewish law. Judaism knows no such distinctions and indeed the very vocabulary employed in drawing such distinctions is foreign to rabbinic literature. Rambam in his commentary on the Mishnah, *Pesahim* 4:9, draws a cogent parallel between food and medication. God created food and water; we are obliged to use them in staving off hunger and thirst. God created drugs and medicaments and endowed man with the intelligence necessary to discover their medicinal properties; we are obliged to use them in warding off illness and disease. Similarly, God provided the materials and the technology which make possible catheters, intravenous infusions, and respirators; we are obligated to use them in order to prolong life.

Judaism does recognize situations in which certain forms of medical intervention are not mandatory. This is so not because such procedures involve expense, inconvenience, or hardship, but because they are not part of an accepted therapeutic protocol. The obligation to heal is limited to the use of a *refu'ah bedukah,* drugs and procedures of demonstrated efficacy. (See R. Jacob Emden, *Mor u-Kezi'ah* 338). Man must use the full range of benefits made available by science; but he is not obliged to experiment with untried and unproven measures. Nor is he obliged to avail himself of therapeutic measures which are in themselves hazardous in the hope of effecting a complete cure. Even *hayyei sha'ah,* a short, transitory period of existence, is of such inestimable value that man is not obliged to gamble with precious moments of life, even in the hope of achieving health and longevity.

The physician's duty does *not* end when he is incapable of restoring the lost health of his patient. The obligation, "and you shall restore it to him" (Deuteronomy 22:2) refers, in its medical context, not simply to the restoration of health but to the restoration of even a single moment of life. Again, *Shabbat* and other laws are suspended even when it is known with certainty that human medicine offers no hope of a cure or restoration to health. Ritual obligations and restrictions are suspended as long as there is the possibility that life may be prolonged even for a matter of moments.

The sole exception to these principles which *Halakhah* recognizes is the case of a *goses,* a moribund patient actually in the midst of death throes.[2] The physiological criteria indicative of such a condition must be spelled out with care. (See Rema, *Even ha-Ezer* 121:7 and *Ḥoshen Mishpat* 221:2). It is surely clear that a patient whose life may be prolonged for weeks and even months is not yet moribund; the death process has not yet started to commence and hence the patient is not a *goses.* The halakhic provisions governing care of a *goses* may most emphatically not be applied to all who are terminally ill.

The aggressiveness with which Judaism teaches that life must be preserved is not at all incompatible with the awareness that the human condition is such that there are circumstances in which man would prefer death to life. The Gemara, *Ketubbot* 104a, reports that Rabbi Judah the Prince, redactor of the Mishnah, was afflicted by what appears to have been an incurable and debilitating intestinal disorder. He had a female servant who is depicted in rabbinic writings as a woman of exemplary piety and moral character. This woman is reported to have prayed for his death. On the basis of this narrative, the thirteenth-century authority, Rabbenu Nissim of Gerondi, in his commentary to *Nedarim* 40a, states that it is permissible, and even praiseworthy, to pray for the death of a patient who is gravely ill and in extreme pain.

Although man must persist in his efforts to prolong life he may, nevertheless, express human needs and concerns through the medium of prayer. There is no contradiction whatsoever between acting upon an existing obligation and pleading to be relieved of further responsibility. Man may beseech God to relieve him from divinely imposed obligations when they appear to exceed human endurance. But the ultimate decision is God's and God's alone. There are times when God's answer to prayer is in the negative. But this, too, is an answer.

In the *Republic* (I, 340), Plato observes that a physician, at the time that he errs in treating a patient, is not worthy of his title. When the physician's knowledge fails him, he ceases to be a practitioner of the healing arts. Our teachers went one step further: They taught that a physician who declines to make use of his skills is not a physician; they admonished that a physician who gives up his patient as hopeless is not a physician. "*And he shall surely heal*—From here it is derived that the physician is granted permission to heal" (*Bava Kamma* 85a). The ḥasidic Seer, the *Ḥozeh* of Lublin, added a pithy comment: "The Torah gives permission to heal. It does not give the physician dispensation to refrain from healing because in his opinion the patient's condition is hopeless."

This lesson is the moral of a story told of the 19th-century Polish scholar, popularly known as Reb Eisel Charif. The venerable Rabbi was afflicted with a severe illness and was attended by an eminent specialist. As the disease progressed beyond hope of cure, the physician informed the Rabbi's family of the gravity of the situation. He also informed them that he therefore felt justified in withdrawing from the case. The doctor's grave prognosis notwithstanding, Reb Eisel Charif recovered completely. Some time later, the physician chanced to come upon the Rabbi in the street. The doctor stopped in his tracks in astonishment and exclaimed, "Rabbi, have you come back from the other world?" The Rabbi responded, "You are indeed correct. I *have* returned from the other world. Moreover, I did you a great favor while I was there. An angel ushered me in to a large chamber. At the far end of the room was a door and lined up in front of the door were a large number of well-dressed, dignified and intelligent-looking men. These men were proceeding through the doorway in a single file. I asked the angel who these men were and where the door led. He informed me that the door was the entrance to the netherworld and that the men passing through those portals were those of whom the Mishnah says, 'The best of physicians merits *Gehinnom.*' Much to my surprise, I noticed that you too were standing in the line about to proceed through the door. I immediately approached the angel and told him: 'Remove that man immediately! He is no doctor. He does not treat patients; he abandons them!' "

To depict any human condition as hopeless is to miss entirely the spiritual dimension of human existence. Dr. John Shepherd, a neurosurgeon at Nassau County Medical Center, claims the cure of at least two comatose patients whose vital signs were even more discouraging than those of Karen Quinlan—but that is not the point. Even were it true that medical diagnoses and prognoses are infallible, the decision to terminate treatment is not a medical decision; it is the determination of a moral question. That the physician possesses specialized knowledge and unique skills is unquestionable. However, his professional training guarantees neither heightened moral sensitivity nor enhanced acumen. He may quite legitimately draw medical conclusions with regard to anticipated effects of the application or withholding of various therapeutic procedures. But the decision to proceed or not to proceed is a moral, not a medical, decision. From the fact that a condition is medically hopeless it does not follow that the remaining span of life is devoid of meaning. *"Nistarim darkhei ha-Shem"*

— "the ways of God are hidden." He has decreed that we must love, cherish and preserve life in all its phases and guises until the very onset of death. While even terminal life is undoubtedly endowed with other meaning and value as well, subservience to the divine decree and fulfillment of God's commandment is, in itself, a matter of highest meaning.

The sanctity of human life is not predicated upon hedonistic proclivity, pragmatic utility or even upon the potential for service to one's fellow man. The telos of human existence is service of God and the performance of His commandments. It is in this explanation of human existence that Me'iri (*Yoma* 85a) finds the rationale underlying the obligation to preserve the life of even the hopelessly ill. Me'iri observes that although the moribund patient may be incapable of any physical exertion he may be privileged to experience contrition and utilize the precious final moments of life for the achievement of true repentance.

One personal experience lives vividly in my mind. My family and I had travelled some distance to attend a family *simḥah* (celebration). Arriving on *erev Shabbat* we were grieved to learn that an elderly relative had experienced renal failure and was in a critical condition. At the hospital I requested and was shown the patient's medical chart. It was readily apparent that the patient was not being treated aggressively and, indeed, none of several available forms of therapy had been instituted. I immediately telephoned the attending physician and demanded an explanation. In reply I was informed that the doctors were unanimous in their opinion that the patient was terminal though they could not predict how long she might survive in a comatose state. The doctor could see no point in prolonging life under such conditions. As a matter of Halakhah I had no choice but to insist upon the administration of therapeutically indicated medication. However, the decision, humanly speaking, was not an easy one. But then an incident occurred which put the entire matter into a different perspective.

Late *Shabbat* afternoon I returned from *minḥah* and although the patient had been totally unresponsive for over thirty-six hours, I walked into the hospital room and said *"Gut Shabbos"* in a loud voice. I was greeted in response by the flickering of an eyelid and, in a weak but clear voice, the words *"Gut Shabbos"* in return. At that moment there flashed across my mind the comments of Rav Akiva Eger (*Oraḥ Ḥayyim* 271:1) who declares that even the simple, standard *Shabbat* greeting expressed by one Jew to another constitutes a fulfillment of the *mitzvah:* "Remember the Sabbath day to keep it holy." At that moment I realized not only intellectually, but also emotionally, that every moment of life is of inestimable value. Here was a dramatic unfolding of the lesson that every moment of life carries with it the opportunity for the performance of yet one more *mitzvah*.

No scientist has ever determined the absolute (as distinct from recordable) threshold of psychic activity. No clinical experiment has ever been conducted to determine at what level of consciousness a comatose patient becomes incapable of remorse and repentance. But, even if possible, such an undertaking would be irrelevant. Me'iri's rationale adds a measure of understanding but does not establish the parameters of the halakhic obligation. Halakhic ramifications frequently remain operative even in situations in which the reasoning upon which they are grounded is not strictly applicable. Halakhah acquires a sancity, *sui generis,* of its own. Human life, regardless of its quality and, indeed, of its potential for even the most minimal fulfillment of *mitzvot,* is endowed with sanctity. (See *Bi'ur Halakhah, Orah Hayyim* 329:4).

The coining of the phrase "death with dignity" by advocates of passive euthanasia was a stroke of genius. Opponents of such practices are immediately disarmed. Everyone respects "rights" and no one decries "dignity." Yet, while repeated use of a glib phrase by the press and media may influence attitudes, the coining of a cliché is not the same as making a case. Is sickness or frailty, however tragic, really an indignity? Is the struggle for life, in any form, an indignity? Is it not specious to insinuate that the attempt to sustain life is aught but the expression of the highest regard for the precious nature of the gift of life and of the *dignity* in which it is held?

There is a definite conflict between the ethical teachings of Judaism and the prevalent moral climate. Unfortunately, Jews are prone to celebrate Jewish thought when it coincides with what chances to be in vogue and to ignore it when it runs counter to ideas or practices heralded by the dominant culture. Judaism has something to say—and to teach—about all moral issues. Jewishness is more than a matter of ethnic identity and Judaism more than perfunctory performance of ritual. Jews who take their Jewishness seriously must necessarily search for the uniquely Jewish answers to the dilemmas of life and death which emerge from the Jewish tradition. Judaism teaches that man is denied the right to make judgments with regard to quality of life. Man is never called upon to determine whether life is worth living—that is a question over which God remains sole arbiter.

NOTES

1. Indeed the Supreme Court of New Jersey, In the Matter of Karen Quinlan, 70 N.J. 10, 355 A 2d, 647, subsequently stated, "Under the law as it then stood, Judge Muir was correct in declining to authorize withdrawal of the respirator" and found it necessary to reevaluate applicable judicial considerations. For the effect of this

decision upon the earlier formulated opinion that there exists no right to die see above, p. 10.

2. Some authorities, most notably *Beit Ya'akov,* no. 59, followed by *Iggerot Moshe, Yoreh De'ah,* II, no. 174, maintain that it is forbidden to prolong the life of a *goses* by any means whatsoever. But the position is by no means universally accepted. *Shevut Ya'akov,* I, no. 13, cites *Yoma* 85a in demonstrating that *Shabbat* laws are superceded for the purpose of even marginal prolongation of life. *Shevut Ya'akov* declares that all accepted therapeutic remedies must be utilized in prolonging the life of a *goses* regardless of how brief a period of time he may be expected to survive. This authority evidently distinguishes between natural remedies of demonstrated efficacy involving readily recognizable causal relationships and non-scientific *segulot* of undemonstrable causal efficacy such as the placing of salt upon the tongue. The latter, according to this analysis, are not required in the case of a *goses* because they are not recognized medical procedures. Alternatively, a distinction must be made between the state of *gesisah* and the actual state of dying, a departure of the soul from the body. See R. Eliezer Waldenberg, *Ẓiẓ Eli'ezer,* XIII, no. 89, sec. 14, who describes the latter as *gemar kelot ha-nefesh* in contradistinction to *gesisah;* in *Assia,* Nisan 5738, p. 18, he uses the prase *sha'at yeẓi'at neshamah* in making the identical distinction. [The distinction drawn by R. Aryeh Lev Grossnass, *Teshuvot Lev Aryeh,* II, no. 37, between one who may survive at least for a short time and one who can live only by means of external aids is without foundation. See G. G. Halibard, "Euthanasia," *The Jewish Law Annual,* I (1978), 197.] The position of *Shevut Ya'akov* is also espoused by *Mishnah Berurah, Bi'ur Halakhah* 329:4, and by the present head of the Jerusalem *Bet Din,* Rabbi Eliezer Waldenberg in his *Ramat Raḥel,* no. 28 and *Ẓiẓ Eli'ezer,* VIII, no. 15, chap. 3, sec. 16; *ibid.,* IX, no. 47; and *Assia,* Nisan 5738, p. 195.

While adjudication of this question is quite properly left to competent rabbinic decisors on a case-by-case basis, it is important to emphasize that withholding of treatment does not at all come into question unless the patient is actually in a state of *gesisah.* A detailed clinical profile of the halakhic criteria which are indicative of this state is beyond the scope of these comments. It should, however, be stated that while the technical criteria must be carefully elucidated, it is clear that a *goses* is by definition a moribund person whose death is imminent. It seems incomprehensible to me that a patient whose physiological state permits survival for an indeterminate period of time and who has, in fact, survived for over fourteen months (at the time of this writing) can be considered a *goses.* It must be remembered that the quality of life which is preserved is not a determinant halakhic factor. Sources for a definition of *gesisah* are to be found in *Shulhan Arukh, Yoreh De'ah* 339:2; Rema, *Even ha-Ezer* 121:7, and *Ḥoshen Mishpat* 211:2, as well as Rambam and *Tosafot Yom Tov* in their respective commentaries on the Mishnah, *Arakhin* 1:3, and in the comments of *Derishah, Tur Yoreh De'ah* 339:5.

Even in the case of a *goses,* the distinction between withholding treatment and an overt act designed to shorten life is a most crucial one. Note should be made of the suggestion that "pulling the plug" be considered a form of withholding treatment. This thesis was advanced by Rabbi Baruch Rabinowitz of Holon in the Sivan 5731 issue of *Assia.* See also R. Aryeh Lev Grossnass, *Teshuvot Lev Aryeh,* II, no. 37; and R. Eliezer Waldenberg, *Ẓiẓ Eli'ezer,* XIII, no. 89, secs. 2–3. Whatever the cogency of the argument, the suggestion is one which has been considered and at present is rejected by recognized halakhic authorities who deem "pulling the plug" to be an act of overt intervention. See R. Simḥah ha-Kohen Kook, *Torah She-be'al Peh,* XVIII (5736), 87; R. Menashe Klein, *Mishneh Halakhot,* VII, no. 287; and

R. Eliezer Waldenberg, *Ziz Eli'ezer,* XIII, no. 89, sec. 9. Cf, however, R. Waldenberg, *Assia,* Nisan 5738, p. 20, where he takes note of the consideration that physiological stress occasioned by removal of the respirator may overtly hasten death.

It is noteworthy that in the Quinlan case the Supreme Court of New Jersey was not at all concerned with the question of whether or not removal of a respirator constitutes an overt act of homicide. The court did indeed state that "the ensuing death would not be homicide but rather expiration from existing natural causes" but hastened to add, "even if it were to be regarded as homicide, it would not be unlawful." It was the court's position that, in the absence of a reasonable possibility of the patient ever emerging from a comatose condition to a cognitive, sapient state, the patient or her guardian may lawfully demand termination of treatment pursuant to the right of privacy. Since the act is lawful, "a death resulting from such an act would not come within the scope of the homicide statutes proscribing only the unlawful killing of another." See In re Quinlan 70 N.J. 10, 51 355 A. 2d 647 (1976). This position is, of course, antithetical to Jewish teaching. Judaism recognizes no right to privacy insofar as termination of human life is concerned. Such right is vested solely in the Creator.

17
Establishing
Criteria of Death
J. DAVID BLEICH

I acknowledge before You, my God and the God of my fathers . . . that my cure is in Your hand and my death is in Your hand. . . . And if my appointed time to die has arrived You are righteous in all that befalls me.
(Confession of the dying)

A man of serious conscience means to say in raising urgent ethical questions that there may be some things that men should never do that, now or in the future, they could do. The good things that men do are made complete only by the things they refuse to do. It would perhaps be better not to raise the ethical issues of medical practice in an age when public policy and research requirements threaten to be overriding than not to raise them in earnest.

(Paul Ramsey, *New England Journal of Medicine,* April 1, 1971)

The task of defining death is not a trivial exercise to be relegated to the purview of the lexicographer. It is perhaps the most pressing concern in the field of bioethics. The formulation of such a definition involves an attempt to arrive at an understanding of the very essence of human life and an endeavor to identify the nature of the ephemeral substance which is lost at the time of death.

The loss of that elusive component which transforms the human organism into a living being effects a change in the moral and legal status of the individual. The traditional view is that death occurs upon the separation of the soul from the body. Of course, the occurrence of this phenomenon does not lend itself to direct empirical observation. Accordingly, traditional definitions of death have focused upon cessation of circulatory and respiratory functions as criteria of the ebbing of life. *Black's Law Dictionary* (rev. 4th ed. 1968), in recording the accepted legal definition, describes death as ". . . total stoppage of the circulation of the blood, and a cessation of the animal and vital functions consequent thereupon, such as respiration, pulsation, etc."

Contemporary medical science has developed highly sophisticated techniques for determining the presence or absence of vital bodily functions. Moreover, improvements in resuscitatory and supportive measures now at times make it possible to restore life as judged by the traditional standards of persistent respiration and continuing heart beat. This can be the case even when there is little likelihood of an individual recovering consciousness following massive brain damage. These new medical realia have led to a reassessment of traditional definitions of death. Some members of the scientific community now advocate that previously accepted criteria of death be set aside and have formulated several proposals for a redefinition of the phenomenon of death.

Chief among these is the now popular concept frequently, though inaccurately, referred to as brain death. According to this view, death is equated with the complete loss of the body's integrating capacities as signified by the activity of the central nervous system and is determined by the absence of brain waves as recorded by an electroencephalogram over a period of time. It is most interesting to note that reports have appeared, both in the popular press and in scholarly publications, of a significant number of instances in which patients have made either partial or complete recoveries despite previous electroencephalogram readings which registered no brain activity over an extended period of time.[1]

Several years ago the Ad Hoc Committee of the Harvard Medical School to Examine the Definition of Brain Death was established. The published report of this committee[2] states that its primary purpose was to "define irreversible coma as a new criterion of death." In order to arrive at a clinical definition of irreversible coma, the Ad Hoc Committee recommends establishment of operational criteria for the determination of the characteristics of a permanently nonfunctioning brain. The three recommended criteria are: (1) lack of response to external stimuli or to internal need; (2) absence of movement or breathing as observed by physicians over a period of at least one hour; (3) absence of elicitable reflexes ("except in some cases through the spinal cord").[3] A fourth criterion, a flat, or isoelectric, electroencephalogram, is recommended as being "of great confirmatory value" but not of absolute necessity. Subsequently, Dr. Henry K. Beecher, the chairman of the Ad Hoc Committee, noted, "Almost everybody else has required the use of the electroencephalogram. We think it adds helpful confirmatory evidence, but we do not think that it is necessary by itself."[4] The procedure advocated by the Ad Hoc Committee calls for repetition of the relevant tests following a lapse of twenty-four hours. Repeated examinations over a period of twenty-four hours or longer are required in order to obtain evidence of the irreversible nature of the coma.

Most revealing is the quite candid statement of the committee chairman: "Only a very bold man, I think, would attempt to define death. . . . I was chairman of a recent *ad hoc* committee at Harvard composed of members of five faculties in the university who tried to define irreversible coma. We felt we could not define death. I suppose you will say that by implication we have defined it as brain death, but we do not make a point of that."[5]

More recently, the adequacy of even this notion of brain death has been challenged in some quarters. Proponents of a broader definition ask, "Why is it that one must identify the entire brain with death; is it not possible that we are really interested only in man's consciousness: in his ability to think, reason, feel, interact with others and control his body functions consciously?"[6] According to this latter view, death is to be equated with irreversible loss of consciousness. If this definition were to gain acceptance, the effect would be that in cases where the lower brain function is intact while the cortex, which controls consciousness, is destroyed, the patient would be pronounced dead.

Much of the debate concerning the definition of death misses the mark. A definition of death cannot be derived from medical facts or scientific investigation alone. The physician can only describe the physiological state which he observes; whether the patient meeting that description is alive or dead, whether the human organism in that physiological state is to be treated as a living person or as a corpse, is an ethical and legal question. The determination of the time of death, insofar as it is more than a mere exercise in semantics, is essentially a theological and moral problem, not a medical or scientific one.

For Jews, questions of this nature can be answered only within the framework of Halakhah. The great strides made in the life sciences in the past number of years have reopened a host of medico-halakhic problems. With the invention and refinement of life-saving apparatus, the life of a terminally ill patient may, in some instances, be prolonged for a significant period of time. As a result, a precise definition of death becomes of crucial importance because only the presence of the criteria of death which are recognized by Halakhah relieves the physician of his obligation to use all available means in order to preserve the life of the patient. The most breathtaking of recent scientific breakthroughs is no doubt the development of the techniques for successful heart transplantation. While discouraging results have resulted in virtual suspension of such transplants, there is reason to anticipate that with further research the difficulties which have been encountered will be overcome. From the perspective of Jewish law there are a number of halakhic and ethical questions which must be analyzed before a definite position can be formulated regarding the permissibility of this or similar procedures. Chief among these problems is the halakhic definition of death, since for medical reasons the donor's heart must be removed without delay if the operative procedure is to be successful.

The surgeon is faced with a dilemma. In order to save the life of his patient, he must remove the donor's heart at the earliest possible moment consistent with the latter's claim to life. When may he proceed? Certainly, all to whom human life is sacred would answer: the instant death occurs. But this answer merely begs the crucial question: when *does* death occur? The sanctity of human life is a cardinal principle of Judaism. It is self-evident that every measure must be taken to preserve the life of every human being. By the same token, the slightest action which might hasten the death of another is proscribed. Hence the extreme importance of determining with exactitude the halakhic definition of death.

In view of the far-ranging significance of this problem, a detailed analysis of the sources from which such a definition must be derived is in order. Moreover, as will be shown, there exists a crucial conceptual difficulty which requires careful analysis; namely, do the hallmarks of death as given by Jewish law constitute a definition of death *per se,* i.e., is the physiological state described by such signs synonymous with death in the eyes of Halakhah, or are such signs merely symptomatic of death, the state of death itself, from the point of view of Halakhah, being beyond analytic definition in empirical terms? This problem requires careful elucidation and examination since it is a question which is not explicitly formulated in responsa literature.

I

It is axiomatic, according to Halakhah, that death coincides with cessation of respiration. The primary source of this definition is to be found in *Yoma* 85a in connection with suspension of Sabbath regulations for the sake of the preservation of human life. The case in point concerns an individual trapped under a fallen building. Since desecration of the Sabbath is mandated even on the mere chance that a human life may be preserved, the debris of a collapsed building must be cleared away even if it is doubtful that the person under the rubble is still alive. However, once it has been determined with certainty that the person has expired, no further violation of the Sabbath regulations may be sanctioned. The question which then arises is how much of the body must be uncovered in order to ascertain conclusively that death has in fact occurred? The first opinion cited by the Gemara maintains that the nose must be uncovered and the victim of the accident be pronounced dead only if no sign of respiration is found. A second opinion maintains that death may be determined by examination of the chest for the absence of a heartbeat. It is evident that both opinions regard respiration as the crucial factor indicating the existence of life; the second opinion simply adds that the absence of a heartbeat is also to be deemed sufficient evidence that respiration has ceased and that death has actually occurred. This is evident from the statement quoted by the Gemara in the name of R. Papa in clarification of this controversy. R. Papa states that there is no disagreement in instances in which the body is uncovered "from the top down." In such cases the absence of respiration is regarded by all as being conclusive. The dispute, declares R. Papa, is limited to situations in which the body is uncovered "from the bottom up" and thus the heart is uncovered first. The controversy in such cases is whether the absence of a heartbeat is sufficient evidence to establish death in and of itself, or whether further evidence is required, i.e., uncovering of the nostrils. The necessity for examination of the nostrils is based upon the assumption that it is possible for life to exist even though such life may be undetectable by means of an examination for the presence of a heartbeat—as Rashi succinctly puts it, "For at times life is not evident at the heart but is evident at the nose."[7] In demonstration of the principle that respiration is the determining factor, the Gemara cites the verse ". . . all in whose nostrils is the breath of the spirit of life" (Gen. 7:22). Both Maimonides[8] and *Shulḥan Arukh*[9] cite the first opinion as authoritative. Hence in terms of normative Halakhah, regardless of whether the head or the feet are uncovered first, death can be established only by examination of the nostrils and determination of the absence of signs of respiratory activity at that site.

However, even according to the accepted view, namely, that determination of death is contingent upon lack of respiration, absence of cardiac activity is a relevant factor. Cessation of respiration constitutes the operative definition of death only because lack of respiration is also indicative of prior cessation of cardiac activity. This may be inferred from Rashi's choice of language. The phrase, "At times life is not evident at the heart but is evident at the nose," would indicate that, hypothetically, if confronted by a situation in which "life" is not evident at the nose for whatever reason, but *is* evident at the heart, cardiac activity would itself be sufficient to negate any other presumptive symptom of death.[10] This view is clearly expressed by R. Zevi Ashkenazi, *Teshuvot Ḥakham Zevi,* no.77. *Hakham Zevi* notes that in some cases a heartbeat may be imperceptible even though the individual is still alive. A weak beat may not be audible or otherwise perceivable since the ribcage and layers of muscle intervene between the heart itself and the outer skin. Respiration is more readily detectable and hence the insistence upon an examination of the nostrils. However, concludes *Hakham Zevi,* "It is most clear that there can be no respiration unless there is life in the heart, for respiration is from the heart and for its benefit." Similarly, R. Moses Sofer, *Teshuvot Ḥatam Sofer, Yoreh De'ah,* no. 338, states that absence of respiration is conclusive only if the patient "lies as an inanimate stone and there is no pulse whatsoever."[11]

These sources indicate clearly that death occurs only upon the cessation of both cardiac and respiratory functions. The absence of other vital signs is not, insofar as Halakhah is concerned, a criterion of death.

II

Although, in theory, the cessation of respiration is the determining criterion in establishing that death has occurred, in practice this principle is considerably modified so that the absence of respiratory activity in itself is not sufficient to establish that death has occurred. Halakhah provides that the Sabbath may be violated in order to save the life of an unborn fetus. Therefore *Shulḥan Arukh*[12] states that if a woman dies in childbirth on the Sabbath a knife may be brought through a public domain in order to make an incision into the uterus for the purpose of removing the fetus. However, R. Moses Isserles (Rema), in a gloss to this ruling, indicates that this provision, while theoretically valid, is nevertheless inoperative in practice. Rema declares that, quite apart from the question of desecration of the Sabbath, it is forbidden to perform a postmortem Caesarean in order to save the fetus, on weekdays as well as on the Sabbath, because we are not competent to determine the moment of maternal death with exactitude.

Since it is forbidden to as much as move a limb of a moribund person lest this hasten his death,[13] there can be no question of an incision into the womb until death has been established with absolute certainty. In view of the fact that by the time the death of the mother can be conclusively determined the fetus is no longer viable, this procedure would be purposeless and consequently would constitute an unwarranted violation of the corpse.

The principle enunciated by Rema[14] is that what may appear to be cessation of respiratory activity cannot be accepted as an absolute criterion of death. Our lack of competence is due to an inability to distinguish between death and a fainting spell or swoon. In the latter cases respiratory activity does occur, although respiration may be so minimal that it cannot be perceived.

In stating that we are incompetent to determine the moment of death with precision and cannot apply the criterion of respiration with reliability, Rema does not spell out clinical signs which may be accepted as conclusive. Nor does he indicate how much time must elapse following apparent cessation of respiration before the patient may be pronounced dead. There is some discrepancy in the writings of later authors with regard to establishing such a time-period. A contemporary authority, Rabbi Jehiel

Michael Tucatzinsky, *Gesher ha-Ḥayyim,* I chap. 3, p. 48, records that the practice in Jerusalem is not to remove the body from the deathbed for a period of twenty minutes following the presumed time of death. Earlier, Rabbi Shalom Gagin, *Teshuvot Yismaḥ Lev, Yoreh De'ah,* no. 9, stated that the custom in Jerusalem is to wait a period of one half-hour. Rabbi Gagin further noted that our incompetence to determine time of death with precision should not necessitate a delay of "more than half an hour or at the most an hour" for final pronouncement of death.[15]

Writing in the Tammuz 5731 issue of *Ha-Ma'ayan,* Dr. Jacob Levy, an Israeli physician and frequent contributor to halakhic journals, argues that, in light of the clinical aids now available to the physician, the considerations which previously necessitated this waiting period are no longer operative. Rema's declaration that the ruling of the *Shulḥan Arukh* is not followed in practice is based upon the fear that a fainting spell or swoon may be misdiagnosed as death. Dr. Levy points out that in many cases the possibility of such errors can be eliminated by use of a sphygmomanometer to determine that no blood pressure can be detected, in conjunction with an electrocardiagram to ascertain that all cardiac activity has ceased. Accordingly, Dr. Levy strongly recommends that rabbinic authorities declare that the original ruling of the *Shulḥan Arukh* now be followed in practice.

Dr. Levy adds that this proposal should not be construed as an abrogation of Rema's ruling, since many authorities recognize that Rema's statement is based upon empirical considerations and admits to exceptions. For example, R. Jacob Reischer, *Shevut Ya'akov,* I, no. 13, in discussing the bizarre case of a pregnant woman who was decapitated on the Sabbath, states unequivocally that the physician who had the presence of mind to incise the abdomen immediately in order to remove the fetus need have no pangs of conscience, since in this instance the mother's prior death is established beyond cavil.[16] Similarly, concludes Dr. Levy, Rema's statement should not be viewed as normative under changed circumstances which enable medical science to determine that death has already occurred. This argument is cogent in view of the fact that Rema himself remarks that it had become necessary to disregard the earlier authoritative decision of the *Shulḥan Arukh* solely because of a lack of medical expertise.[17]

Granted that with the use of clinical aids one can establish conclusively that all cardiac activity has ceased, Dr. Levy's contention that no further waiting period is needed is borne out by *Ḥakham Ẓevi's* previously cited statement, "There can be no respiration unless there is life in the heart."

Ḥakham Ẓevi's original ruling elicited the sharp disagreement of R. Jonathan Eybeschuetz and sparked a controversy which has become classic in the annals of Halakhah. The dispute centered around a chicken which, upon evisceration, proved to have no discernible heart. The chicken was brought to *Ḥakham Ẓevi* for a determination as to whether the fowl was to be considered *terefah* because of the missing heart. *Ḥakham Ẓevi* ruled that it is empirically impossible for a chicken to lack a heart because there can be no life whatsoever without a heart. The chicken clearly lived and matured; hence it must have had a heart which somehow became separated from the other internal organs upon the opening of the chicken and was inadvertently lost. The impossibility of life without a heart, in the opinion of *Hakham Zevi,* is so obvious a verity that he declares that even the testimony of witnesses attesting to the absence of the heart and the impossibility of error is to be dismissed as blatant perjury. R. Jonathan Eybeschuetz, in a scathing dissenting opinion, argues that such a possibility cannot be dismissed out of hand. In his commentary to *Yoreh De'ah, Kereti u-Feleti* 40:4, R. Jonathan Eybeschuetz contends that the functions of the heart, including the pumping of blood, might well be performed by an organ whose external form is quite unlike that of a normal heart and which may even be located in some other part of the body. This organ might be indistinguishable from other, more usual tissue, and hence the observer might have concluded that the animal or fowl lacked a "heart."

There is nothing in this opinion which contradicts the point made on the basis of *Hakham Zevi's* responsum with regard to determination of the time of death. R. Jonathan Eybeschuetz concedes that life cannot be sustained in the absence of some organ to perform cardiac functions. R. Jonathan Eybeschuetz argues only that, in the apparent absence of a recognizable heart, cardiac functions may possibly be performed by some other organ; he does not at all assert that life may continue following cessation of the functions normally performed by the heart.

However, at least one authority indicates that life can continue, at least theoretically, after the heart has been removed. Specifically rejecting the opinion of authorities who have concluded that "it is impossible to exist even for a moment" without a functioning heart, *Mishkenot Ya'akov, Yoreh De'ah,* no. 10, declares that such a contingency is a distinct possibility. According to this opinion it may perhaps be the case that a waiting period of some duration, as demanded by Rema, cannot be waived even when heart stoppage is confirmed by clinical apparatus, since cessation of cardiac activity does not, in and of itself, indicate that death has occurred. Acceptance of Dr. Levy's thesis would quite probably involve rejection of the opinion of *Mishkenot Ya'akov* in favor of the view expressed by *Hakham Zevi.*

III

There is, as previously noted, one fundamental problem with regard to a clear analysis of the halakhic position which views time of death as being simultaneous with cessation of respiration. Is cessation of respiration to be equated with death itself, or is it merely a physiological symptom enabling us to ascertain the time of death? Couched in different terminology, are respiration and life itself one and the same, so that the absence of respiratory activity, by definition, constitutes the state of death? Or is life some ephemeral and indefinable state or activity which cannot be empirically perceived but of which absence of respiration is a reliable indication?

There is some *prima facie* evidence indicating that lack of respiration and the state of death are, by definition, synonymous. The Sages inform us that the soul departs through the nostrils, thereby causing respiration to cease and death to occur. *Pirkei de-Rabbi Eli'ezer,* ch. 52,[17a] observes that after sneezing one should give thanks for having been privileged to remain alive.[18] The *Yalkut,* noting that the first mention of sickness in Scripture occurs in Genesis 48:1, remarks that prior to the time of Jacob sickness was unknown. It is the view of the Sages that illness became part of man's destiny in answer to Jacob's plea for prior indication of impending death in order that he might make a testament before dying. Before the days of Jacob, according to the *Yalkut,* an individual simply sneezed and expired without any indication whatsoever that death was about to overtake him. The *Yalkut* can readily be understood on the basis of the verse ". . .and He blew into his nostrils the soul of life" (Gen. 2:6). In the narrative concerning the creation of Adam, the soul is described as having entered through the nostrils. According to the *Yalkut,* the soul departs through the same aperture through which it entered; hence terminal sneezing is associated with the soul's departure from the body. Apparently, then, respiration and life both cease with the departure of the soul.

Likewise, we find that the nose is deemed to be the site of the soul's departure from the body with regard to the provisions surrounding the *eglah arufah* (the broken-necked heifer). Biblical law (Deut. 21:1–9) provides that if homicide is committed outside a city and the identity of the murderer is unknown it becomes incumbent upon the elders of the city closest to the site where the corpse is found to perform the ritual of breaking the neck of a calf in expiation of the untraced murder. In the event that the body be found in a spot virtually equidistant between two cities, the Mishnah, *Sotah* 45b, cites the opinion of R. Akiva who states that the distance to the neighboring cities is to be measured from the nose in order to determine which is closest. In explaining R. Akiva's opinion, which in this case is authoritative, the Gemara states that his view is predicated upon the premise that "primary life—*ikar hiyuta*—is in the nose." This would seem to indicate that death and cessation of respiration are synonymous.

There is, however, evidence from the Talmud itself that at least in rare instances individuals have lived despite previous cessation of respiration. *Semahot,* chap. 8, records that in times when burial was made in cavernous crypts, it was customary to visit the crypt during the first three days following interment in order to examine the burial site for signs of life.[19] It is recorded that on one occasion a person so buried was later found to be alive. Moreover he is reported to have sired a number of children before his ultimate death some twenty-five years later.[20]

In any event, if life may at times continue after respiration has ceased, it would then appear that absence of respiration is at best a sign that death may be presumed to have occurred but is not, in itself, one and the same as death. This is indeed the conclusion drawn by R. Shalom Mordecai Schwadron, the author of *Teshuvot Maharsham.* In vol. VI, no. 124 of his responsa, this authority states that the dictum "primary life is in the nose" indicates that in ordinary situations, where there is no evidence to the contrary, one may rely upon examination of the nostrils, since in virtually all instances life has completely ebbed prior to cessation of respiration. Instances where this is not the case are so extremely rare that such contingencies need not be considered. Yet, maintains *Maharsham,* if any sign of life is observed in other limbs, examination of the nose may not be accepted as conclusive. In the case presented for his consideration, he indicates that a noise apparently emanating from the body after breathing had ceased would necessitate further delay in order to determine with certainty that death had indeed occurred.

Maimonides, *Guide for the Perplexed,* Book 1, chap 42, describes the occurrence of such a phenomenon in support of his contention that the term *mavet* is a homonym and that in Biblical usage this term in certain places means "severe illness" rather than "death." In the narrative concerning Nabal's demise Scripture reports, ". . . and his heart died within him and he became hard as stone" (I Sam. 25:37), and then goes on to state, "And it came to pass after ten days and the Lord smote Nabal and he died" (I Sam. 25:38). Maimonides cites Andalusian authors who interpret the phrase "and his heart died within him" of the earlier passage as meaning "that his breath was suspended, so that no breathing could be perceived at all, as sometimes an invalid is seized with a fainting fit and attacks of asphyxia, and it cannot be discovered whether he is alive or dead, and in this condition the patient may remain one day or two."[21]

It would appear that a divergent view is espoused by *Ḥatam Sofer,* who indicates that death is synonymous with cessation of respiration. *Teshuvot Ḥatam Sofer, Yoreh De'ah,* no. 338, states that the commandment "And if a man have committed a sin worthy of death, and he be put to death . . . his body shall not remain all night upon the tree, but thou shalt surely bury him the same day . . ." (Deut. 21:23) implies a clearly defined definition of death. Halakhah deems cessation of respiratory activity to constitute such a definition. This tradition, according to *Ḥatam Sofer,* was either (1) received from the scientists of antiquity, even though it has been "forgotten" by contemporary physicians, or (2) received by Moses on Mt. Sinai, or (3) derived from the verse "all which has the breath of the spirit of life in his nostrils" (Gen 2:6). "This necessarily is the *shi'ur* [the term *shi'ur* should in this context be understood as meaning "clinical symptom of death"] received by us with regard to all corpses from the time that the congregation of the Lord became a holy nation." *Hatam Sofer,* while not spelling out the issue at stake, quite obviously views cessation of respiration as itself constituting death rather than as being merely symptomatic of death. However, in developing this thesis, *Hatam Sofer* appears to broaden his definition of death by requiring the presence of yet another necessary condition. *Hatam Sofer* cites the previously mentioned phenomenon described by the Andalusians and accounts for the situation described by them by stating that although in the incident described respiration had ceased, nevertheless the pulse was still detectable either at the temples or at the neck. Without making an explicit statement to this effect, *Hatam Sofer* here seems nevertheless to amend his definition of death and now appears to state that death occurs only if both pulse beat and respiration have ceased.[22] This definition of death is thus compatible with the previously cited view supported by *Yoma* 85a that death is to be identified with absence of respiration coupled with prior cessation of cardiac activity. Although death occurs only upon the conjunction of both physiological occurrences, cessation of respiration is accepted as the sole operational definition because, in the vast majority of cases, it is indicative of prior cardiac arrest. *Hatam Sofer* summarizes his position in the statement, "But in any case, once he lies like an inanimate stone, there being no pulse whatsoever, and if subsequently breathing ceases, we have only the words of our holy Torah that he is dead." Accordingly, concludes *Hatam Sofer,* the corpse must be buried without delay and a *kohen* dare not defile himself by touching the corpse after these signs of death are in evidence. Cases such as those described in *Semahot* 8:1 are extremely unusual, to say the least, and are dismissed by *Hatam Sofer* as being comparable to the celebrated story of Honi the Circle-Drawer (*Ta'anit* 23a), who slept for seventy years. Oddities such as these occur with such great rarity that Halakhah need not take cognizance of such contingencies.[23] In the same vein, R. Hayyim Joseph David Azulai, *Teshuvot Hayyim Sha'al,* II, no. 25, declares that when the statutory signs of death are present, it is incumbent upon us to execute burial without delay, "and if in one of many tens of thousands of cases it happens that he is alive, there does not [devolve] upon us the slightest transgression, for so has it been decreed upon us . . . and if we err in these signs [of death], such was His decree, may He be blessed."

IV

Currently, in an age of medical progress, the paramount question is not simply whether burial should be delayed on the chance that life may yet exist, but rather to what extent it is mandatory to engage in attempts at resuscitation. In terms of definitive Halakhah, there is no question whatsoever that the physician is obligated to utilize all means available to him in order to revive the patient. This may be established in several ways. It goes without saying that according to the authorities who deem the cessation of respiration to be merely symptomatic of the absence of life, there obviously exists such an obligation as long as there is any prospect of resuscitation, no matter how remote the chances of success may be. Such an obligation most certainly exists if any other clinical signs of life, such as brain activity as recorded by an electroencephalogram, are in evidence. Secondly, in light of Rema's ruling that we are incompetent to apply the criterion of respiration, there exists a *safek,* or doubt, as to the presence of death during the twenty, thirty or sixty minutes following what appears to us to be cessation of respiration. There obviously devolves upon the physician a definite obligation to resuscitate the patient within this period even if this involves violation of the Sabbath laws or of other Biblical prohibitions. The question, then, requires analysis only with regard to the position of those authorities who maintain that death is to be defined as the cessation of both respiration and cardiac activity. In light of Rema's ruling, the question becomes actual only after the requisite period of time has elapsed following the cessation of respiratory activity so that death may be established with certainty. Despite these considerations, it may be argued that if any clinical signs of life are present the patient may not be presumed to have actually died. A contemporary authority, Rabbi Eliezer Waldenberg, *Ẓiẓ Eli'ezer,* X, no. 25, chap. 4, sec. 5, asserts that inherent in *Ḥatam Sofer's* position is the assumption that whenever other clinical signs of life are evident, respiration is indeed taking place, albeit unperceived by us. Accordingly, the physician is obligated to use all available means to preserve life, even in the absence of perceivable respiration. In a similar vein, Rabbi Moses Sternbuch, in a recently published booklet, *Ba'ayot ha-Zeman be-Hashkafat ha-Torah,* I, 9, states that the Talmudic source (*Yoma* 85a) advisedly employs the example of a person crushed under a heap of rubble as a paradigm case because in situations where artificial respiration or similar measures are possible the person cannot be considered to be dead simply because breathing has ceased. Nevertheless, adds Rabbi Sternbuch, when such measures are of no avail, the time of death must be retroactively established as coinciding with cessation of respiration.[24]

The question thus becomes purely theoretical. As noted, *Ḥatam Sofer* maintains that death is to be defined as the total absence of respiration and cardiac activity to the exclusion of other clinical signs. It follows from this position that if it could be determined with absolute certainty that these activities had indeed ceased — and it must be borne in mind that the previously cited authorities maintain that such a determination is impossible — subsequent resuscitation, if accomplished, would, in fact, constitute a form of "resurrection" of the dead. Is there any obligation upon the physician to restore life to the dead, or are his obligations limited to healing the living? If it could be conclusively determined that the patient has already expired, may Sabbath laws and other halakhic proscriptions be set aside in order to effect resuscitation?

This question in one of its guises is raised by *Tosafot, Bava Meẓi'a* 114b, who questions the permissibility of Elijah's resuscitation of the son of the widow of Zarephath. The Talmudic view is that Elijah and Phinehas were one and the same person. Since Phinehas was a priest, he was forbidden to defile himself by physical contact with the dead. How, then, was he permitted to revive the son of the widow of Zarephath?

Several commentaries, by virtue of their answers to the query presented by *Tosafot,* indicate that, in their opinion, there is no obligation whatsoever to resurrect the dead. The *Shitah Mekubezet* parallels the previously cited view of Maimonides in stating that the child was not dead but merely in a swoon. Rosh,[25] Radbaz[26] and Abrabanel[27] all state that Elijah's act was a form of *hora'at sha'ah*—an action having express divine sanction limited to the specific case at hand—and from which no normative halakhic practice can be deduced.

Tosafot answers that since Elijah was certain of the success of his endeavor, violation of the priestly code was permissible for the sake of preservation of human life. *Ḥemdat Yisra'el,*[28] in quoting *Tosafot's* line of reasoning, points out that we do not find any source indicating an obligation to resurrect the dead; the obligation to preserve human life extends only to those yet living, not to those already deceased. Furthermore, if the halakhic category of preservation of life encompasses resurrection of the dead, then the obligation should logically extend even to cases of doubtful success, no matter how remote such chances may be, as is the rule with regard to preservation of the life of those living. Accordingly, all halakhic restrictions should be suspended even in cases of doubt. If so, *Tosafot's* insertion of the words "since he was certain of being able to resurrect life" is incomprehensible. It has been suggested[29] that there is an obligation to resuscitate or "resurrect" the dead, but that this obligation is not encompassed within the general obligation to preserve life. Rather, according to this interpretation, the obligation to restore life to one who has already died is based upon the rationale adduced by the Gemara, *Yoma* 85b, "Better to desecrate one Sabbath on his behalf in order that he may observe many Sabbaths." The concern then is to enhance the total number of *mitzvot* performed. Since this is the sole halakhic consideration mandating resuscitation of one already dead, *Tosafot* reasons that no halakhic prohibition may be violated in the process unless there is absolute certainty with regard to the success of such efforts.[30]

In sharp disagreement with this interpretation of *Tosafot,* R. Jehiel Jacob

Weinberg asserts that *Tosafot* does not mean to invoke the commandment regarding preservation of human life; rather, asserts R. Weinberg, *Tosafot* regards resuscitation as a form of "honor of the deceased" since there can be no greater honor than resuscitation. Halakhah stipulates that a priest may defile himself in order to accord the honor of burial to a corpse which would otherwise remain uninterred (a *met mitzvah*). According to this interpretation, *Tosafot* reasons that priestly defilement is also permissible under the same conditions in order to accord the deceased the "honor" of resurrection. Since Elijah alone was capable of reviving the dead child, Elijah was permitted to defile himself for this purpose. However, such defilement is permitted only if success is assured since defilement is sanctioned only when resultant honor to the deceased is a certainty. Thus, according to Rabbi Weinberg's analysis of *Tosafot*, other commandments may not be violated even if success could be predicted with certainty, since only the prohibition against priestly defilement may be set aside in order to honor the dead; whereas, according to *Ḥemdat Yisra'el*, all prohibitions, e.g., desecration of the Sabbath, are suspended under such circumstances.[31]

It should be reiterated that the foregoing discussion is purely theoretical. In terms of practical Halakhah, both Rabbi Waldenberg and Rabbi Sternbuch stress that the exact moment of death cannot be determined with precision. Accordingly, when there is a possibility of resuscitation, everything possible must be done to restore the patient to life.[31a] In application, it is only *irreversible* cessation of respiratory and cardiac activity accompanied by total absence of movement which constitute the halakhic criteria of death.

V

It must be emphasized that in all these questions involving the very heart of a physician's obligations with regard to the preservation of human life, halakhic Judaism demands of him that he govern himself by the norms of Jewish law whether or not these determinations coincide with the mores of contemporary society. Brain death and irreversible coma are not acceptable definitions of death insofar as Halakhah is concerned. The sole criterion of death accepted by Halakhah is total cessation of both cardiac and respiratory activity. Even when these indications are present, there is a definite obligation to resuscitate the patient, if at all feasible. Jewish law recognizes the malformed, the crippled, the terminally ill and the mentally retarded as human beings in the full sense of the term. Hence the physician's obligation with regard to medical treatment and resuscitation is in no way diminished by the fact that the resuscitated patient may be a victim of brain damage or other debilitating injury.

Of late, there has been increased discussion of a patient's right to "die with dignity" and a general urging that physicians not overly prolong the lives of comatose patients who are incurably ill. It is exceedingly difficult to argue against an individual's right to "die with dignity." This phrase, so pregnant with approbation, bespeaks a concept which is rapidly joining motherhood, the Fourth of July and apple pie as one of the great American values.

Certainly one has a right to dignity both in life and in death. But is death, properly speaking, a *right?* Suicide is forbidden both by religious and temporal law. It is proscribed because Western culture has long recognized that man's life is not his own to dispose of at will. This fundamental concept is expressed most cogently by Plato in his *Phaedo.* Socrates, in a farewell conversation with his students prior to his execution, speaks of the afterlife with eager anticipation. Thereupon one of his disciples queries, if death is so much preferable to life, why did not Socrates long ago take his own life? In a very apt simile, Socrates responds that an ox does not have the right to take its own life because it thereby deprives its master of the enjoyment of his property.[32] Man is the chattel of the gods, says Socrates. Just as "bovicide" on the part of the ox is a violation of the proprietor-property relationship, so suicide on the part of man constitutes a violation of the Creator-creature relationship.

Man does not possess absolute title to his life or to his body. He is but the steward of the life which he has been privileged to receive. Man is charged with preserving, dignifying, and hallowing that life. He is obliged to seek food and sustenance in order to safeguard the life he has been granted; when falling victim to illness and disease he is obligated to seek a cure in order to sustain life. Never is he called upon to determine whether life is worth living—this is a question over which God remains sole arbiter.

Surely, even on the basis of humanistic assumptions, one must recognize that human life must remain inviolate. As long as life is indeed present, the decision to terminate such life is beyond the competence of man. In pragmatic terms, a decision not to prolong life means precluding the application of some new advance in therapeutics that would secure a remission or cure for that patient should a breakthrough occur. But, more fundamentally, man lacks the right to assess the quality of any human life and to determine that it is beneficial for that life to be terminated; all human life is of inestimable value. If the comatose may be caused to "die with dignity," what of the mentally deranged and the feeble-minded incapable of "meaningful" human activity? Withdrawal of treatment leads directly to overt acts of euthanasia; from there it may be but a short step to selective elimination of those whose life is deemed a burden upon society at large.

Undoubtedly, caring for a patient *in extremis* places a heavy burden upon the family, the medical practitioner and hospital facilities. It is natural for us, both individually and collectively, to harbor feelings of resentment because of the toll exacted from us. But we must recognize that preservation of any value demands sacrifices. Above all, we must be on guard against self-interest cloaked in altruism, against allowing self-serving motives to find expression in the language of idealism.

Attempts have been made in the past to make the right to life subservient to other values. The results have been tragic. Hannah Arendt and others have pointed out that in the scale of values accepted in Germany during the World War II era, obedience to law took priority over the sanctity of human life. Yet we have refused to accept this argument as a valid line of defense, because we believe it to be self-evident that the right to life is a right which has been endowed upon all men by their Creator. A person's right to life, as long as it does not conflict with another's right to life, is inviolate. And the right to life precludes the right to hasten death either overtly or covertly. The teachings of Judaism in this regard are nowhere expressed more eloquently than in the *Siddur:*

> My God, the soul which You have placed within me is pure. *You* have created it; *You* have fashioned it; *You* have breathed it into me and *You* preserve it within me; *and You will at some time take it from me* and return it to me in the time to come. As long as the soul is within me I will give thanks unto You . . .

NOTES

1. *Jerusalem Post,* November 14, 1968; *Hirntod* (Stuttgart, 1969), pp. 63, 66, 98, and 106. See Jacob Levy, *Mavet Moḥi, Ha-Ma'ayan,* Nisan 5732, p. 25; J. B. Brierly, J. H. Adams, D. I. Graham, *et al.,* "Neocortical Death after Cardiac Arrest," *Lancet* 2:560–65, 1971; Hadassah Gillon, "Defining Death Anew," *Science News* 95 (January 11, 1969), p. 50; Harold L. Hirsch, *Case and Comment,* September-October 1974; *Rochester Democrat and Chronicle,* March 19, 1975, p. 19. Cf. also Henry K. Beecher, "Definitions of 'Life' and 'Death' for Medical Science and Practice," *Annals of the New York Academy of Sciences,* vol. 169, art. 2 (January 21, 1971), pp. 471–472; E. Bental and U. Leibowitz, "Flat Electroencephalograms During 28 Days in Case of 'Encephalitis,' " *Electroenceph. Clin. Neurophysiology,* XIII (1961), 457–460; R. G. Bickford, B. Dawson and H. Takeshita, "EEG Evidence of Neurologic Death," *Electroenceph. Clin. Neurophysiology,* XVIII (1965), 513–514; T. D. Bird and F. Plum, "Recovery from Barbiturate Overdose Coma with Prolonged Isoelectric Electroencephalogram," *Neurology,* XVIII (1968), 456–460; R. L. Tentler *et al.,* "Electroencephalographic Evidence of Cortical 'Death' Followed by Full Recovery: Protective Action of Hypothermia," *Journal of the American Medical Association,* CLXIV (1957), 1667–1670; P. Braunstein, J. Korein *et al.,* "A Simple Bedside Evaluation of Cerebral Blood Flow in the Study of Cerebral Death." *The American Journal of Roentgenology Radium Therapy and Nuclear Medecine,* CXVIII (1973), 758; and P. Braunstein, I. Kricheff, *et al.,* "Cerebral Death: A Rapid and Reliable Diagnostic Adjunct Using Radiosotopes," *Journal of Nuclear Medecine,* XIV (1973), 122.

2. "A Definition of Irreversible Coma," *Journal of the American Medical Association,* vol. 205, no. 6 (August 5, 1968), pp. 337–40.

3. This modification appears in Beecher, *Annals,* p. 471.

4. *Loc. cit.*

5. *Loc. cit.*

6. Robert M. Veatch, "Brain Death: Welcome Definition or Dangerous Judgment?" *Hastings Center Report,* II, no. 5 (November 1972), p. 11.

7. There is no opinion recorded in the Babylonian Talmud—majority or minority—which *requires* examination of the heart. See, however, Palestinian Talmud, *Yoma* 8:5, where the correct textual reading is the subject of dispute. According to the version of *Korban ha-Edah,* one *Amora* requires examination of the heart. *P'nei Moshe,* in accepting a variant reading, rejects this contention.

8. *Mishneh Torah, Hilkhot Shabbat* 2:19.

9. *Oraḥ Ḥayyim* 329:4.

10. See R. Eliezer Waldenberg, *Ẓiẓ Eli'ezer,* X, no. 25, chap. 4, sec. 7. Cf. also *Ẓiẓ Eli'ezer,* IX, no. 46, sec. 5, who cites medieval writers on physiology—among them *Sha'ar ha-Shamayim,* a work which is attributed to the father of Gersonides— who declare that life is dependent upon nasal respiration because warm air from the heart is expelled through the nose and cold air, which cools the heart, enters through the nose. It was thus clearly recognized that respiration without cardiac activity is an impossibility.

11. However, according to the previously cited reading and interpretation of *Korban ha-Edah,* there is one opinion in the Palestinian Talmud which requires examination for presence of a heartbeat to the exclusion of examination for respiration. The most plausible explanation of this ruling is that it is based upon the empirical belief that the presence of a heartbeat is more readily detectable than respiration and hence absence of a heartbeat is deemed to be a more reliable clinical symptom of respiratory stoppage than absence of perceived respiration.

12. *Oraḥ Ḥayyim* 330:5.

13. *Yoreh De'ah* 339:1.

14. *Koret ha-Berit,* no. 330, sec. 15, infers from the phraseology adopted by Rema that the latter does not at all disagree with the *Shulḥan Arukh* but simply endeavors to provide the rationale underlying the prevalent custom. See *Ẓiẓ Eli'ezer,* X, no. 25, chap. 4, sec. 4.

15. A waiting period of "at least one full hour" before moving the deceased is also cited by Hyman Goldin, *Ha-Madrikh,* p. 111, in the name of *Derekh ha-Ḥayyim.* Although there are several works bearing this title which discuss laws of mourning and related topics, none of them appears to contain a source for this citation.

It is interesting to note that the previously cited report of the Ad Hoc Committee of the Harvard Medical School requires "observations covering a period of at least one hour by physicians" to satisfy the criteria of no spontaneous muscular movements or spontaneous respiration as one of the characteristics of irreversible coma.

16. See also R. Ephraim Oshry, *She'elot u-Teshuvot mi-Ma'amakim,* II, no. 10.

17. Also, the phraseology used by Rema is different from that which is usually employed by Rema in disagreeing with a ruling of *Shulḥan Arukh.* See numerous sources cited by R. Solomon Schneider, *Ha-Ma'or,* Kislev-Tevet 5735.

17a. See also *Yalkut Shimoni,* Lekh Lekha, no. 77.

18. Cf. R. Baruch ha-Levi Epstein, *Torah Temimah,* Gen. 7:22.

19. It should be noted that both *Ḥatam Sofer* and Rabbi Gagin in his previously cited responsum, *Yismaḥ Lev, Yoreh De'ah,* no. 9, state that this procedure was by no means obligatory; the practice was merely sanctioned as not constituting *darkei ha-Emori,* a forbidden pagan practice.

20. Indeed, Moses Mendelssohn sought to use this source as a basis for permitting delayed burial in contravention of the halakhic requirement of immediate burial. Mendelssohn contended that such delay is necessary in order to ascertain that death has actually occurred. See *Ha-Me'assef* (1785), pp. 152–55, 169–74, and 178–87. This material was reprinted in *Bikkurei ha-Ittim* (1824), p. 219–24 and 229–38. Mendelssohn's advocacy of delayed burial and the ensuing controversy are discussed in detail by Alexander Altmann, *Moses Mendelssohn: A Biographical Study* (University Ala., 1973), pp. 288–93. See also *Teshuvot Hatam Sofer, Yoreh De'ah,* no. 338.

21. This exposition of Maimonides' position follows the interpretation advanced by Abrabanel in the latter's commentary on the text of the *Guide* and appear to be the most facile analysis of Maimonides' comments. Cf., however, Shem Tov, who sees the Andalusians as denying the miraculous resurrection of the son of the woman of Zarephath (I Kings 17:17) and claims that Maimonides himself accepted the position of the Andalusians. Narboni and Ibn Kaspi also ascribe such views to Maimonides. Ibn Kaspi attempts to show that Maimonides was herein following the Talmudic interpretation of this narrative. According to Ibn Kaspi, the Talmudic exposition does not consider the described phenomenon to be a case of resurrection. Maimonides was severely (and, according to Abrabanel, erroneously) attacked by others for denying that the son of the woman of Zarephath was resurrected since these authorities view Maimonides' position as being contradictory to the rabbinic interpretation of the relevant passages. Cf. the letter of R. Judah ibn Alfakhar to R. David Kimḥi in *Koveẓ Teshuvot ha-Rambam* (Lichtenberg, Leipzig, 1859), p. 29, and *Teshuvot Rivash,* no. 45. Cf. also *Teshuvot Hatam Sofer, Yoreh De'ah,* no. 338, who interprets Maimonides as accepting the resurrection of the son of the woman of Zarephath literally but denying Elisha's resurrection of the son of the Shunammite. (II Kings 4:34–35).

22. Rabbi Moses Sternbuch, *Ba'ayot ha-Zeman be-Hashkafat ha-Torah,* I, 10, asserts that according to *Hatam Sofer,* absence of respiration is sufficient to establish death unless the person is in a swoon. However, in a state of swoon it is possible for the person to be alive and yet not to breathe. Hence the possibility of a swoon must be ruled out before lack of respiration may be accepted as conclusive evidence that death has occurred. Rabbi Sternbuch evidently interprets *Hatam Sofer* as believing that lack of respiration is merely symptomatic of death rather than constituting death in and of itself.

23. Rabbi I. Y. Unterman, *"Ba'ayot Hashtalat ha-Lev le-Or ha-Halakhah,"* *Torah she-be-'al Peh* (5729), p. 13 and *No'am,* XIII (5730), p. 3, points out that *Hatam Sofer* is speaking specifically of a patient suffering from a lingering illness and whose condition has steadily deteriorated. These symptoms, declares R. Unterman, cannot be regarded as definitive signs of death with regard to one who has experienced a sudden seizure. In such cases, all resources of medical science must be employed to save human life. Although he does not elaborate, R. Unterman presumably means that we may not accept our inability to detect these signs of life as conclusive evidence of their absence. R. Waldenberg, *Ẓiẓ Eli'ezer,* X, no. 25, chap. 4, no. 5, quite obviously disagrees with this view. *Ẓiẓ Eli'ezer* cites the symptoms advanced by *Hatam Sofer* as reliable criteria of death in all instances. R. Waldenberg explains the numerous cases in which the patient has been restored to life following cessation of respiration as instances wherein respiration was indeed present but not perceived. The physician may, nevertheless, rely upon his determination that respiration has ceased in pronouncing death. Nevertheless, "if it is possible for him to conduct further tests in the anticipation that he may perhaps find life, certainly it is incumbent upon him to do so; however, as to the primary determining factor, with regard to this we have only the words of our Torah and the

tradition of our fathers . . .''

24. This is also the position of R. Solomon Zalman Auerbach. See R. Gavriel Krauss, *Ha-Ma'ayan,* Tishri 5729, p. 20.

25. Quoted by *Shitah Mekubezet, Bava Mezia* 114b.

26. Vol. V, no. 2203.

27. Commentary of the *Guide,* I, 42. Puzzling is the parallel cited by Abrabanel concerning the slaying of Zimri and Cozbi by Phineas (Num. 25:6–8), a deed which necessarily involved the latter's defilement. The rabbinic view is that since Phineas was born before the consecration of Eliezer, he was not a priest by virtue of genealogical descent and, accordingly, required personal consecration to achieve priestly status. Rabbinic tradition views the verse "Behold I give him my covenant of peace" (Num. 26:12) as recording that this status was accorded him as a reward for his zeal in the matter of Zimri. Thus, at the time of the slaying, Phineas had not yet attained the status of a priest and was not bound by the priestly prohibition regarding defilement (See *Zevahim* 101b).

28. R. Meir Dan Plocki, *Hemdat Yisra'el, Maftehot ve-Hosafot,* p.33. This position is also stated emphatically by R. Moses Feinstein, *Iggerot Moshe, Yoreh De'ah,* II, no. 174. Rabbi Feinstein suggests that the preservation of life referred to by *Tosafot* is either the life of the child's grief-stricken mother or perhaps that of Elijah himself.

29. See R. Jehiel Jacob Weinberg, *No'am* IX, (5726), p. 214, reprinted in *Seridei Esh,* III, no. 127, p. 350. Rabbi Weinberg cites this exposition as that of *Hemdat Yisra'el* and after disagreeing substitutes his own interpretation. However, an examination of *Hemdat Yisra'el, loc. cit.,* shows that R. Plocki offers an interpretation similar to that advanced by R. Weinberg himself.

30. A similar view is expressed by R. Naphtali Zevi Judah Berlin, *Ha'amek She'elah,* no. 166, sec. 17. R. Berlin asserts that the ruling of *Ba'al Halakhot Gedolot* permitting desecration of the Sabbath on behalf of an embryo even within the first forty days of gestation applies only to cases where the medical efficacy of the therapeutic technique is a known certainty. The argument is that such activity can be sanctioned within the first forty days of gestation only upon application of the principle "Better to desecrate a single Sabbath on his behalf so he may observe many Sabbaths," which is operative only if there exists positive knowledge of the capacity for such future observance, rather than upon the general obligation to preserve human life which would mandate suspension of Sabbath laws even if the outcome is doubtful.

31. For another interpretation of *Tosafot's* comments see Rabbi I. Y. Unterman, *Ha-Torah ve-ha-Medinah,* IV, 25 f. R. Unterman cites Rema, *Yoreh De'ah* 155:3, who rules that untested or unknown modes of therapy may not be employed even in face of danger to life when such therapy involves an otherwise forbidden act. The action of Elijah, argues R. Unterman, constituted an "unknown" form of therapy and hence was permissible only by virtue of the certainty of its success.

31a. See also *Ziz Eli'ezer,* IX, no. 46, sec. 4; R. Unterman, *Torah she-be-al Peh,* XI (5729), 13; and above n. 24.

32. In halakhic literature this concept is developed by Radbaz in his commentary on Rambam, *Hilkhot Sanhedrin* 18:6. It is a basic halakhic principle that, while a defendant's testimony is accorded absolute credibility with regard to establishing financial liability, a confession of guilt is never accepted as evidence of criminal culpability. Citing the verse "Behold, all souls are Mine" (Ezek. 18:4), Radbaz explains that while material goods belong to man and may be disposed of at will, the human body is the possession of God and may be punished only by Him. See also Rambam, *Hilkhot Roze'ah* 1:4 and *Shulhan Arukh ha-Rav,* VI, *Hilkhot Nizkei Guf* 4.

18
The Halakhic Definition of Death
AARON SOLOVEICHIK

The basic halakhic source for the definition of death is a passage in the Talmud. The Mishnah states as follows:

> If debris of a collapsing building falls on someone and he is found alive, the finder should remove the debris (even on the Sabbath); but if he is dead, the finder should leave him. [1]

Commenting on this Mishnah, the Gemara states: "How far does one search (to ascertain whether he is dead or alive)? Until his nose. Some say up to his heart. Rav Papa says: the disagreement is only where the finder searches from the feet upward, but if he started examining the victim from the head downward, everyone agrees that immediately upon finding the victim devoid of breathing, the latter must be left where he was found (until after the Sabbath)." [2]

Maimonides rules as follows: "If upon examination, no sign of breathing can be detected at the nose, the victim must be left where he is because he is already dead." [3]

Maimonides thus explicitly codifies the ruling in accordance with the first opinion recorded in the Gemara, that is to say the victim is to be considered dead upon a determination that he is devoid of breathing. This is also the ruling of Jacob ben Asher *(Tur)* and Joseph Caro, author of the *Shulḥan Arukh*. [4] The only early authority who follows the second opinion recorded in the Gemara, i.e., that the victim is to be considered dead when it is determined that his heart has stopped, is Baḥya ben Asher (Rabbenu Baḥya) as stated in his commentary on the Pentateuch.

The *Shulḥan Arukh* states that "even if the victim was found so severely injured that he cannot live for more than a short while, one must probe the debris until one reaches his nose. If one cannot detect signs of respiration at the nose, he is certainly dead whether the head was uncovered first or whether the feet were uncovered first." It thus seems that cessation of respiration is the determining physical sign for the ascertainment of death. However, there are two halakhic rulings which appear to be inconsistent with the proposition that cessation of respiration marks the termination of life. One ruling is by Maimonides who states the following: "Whosoever closes the eyes of a dying person while the soul is departing is shedding blood. One should wait a while; perhaps he is only in a swoon."[5] Maimonides is obviously referring to a person in whom respiration has ceased completely for if not, even if one waited a while, one would not be able to consider the person to be dead.

If that is the case, why can we not treat the dying person as dead without waiting a while (approximately half an hour) inasmuch as the respiration has ceased? It can, therefore, be deduced from this Maimonidean ruling that a dying person cannot be considered completely dead immediately upon the cessation of respiration. The rationale behind this ruling is that a dying person may become completely devoid of respiration and pulsation, yet other bodily activities, including that of the brain, continue to function for a short period of time. There have been cases in which a person had suffered a severe heart attack as a result of which he had no heart pulsation or breathing for a period of five minutes but was completely resuscitated with the aid of machines (pacemaker and respirator). One cannot argue that such an individual was completely dead and was then resurrected. Doctors are not endowed with the power of resurrecting the dead.

We can, therefore, conclude that the ruling cited by Maimonides[6] strongly implies that the absence of spontaneous respiration does not in itself determine death. Furthermore, in his commentary on the Mishnah, Maimonides makes a statement which confirms the thesis that cessation of respiration *per se* does not constitute death. The Mishnah reads as follows:

> A man does not convey uncleanness (as a corpse) until his soul is gone forth. Even if his arteries are severed or even if he is on the verge of death, he still makes levirate marriage obligatory and liberates from levirate marriage; he qualifies (his mother) from eating *terumah* (heave offering). Similarly, cattle and beasts do not convey uncleanness until their soul is gone forth. If their heads have been cut off, even though they (the animals) are moving convulsively, they are unclean — like the tail of a lizard which moves convulsively (after it is cut off).[7]

Maimonides makes the following comment on the above Mishnah:

> Spasmodic jerking of the muscles can take place in a heretofore living

organism even after the death of the organism. This type of locomotion is not indicative of life because the power of locomotion that is spread in the limb does not originate in one center but is independently spread through the body.

It follows from this Maimonidean assertion that if the central control (actual or potential) is still operating within the organism, then the latter is not dead even though spontaneous respiration and cardiac pulsations have ceased. The reason is that central control (of movement) is a basic life function. Consequently, a person cannot be declared dead as long as a basic life function is still operating. This means that as long as the brain is capable of producing electric waves, the person is not dead even if spontaneous respiration has ceased. These two rulings of Maimonides are apparently inconsistent with a third ruling in which Maimonides states that "if upon examination, no sign of breathing can be detected at the nose, the victim (in the rubble of a collapsed building) must be left where he is (until after the Sabbath) because he is already dead."[8]

The second source which seems to be inconsistent with the proposition that cessation of respiration marks the termination of life is the ruling of R. Moses Isserles (Rema), in his gloss on Caro's *Shulḥan Arukh*. *Shulḥan Arukh* states the following:

> If a woman is sitting on the birthstool and she dies, one may bring a knife on the Sabbath even through a public domain, and one incises her womb and removes the fetus since one might find it alive.[9]

Rema adds this statement:

> However, today we do not conduct ourselves according to this rule even during the week because we are not competent to precisely determine the moment of maternal death.

Magen Avraham, in his commentary,[10] explains the assertion of Rema on the basis of the fact that if the fetus is to be saved it must be removed from the mother's womb immediately upon the death of the mother. This cannot be done because cessation of breathing and cessation of the heartbeat are not conclusive evidence of the death of the mother. A short time must elapse from the apparent death of the mother (i.e. from the time breathing and the heartbeat stop). By that time, it is too late to save the fetus.

This line of reasoning seems to be inconsistent with the ruling of the *Shulḥan Arukh* elsewhere in which it is stated:

> even if the victim was found so severely injured that he cannot live for more than a short while, one must continue to probe the debris until one reaches the nose. If one cannot detect signs of respiration at the nose, he is

certainly dead, whether the head was uncovered first or whether the feet were uncovered first.[11]

Let us examine the Talmudic discussion[12] in which two sages disagree in regard to a person who was found on the Sabbath beneath a heap of stones (i.e., a collapsed building) and the debris was uncovered from the victim's feet up to and above the heart and no heartbeat was detected. Is the finder to anticipate that the victim is alive and, consequently, should the finder then continue to desecrate the Sabbath further by removing the debris? Or is the finder to assume that the victim is dead? Consequently, may the Sabbath no longer be desecrated and must the victim be left under the debris until after the Sabbath? The first sage cited by the Talmud asserts that the finder cannot consider the victim to be dead until he examines his nose and finds no breath emanating from it. The second sage, however, says that immediately upon detecting the absence of the heartbeat, the finder is to consider the victim to be dead. Consequently, the finder may no longer desecrate the Sabbath on the victim's behalf.

R. Papa states [13] that if the finder uncovers the debris from the head of the victim proceeding downward, both sages would agree that immediately upon detecting cessation of respiration in the victim, the finder is to consider the victim to be dead and cease the desecration of the Sabbath on the victim's behalf. This means both sages agree that cessation of respiration is a sign of death. The second sage, however, is of the opinion that the lack of a heartbeat is also a sign of death whereas the view of the first sage is that only a lack of spontaneous breathing is a sign of death.

Maimonides, *Tur* and *Shulḥan Arukh* rule in accordance with the opinion of the first sage whereas Rabbenu Baḥya rules according to the second sage. Rabbenu Baḥya, in his commentary on the scriptural verse "and thou shalt love the Lord thy God with all thine heart," states the following:

> . . . the heart is the seat of the soul and the heart. And because it is the first organ in the creation of man and the last to die of all the organs of the body, Scripture states *with all thine heart,* that is to say until the last moment of death.[14]

It is possible to interpret the Talmudic discussion in three different ways. Firstly, one can say that the disagreement between the two sages concerns the question of whether or not cessation of the heartbeat *per se* constitutes death. The first sage would then be of the opinion that the scriptural verse "all in whose nostrils was the breath of the spirit of life"[15] implies that cessation of respiration constitutes death and the complete termination of life. Cessation of the heartbeat, according to the first sage, does not constitute death. According to the view of the second sage, cessation of the heartbeat constitutes death. The scriptural verse implies that absence of spontaneous respiration is symptomatic of death, not that lack of breath *per se* constitutes death. In view of the fact that cessation of the heartbeat virtually always accompanies cessation of respiration, the absence of breathing serves as an indication that the heart has also ceased beating. This seems to be Rabbenu Baḥya's analysis of this Talmudic discussion. Rabbenu Baḥya rules in accordance with the opinion of the second sage. However, those rabbinic authorities who rule in accordance with the opinion of the first sage might still agree with Rabbenu Baḥya's view that the disagreement between the first and the second sage in the Talmudic discussion concerns the question as to whether lack of respiration or lack of a heartbeat *per se* is indicative of the end of life.

A second interpretation of this Talmudic discussion is that lack of spontaneous respiration *per se* does not constitute death. However, if a person is found beneath a heap of stones and his nose is examined and found to be devoid of breath, a conclusive presumption is established that the victim is devoid not only of respiration but of all basic bodily functions. This is the opinion of the first sage. According to the second sage, the same conclusive presumption is established by a determination that the victim is devoid of a heartbeat. From the language of Rashi's commentary, it appears that he adopted this interpretation. Rashi comments:

> If the victim resembles a dead person whose limbs are motionless like a stone, how far may the finder probe the debris (on the Sabbath) to know the truth? Up to the nose! And if there is no life in his nose in that there is no air emanating therefrom, he is certainly dead and must be left there (until after the Sabbath).[16]

According to Rashi, the absence of respiration is considered to be a sign of death only if the victim is motionless like a stone. But if the limbs of the victim move even the slightest bit, the victim is not dead. If cessation of respiration *per se* constitutes death, it should follow that even if the victim is not motionless he would be considered as dead.

A third interpretation of the Talmudic discussion in *Yoma* 85a may be advanced in order to resolve the apparent inconsistencies in Maimonides' code cited above. It will also serve to resolve the apparent inconsistency between the ruling in *Shulḥan Arukh* 329 that cessation of respiration is the conclusive sign and the gloss of Rema on *Shulḥan Arukh* 330:5 that today we are not competent to determine the exact moment of maternal death and, therefore, are not allowed, even on weekdays, to incise the womb of a woman whose breathing has stopped. According to the third interpretation, death is defined as the termination of all basic life functions. This includes every bodily function that emanates from a controlling center such as the brain. Brain function must also have terminated before a person is halakhically dead. As long as any function that is not of a local nature (e.g.

reflex twitching after decapitation) but which emanates from a controlling center is still operative, the person is not dead.

Thus, if a person has suffered a severe concussion of the brain and as a result has no spontaneous respiration or heartbeat, but the brain still produces electrical activity as recorded on an electroencephalogram, the person is not considered to be dead. Nevertheless, the scriptural phrase "all in whose nostrils was the breath of the spirit of life" implies that respiration is the mainstream of life. The rationale of this verse seems obvious. Oxygen enters the body via the lungs and is assimilated into the blood stream. Blood is the basic element of animal life as written in the Bible, "For the life of the flesh is in the blood." [17]

There is no contradiction between these two principles. The verse "all in whose nostrils was the breath of the spirit of life" implies that if respiration ceases, the process of death has commenced. Death is not a phenomenon which always takes place in a split second. Death is a process which begins the moment spontaneous respiration ceases. The process of death ends when all bodily functions emanating from a controlling center end. This means that when a person in whom death is imminent becomes devoid of respiration but other bodily functions such as the brain are potentially operative, such a person is no longer completely alive but he is not yet dead: death has begun but the death process is not complete until the brain and heart completely cease to function. During this period, a person is in a state of semi-living, not fully alive but not fully dead. Anyone who kills such a person or who hastens his death is, therefore, guilty of murder. This is the reason why Maimonides rules [18] that one is not allowed to move a dying person while his soul is departing until after one waits awhile. Maimonides refers to a person who is motionless and who has no spontaneous heartbeat or respiration. One must wait half an hour because his brain may still be operative and the patient potentially resuscitable. This "dying" person is in a semi-living state and, therefore, one is prohibited from doing anything which may hasten his death.

On the other hand, the person who was found beneath a heap of stones and was examined and found to be devoid of respiration is considered semi-alive and semi-dead without possibility of resuscitation. That is why the finder may not desecrate the Sabbath to extricate him once he is declared dead. Sabbath laws are only set aside to save or prolong the life (even for only a very short time) of a fully living person but not for one in whom the death process has already begun (i.e. spontaneous respiration has ceased). Naturally, if there is even the remotest possibility of resuscitation, one is obligated to desecrate the Sabbath and attempt such resuscitation. However, the Talmudic discussion [19] does not refer to such a case.

This interpretation allows us to understand the remark of Rema [20] that nowadays we are not competent to determine precisely the moment of maternal death and are, therefore, not allowed even on weekdays to incise the womb of the woman who just died for the purpose of saving the fetus. The reason is that it is possible that the mother is not completely dead but is in a semi-living state which would be prematurely terminated by an incision in her abdomen.

From the point of view of the halakhic definition of death, a person who is in the so-called "brain death" state but whose heart and breathing are still functioning is certainly not dead. Such a person is considered alive even according to the first interpretation of the Talmudic discussion which is the view of Rabbenu Baḥya. A person who has no spontaneous respiration or heartbeat but who still has electrical brain wave activity is considered dead according to this interpretation. However, according to the second interpretation which is the view of Rashi, and according to the third interpretation which is the view of Maimonides, *Shulḥan Arukh* and Rema, such a person is not considered dead. According to Rashi, such a person is fully alive but according to Maimonides, *Shulḥan Arukh* and Rema, he is considered semi-alive and semi-dead.

NOTES

1. *Yoma 83a.*
2. *Ibid.* 85a.
3. *Mishneh Torah, Hilkhot Shabbat* 2:19.
4. *Shulḥan Arukh, Oraḥ Ḥayyim* 329:4.
5. *Mishneh Torah, Hilkhot Avelut* 4:5.
6. *Ibid.*
7. *Oholot* 1:6.
8. *Mishneh Torah, Hilkhot Shabbat* 2:19.
9. *Shulḥan Arukh, Oraḥ Ḥayyim* 330:5.
10. *Ibid.*
11. *Ibid.* 329.
12. *Yoma* 85a.
13. *Ibid.*
14. Deut. 6:5.
15. Genesis 7:22.
16. Rashi *Yoma* 85a *s.v. Ad hekhan hu bodek.*
17. Levit. 17:11.
18. *Mishneh Torah, Hilkhot Avelut* 4:5.
19. *Yoma* 85a.
20. In *Shulḥan Arukh, Oraḥ Ḥayyim* 330:5.

19
Neurological Criteria of Death and Time of Death Statutes

J. DAVID BLEICH

"But your blood of your lives will I require; from the hand of every beast will I require it; and from the hand of man, from the hand of a person's brother, will I require the life of man" (Genesis 9:5). This earliest and most detailed Biblical prohibition against homicide contains one phrase which is an apparent redundancy. Since the phrase "from the hand of man" pronounces man culpable for the murder of his fellow-man, to what point is it necessary for Scripture to reiterate "from the hand of a person's brother will I require the life of man?" Fratricide is certainly no less heinous a crime than ordinary homicide. R. Jacob Zevi Mecklenburg, in his commentary on the Pentateuch, *Ha-Ketav ve-ha-Kabbalah,* astutely comments that while murder is the antithesis of brotherly love, in some circumstances the taking of the life of one's fellow man may be perceived as indeed being an act of love par excellence. Euthanasia, designed to put an end to unbearable suffering, is born not of hatred or anger, but of concern and compassion. It is precisely the taking of life even under circumstances in which it is manifestly obvious that the perpetrator is motivated by feelings of love and brotherly compassion which the Torah finds necessary to brand as murder, pure and simple. Despite the noble intent which prompts such an action, mercy killing is proscribed as an unwarranted intervention in an area which must be governed only by God Himself. The life of man may be reclaimed only by the Author of life. As long as man is yet endowed with a spark of life—as defined by God's eternal Law—man dare not presume to hasten death, no matter how hopeless or meaningless continued existence may appear to be in the eyes of a mortal perceiver.

Various states have enacted legislation supplanting the classical definition

Reprinted from *Tradition* (Summer, 1977). Copyright © 1977 by the Rabbinical Council of America.

of death with more flexible criteria. The new statutes are designed to establish "brain death" as the legal criterion of the termination of life. In particular, the 1975–1976 legislative session saw attempts to pass a law in the State of New York establishing a new legal definition of death embodying the criteria of "brain death." Although the bill was not passed during the 1976 session of the legislature due to the hectic atmosphere of the closing days of the legislative session, the bill was reintroduced in 1977 and will undoubtedly be reintroduced in future sessions. This activity has led to the reopening of discussion concerning a precise definition of the time of death according to Jewish law. Some sectors of the Jewish community are particularly alarmed because of the possible violation of the religious and civil liberties of Jews who deem action compatible with the provisions of the proposed legislation to be tantamount to homicide according to Jewish law.

In the spring of 1976, a short statement authored by Rabbi Moses Feinstein, dated 5 Iyyar 5736, dealing with criteria of death according to Jewish law, was circulated by the Rephael Society, the medical section of the Association of Orthodox Jewish Scientists. Accompanying this document was a statement by Rabbi Moses Tendler going somewhat beyond the position of Rabbi Feinstein. An article by this writer espousing a view at variance with that expressed in those statements appears in the Tevet 5737 issue of *Ha-Pardes*. A position similar in its essential points to that of this writer was presented by Rabbi Aaron Soloveichik in the course of a public lecture, the second annual Harold Rosenbaum Memorial Lecture, held at Yeshiva University on November 18, 1973, under the sponsorship of the Rephael Society. (A somewhat shortened version of that paper may be found in this volume, chapter 18.)

Rabbi Feinstein points to the fact that the traditionally accepted criterion of death is the total absence of respiration. The crucial question is whether a patient maintained on a respirator may be deemed dead even though other vital signs may be present. Rabbi Feinstein opines that total irreversible cessation of independent respiratory activity is sufficient to establish that death has occurred. The practical problem is that of determining that total cessation of independent respiration has indeed occurred. Even though the patient is maintained on an artificial respirator, it is quite possible that at least minimal respiration would be possible without the aid of a respirator. If the patient is capable of even minimal breathing, Rabbi Feinstein declares that it is mandatory to provide every possible mechanical assistance and it is, accordingly, forbidden to remove the respirator. In usual medical practice, it is not uncommon to remove or turn off the respirator in order to determine whether or not the patient retains any respiratory potential. Rabbi Feinstein refuses to sanction this practice since it may cause the demise of a weakened patient capable of some minimal respiration but requiring the assistance of a mechanical respirator in order to sustain life.

Rabbi Feinstein states, however, that once the respirator has been turned off for any reason, the respirator may be withheld and the patient monitored for signs of breathing. If the patient is carefully observed for a period of approximately fifteen minutes during which time absolutely no breathing motion is manifest, the patient, in Rabbi Feinstein's opinion, may be pronounced dead. If, however, any signs of independent breathing, no matter how feeble, are perceived, the respirator must be reactivated.[1]

Rabbi Feinstein adds that this procedure may be followed only in the case of a patient suffering from a lingering and debilitating illness. Absence of respiration may not be accepted as conclusive evidence of death in cases of accident or traumatic injury or in cases of drug-induced coma, since in such cases cessation of respiration may be reversible. Accordingly, in such cases the respirator must be immediately restored even if it becomes disconnected. In the case of a traumatic injury, Rabbi Feinstein states that total cessation of independent respiration may be relied upon as an indication that death has occurred only if it can also be determined by means of radioisotope scanning techniques that cessation of circulation of blood has taken place. If, however, it is found that blood continues to flow to the brain, the patient should be considered to be alive, despite the absence of other vital signs. In the case of patients who have ingested toxic substances such as sleeping tablets or other drugs, no determination of death can be made on the basis of absence of spontaneous respiration until blood tests reveal that toxic substances have been eliminated from the body.

Rabbi Feinstein's position presents a number of difficulties:

1. His statement appears to contradict his previously held opinion as expressed in *Iggerot Moshe, Yoreh De'ah,* II, no. 146. The Mishnah, *Yevamot* 121a, records an incident related by R. Meir concerning an individual who fell into a well and emerged some three days later. In explaining this phenomenon, Rashi comments, "R. Meir is of the opinion that a person may live and remain in water for one or two days." Although his explanation is at variance with commonly accepted scientific postulates, Rabbi Feinstein, following Rashi, understands this incident as demonstrating that in some rare instances a person may survive for at least a limited period of time even without breathing.[2] In the same responsum he asserts that life may be present even in the absence of both perceivable respiratory and cardiac activity and, accordingly, a patient should not be pronounced dead if there are clinical indications of the presence of any vital forces.

2. Rabbi Feinstein states that although a patient incapable of spontaneous respiratory activity need not be placed on the respirator, the patient may not be removed from the respirator

for purposes of determining that he indeed cannot breathe spontaneously. Rabbi Feinstein gives no reason for this distinction. Rabbi Tendler, however, indicates that removal of the respirator may induce physiological stress of a nature which can readily hasten the demise of a respirator patient. If this is indeed the reasoning underlying Rabbi Feinstein's statement, it is difficult to understand why the patient who has been subjected to such stress in disconnecting him from the respirator for purposes of suction or for purposes of servicing the respirator, should not be immediately replaced on the respirator. The physiological stress which may hasten death is the result of human action; the person performing the action is certainly obligated to do everything possible to mitigate the potentially fatal result of the action for which he bears responsibility. To cite a parallel in another area of Jewish law, cooking on *Shabbat* is a culpable offense only if the food is heated to a specified temperature. A person who places a pot of water on the stove on *Shabbat* is surely obligated to remove the pot before it cooks in order to absolve himself of culpability. It would appear that the person disconnecting the respirator—even if he does so for the benefit of the patient or for purposes of servicing the respirator—is likewise obligated to rectify as far as possible any physiological stress caused the patient through his action.

One other point should be noted. Although the opinion is far from unanimous, Rabbi Feinstein, *Iggerot Moshe, Yoreh De'ah,* II, no. 174, has ruled that according to Rema, *Yoreh De'ah* 339:1, it is not necessary to prolong the life of a *goses*. Nevertheless, overt intervention for the purpose of hastening death is strictly forbidden. A distinction is drawn between passive nonintervention and active intervention. Removal of a respirator is regarded as an overt act by most contemporary authorities whereas not returning the patient to the respirator is passive in nature. If not only medicaments but also oxygen need not be administered to a *goses,* it would follow that a *goses* need not be attached to a respirator. This consideration is, however, germane only in the case of a patient actually in a state of *gesisah.*

3. Rabbi Feinstein, in this statement, as opposed to his responsum in *Iggerot Moshe,* does not take cognizance of spontaneous cardiac activity as an indication of life.[3] This appears to be contradicted by *Ḥatam Sofer, Yoreh De'ah,* no. 338, and *Ḥakham Ẓevi,* no. 77. This point will be developed more fully in the ensuing discussion.

Rabbi Feinstein is firm in his opinion that the irreversible cessation of spontaneous respiration is halakhically both a necessary and sufficient condition of death. Radioisotope scanning in cases of traumatic accident is required by him only as confirmatory evidence of the irreversible nature of respiratory cessation. In oral communications Rabbi Feinstein has repeatedly stated that he, in no way, is prepared to accept any form of "brain death" as compatible with the provision of *Halakhah,* a position which is formulated explicitly and unequivocally in *Iggerot Moshe, Yoreh De'ah,* II, no. 146.[4]

Moreover, it should be noted that the practical effects of Rabbi Feinstein's position, as expressed in this statement, are extremely limited. Modern-day respirators are not prone to malfunctions and need not be disconnected for servicing. While respirators are indeed frequently turned off for short intervals, this is done not as a matter of medical or mechanical necessity but to determine whether or not the patient is capable of independent respiration or in order to facilitate suctioning. The latter may readily be accomplished without turning off the respirator. Scrupulous observance of the injunction against unnecessarily disconnecting the respirator would, to a very large extent, preclude utilization of Rabbi Feinstein's criterion of death.

Rabbi Tendler is prepared, at least hypothetically, to accept additional criteria as well. Rabbi Tendler states, ". . . if blood flow studies are refined sufficiently to give full confidence in their results, evidence that the region of the medulla is not being perfused would in my opinion be a fully valid indication that death had occurred." In the absence of reliable blood flow tests, Rabbi Tendler endorses the criteria set forth by the Ad Hoc Committee of the Harvard Medical School.[5] The Harvard Committee seeks to define irreversible coma as a criterion of death. The Harvard recommendations serve to establish operational criteria for determination of the characteristics of a permanently non-functional brain, or what is referred to colloquially as "brain death." The recommended criteria are: 1) lack of response to external stimuli or internal need; 2) absence of movement or breathing as observed by physicians over a period of at least one hour; 3) absence of elicitable reflexes. A fourth criterion, a flat or isoelectric electroencephalogram is recommended as being "of great confirmatory value" but not of absolute necessity. The procedure advocated by the Harvard Committee calls for repetition of the relevant tests following a lapse of twenty-four hours.

This writer, in *Ha-Pardes,* Tevet 5737, addresses himself to the clarification of two questions upon which are contingent the acceptability of currently proposed criteria: 1) Is there any form of "brain death" which conforms to halakhic criteria of death? 2) Is the absence of spontaneous respiration a sufficient criterion of death in the presence of ongoing cardiac activity?

1. A discussion of the compatibility of the criterion of brain death with the provisions of Jewish Law was first presented in the Tishri

5731 issue of *Ha-Darom* by Rabbi Gedalia Rabinowitz and Dr. M. Koenigsberg. The authors predicated their argument upon the Mishnah, *Oholot* 1:6: "And likewise cattle and wild beasts . . . if their heads have been severed, they are unclean (as carcasses) even if they move convulsively like the tail of a newt (or lizard) that twitches spasmodically (after being cut off)." Rabbi Rabinowitz and Dr. Koenigsberg argue that "brain death" is to be equated with decapitation which the Mishnah accepts as synonymous with death. This position was sharply opposed by Dr. Ya'akov Levy, an Israeli physician who has written extensively on topics of medical Halakhah, in a letter which appeared in the Nisan 5731 issue of *Ha-Darom* as well as in articles in the Tishri 5730 and Nisan 5732 issues of *Ha-Ma'ayan.*[6]

Dr. Levy also contributed an article to the 5730 issue of *No'am* in which he demonstrates that neurological criteria of death do not satisfy the halakhic definition.

This writer, in *Ha-Pardes,* Tevet 5737, has argued that the currently proposed criteria differ significantly from decapitation as described in the Mishnah. Decapitation involves destruction of the entire brain. It might be argued with cogency that total cessation of circulation of blood to the brain will result in destruction of brain tissue. *Total* destruction of the brain might then be equated with decapitation,[7] and the patient pronounced dead after total destruction has occurred.[8]

However, in point of fact, there is at present no clinical method of determining that total destruction of brain tissue has occurred. Radioisotope techniques, when and if sufficiently refined, may be employed only to determine that perfusion of the brain has ceased. Cellular decay of the brain does indeed commence upon cessation of blood flow but requires an indeterminate period of time to become complete. Cessation of circulation to the brain cannot, in itself, be equated with total cellular destruction of the brain.

Moreover, radioisotope scanning techniques cannot, in their current state of refinement, be utilized in order to determine that even perfusion to the brain has totally ceased. Investigators responsible for the development of these techniques claim only that such methods may be used to indicate cessation of circulation to the cerebrum, which is the seat of the so-called "higher functions" of the human organism and are careful to describe the phenomena which they report as "cerebral death" rather than as "brain death."[9] These phenomena are entirely compatible with continued circulation and perfusion of the medulla and the brain stem. In fact, radioisotope techniques do not even demonstrate total cessation of circulation to the cerebrum, but only that effective circulation has decreased below the level necessary to maintain its integrity. Even if scanning methods currently used are accurate, they do not indicate that all circulation to even a part of the brain, i.e., the cerebrum, has been interrupted, but only that the rate of flow is below that necessary to maintain viability. Thus, in a summary of findings which forms part of a recent study, these techniques are described as "indicative of significant circulatory *deficit* to the cerebrum."[10]

The Harvard criteria are even less satisfactory than blood flow tests as halakhic criteria for establishing that cellular decay of the brain has taken place. The Harvard criteria serve to establish only the dysfunction of a limited part of the brain; they do not constitute evidence that even a portion of the brain has been destroyed. *Oholot* 1:6 can be cited only to substantiate an argument that destruction of the *entire* brain is tantamount to death.[11]

2. This writer's article contains a citation of sources which demonstrate that the absence of spontaneous respiration cannot be viewed as a criterion of death in the presence of spontaneous cardiac activity. *Ḥatam Sofer, Yoreh De'ah,* no. 338, states that a patient may be pronounced dead only if three criteria are manifest: 1) the patient lies as an "inanimate stone"; 2) no pulse beat is discernible; and 3) respiration has ceased. *Ḥatam Sofer* adds the forceful statement: "These are three clinical symptoms of death which have been transmitted to us from the time that the nation of God became a holy people. All the forces in the universe will not cause us to deviate from the position of our Holy Torah."

It is clear that *Ḥatam Sofer* refuses to accept absence of spontaneous respiration as an indication of death unless accompanied by both total absence of movement and absence of heartbeat as evidenced by pulsation. *Ḥatam Sofer's* position is readily deducible from the comments of Rashi, *Yoma* 85a, who, in his comments upon the stated requirement for an examination of the nostrils in order to determine that cessation of respiration has occurred, remarks that such examination is to be made if the person is "like a corpse which does not move its limbs." The clear implication of this statement is that, in the presence of such movement, absence of respiration is not a determining criterion of death.

Rashi's position may, in turn, be inferred from the Mishnah, *Oholot* 1:6. Were it to be the case that absence of respiration is, in all cases, in and of itself, a fully reliable criterion of death the clarificatory clause, "even if they move convulsively like the tail of a newt that twitches spasmodically"

which serves to establish a novel halakhic category, viz., *pirkus* or convulsive movement, would be totally superfluous. It is manifestly evident
that following decapitation there can be no respiration. At the very most the
Mishnah need but have stated "even if they move convulsively they are
unclean [as carcasses] because respiration has ceased." It is evident that the
Mishnah seeks to differentiate between two types of movement; movement
which is devoid of vital significance, and movement which is indicative of
life. The residual movement of a decapitated person or animal is described
as a mere spasm and hence not indicative of life; the inference being that
other forms of movement are indeed indicative that life is still present. Since
muscular movement is, under ordinary circumstances, an indication of life,
it follows *a fortiori* that spontaneous cardiac activity is an absolute criterion
of life. The beating of the heart in addition to being a form of muscular
movement in the literal sense is certainly a more significant vital sign than
ordinary forms of muscular movement.

It may be inferred from yet another statement of Rashi that death may be
deemed to have occurred only upon cessation of cardiac activity. In
commenting upon the requirement that the nostrils be examined for signs of
breathing, Rashi states that this is necessary "for at times life is not perceivable at the heart, but is perceivable at the nose." In these comments
Rashi takes pains to explain that absence of a perceivable heartbeat is not,
in itself, evidence of death, not because the heartbeat is irrelevant, but
because nonperception of a heartbeat is, in itself, inconclusive. Respiration
is more readily perceivable than a heartbeat and hence the negative finding
of an examination for respiration is a more reliable indicator. It is quite
understandable that a faint heartbeat may not be detected (particularly
without the aid of a stethoscope) because of the intervening rib cage, muscle
tissue and fat, whereas even faint respiration can be perceived by placing a
feather or straw to the nose of a patient. Conversely, in the absence of
mechanical assistance, there can be no heartbeat after respiration has
ceased. Thus, the absence of perceived respiration is an indicator not only
of the cessation of respiratory activity but of the cessation of cardiac activity as well. Indeed, *Ḥakham Ẓevi,* no. 77, citing these comments of
Rashi, states unequivocally that respiration, in itself, is not the criterion of
life, but is simply an indication that the heart is yet beating.[13] It then certainly follows that the patient cannot be pronounced dead other than upon
the irreversible cessation of both cardiac and respiratory activity. The
presence of a heartbeat is thus a conclusive indication of life even in the
absence of brain function or spontaneous respiration.[14]

Rabbi Aaron Soloveichik draws attention to a statement of Rabbenu
Baḥya in which this authority unequivocally declares that cardiac activity
and not respiration is the primary criterion of life. In his commentary on
Deuteronomy 6:5 Rabbenu Baḥya states, ". . . and because (the heart) is

the first organ in the creation of man and the last among the organs of the body to die therefore (Scripture) states 'with all your heart,' i.e., until the last moment of death.''

One further point germane to the clarification of acceptable criteria of death is raised by Rabbi Aaron Soloveichik. On the basis of these sources it would appear that, in the absence of other bodily movement, the patient may be pronounced dead immediately upon the irreversible cessation of both cardiac and respiratory activity and that no further indicators are necessary. One must be mindful that Rema, *Orah Hayyim* 330:5, states that we are not competent to determine with precision that respiration has indeed ceased.[15] Rabbi Aaron Soloveichik has, however, taken the more extreme position that if brain function, as recorded by an electroencephalogram, continues to be manifest, the patient must be considered to be alive even if no other vital signs are present. This position is, in terms of halakhic import, compatible with that of *Mishkenot Ya'akov, Yoreh De'ah,* no. 10, who asserts that some residual life may be present even after the heart is removed or ceases to function. Rabbi Soloveichik, however, bases his argument on the contention that brain waves which can be recorded on an electroencephalogram constitute "movement." Since "movement" is present, the patient cannot be considered to be as an "inanimate stone" and hence one of the necessary criteria of death as enumerated by *Hatam Sofer* is absent.

It is, however, not clear that subvisual motion is considered "movement" from the point of view of Halakhah. In other areas of ritual law, it is well-established that Halakhah concerns itself only with readily perceivable phenomena.[16] It may be the case that brain waves are too ephemeral to be considered "movement" in the eyes of Halakhah.

Rabbi Feinstein, *Iggerot Moshe, Yoreh De'ah,* II, no. 146, discusses the different but related case of a patient who manifests no perceivable heartbeat but evidences cardiac activity as recorded by an electrocardiogram. Rabbi Feinstein (in this responsum) declares that the patient must be considered to be alive, not because he manifests "movement" as recorded by an electrocardiogram, but because life may be present even in the absence of both perceivable respiration and cardiac activity. *Semahot* 8:1 reports the bizarre incident of a person who was interred in a crypt after having been pronounced dead on the basis of accepted criteria of death, but was subsequently found to be alive on the third day following interment. The individual is reported to have enjoyed another twenty-five years of life and to have sired children. Rabbi Feinstein understands this source as demonstrating that life may be present even in the absence of observable cardiac or respiratory activity. He explains that ordinarily this possibility need not be taken into consideration since the likelihood of this occurring is extremely remote. However, he maintains, if residual vital forces are in any

way manifest, e.g., cardiac activity as evidenced by means of an electrocardiogram (or, arguably, brain waves as recorded by an electroencephalogram), the patient must be deemed to be alive. This line of
reasoning appears to be similar to that of *Mishkenot Ya'akov*.

In terms of practical application, the matter is entirely academic, insofar
as electroencephalographic findings are concerned since, in point of fact,
brain waves cease to be discernible almost immediately following cessation
of cardiac activity. The theoretical point is, of course, of paramount
significance with regard to the question at hand. The consideration of
factors such as brain waves as criteria of life can be entertained only because
absence of respiration does not, in itself, always establish conclusively that
death has occurred.

Rabbi Soloveichik presents a somewhat different argument which serves
to establish the same point. Rabbi Soloveichik cites Rambam's commentary
on *Oholot* 1:6 to demonstrate that even cessation of both cardiac and
respiratory activity is not in itself an absolute sign that death has occurred.
In commenting on the phrase "even if they move convulsively like the tail of
a newt," Rambam comments that such convulsive movements are not
indicative of life because this "power of locomotion is not diffused among
all the organs from a single root or source." Rabbi Soloveichik infers from
this comment that as long as there is present any vital activity which is not
local in nature the patient is alive. Movement directed by the central nervous system is in the nature of locomotion which is "diffused among all the
organs." The patient must therefore be considered to be alive on the basis
of brain activity alone even if no respiration or pulsation is present. Thus,
concludes Rabbi Soloveichik, the patient may be considered dead only in
the absence of all three vital activities, i.e., only after respiratory, cardiac
and neurological activity have completely and irreversibly ceased.

It is unlikely that Jewish opinion will succeed in stemming the legislative
tide indefinitely. It is also unrealistic to believe that time of death statutes
will *accurately* reflect even the most liberal of halakhic opinions. Moreover,
no responsible rabbinic authority would want his view to prevail on the
basis of the coercive power of the secular state. There is, moreover, one
point on which all can agree, *viz.*, that no person should be compelled to
act, or to be the object of an act, which is to him morally odious. It is to this
end that spokesmen representing various sectors of the Jewish community
have vigorously advocated that such legislation, if enacted, contain a
provision allowing for exemption from newly legislated legal definitions of
death for reasons of conscience, a provision strongly endorsed in a
statement issued by Rabbi Feinstein on 8 Shevat 5737. If passed, the newly
enacted criteria would not apply in determining the time of death in face of
the announced opposition of the patient or of his next of kin. Thus, civil
and religious liberties would be preserved for all.

NOTES

1. The basis for establishing a fifteen-minute monitoring period is not readily apparent. Support for a period of twenty minutes, thirty minutes, or one hour may be found in earlier sources, see J. David Bleich, *Contemporary Halakhic Problems* (New York, 1977), p. 380.

2. This phenomenon is difficult to understand since it is generally assumed that resuscitation is impossible if the brain has been deprived of oxygen for a period of approximately four to six minutes. Although it is difficult to account for survival despite such long term submersion, the concept is partly explainable in terms of a phenomenon known as the mammalian diving reflex. While contemporary science knows of no successful attempts at resuscitation after "one or two days," recent scientific studies have led to a startling discovery. Drowning victims, submerged in cold water for much longer than six minutes, have been resuscitated and show no lasting ill-effects. This phenomenon is attributed to a combination of coldness, which decreases the body's need for oxygen and a response previously known to exist in diving mammals known as the diving reflex. Absence of respiration combined with cold water in the face triggers a reflex which slows the heartbeat and the flow of blood to tissues relatively resistant to oxygen deprivation. Oxygenated blood is husbanded and sent to the heart and brain for a longer period of time.

Scientists have long been aware of the ability of air-breathing diving animals, such as seals, to remain submerged for periods of up to thirty minutes without replenishing their air supply. This phenomenon was observed in diving ducks as early as 1870 by the French physiologist, Paul Bert. By 1894, it was recognized that this phenomenon is due to the presence of an oxygen-conserving reflex. Studies conducted during the 1930s indicate that during submersion this reflex mechanism causes redistribution of the blood flow. As a result, virtually no blood flows to tissues such as skin or muscle which are resistant to asphyxia but continues to flow unabated to tissues most sensitive to lack of oxygen, viz., the heart and brain. Oxygen consumption is thus reduced to a minimum during submersion and hence conserved. This phenomenon is the result of sympathetic vasoconstriction which virtually cuts off blood flow to the major portion of the body while maintaining the flow of blood to the heart and brain. See Lawrence Irving, "On the Ability of Warm Blooded Animals to Survive without Breathing," *Science Monthly,* 1934, 38:422; L. Irving, D.Y. Solandt, O.M. Solandt, and K.C. Fisher, "The Respiratory Metabolism of the Seal and its Adjustment to Diving," *J. Cell. Comp. Physiol.,* 1935, 7:137, and L. Irving, P.F. Solander and S.W. Grinell, "Respiratory Metabolism of the Porpoise", *Science,* 1940, 91:455. Subsequent studies culminating in a report in the September 9, 1972 issue of the *Medical Journal of Australia* confirm the existence of a comparable diving reflex in man which similarly serves to conserve oxygen and thereby enables survival under water.

The diving reflex is triggered by the sensory stimulus of cold water upon the face. Indeed bradycardia, the slowing of heartbeat associated with the diving reflex, can be induced by immersing the face in a bowl of cold water. These studies indicate that this response is influenced by hypothermia at temperatures below 20° C. and becomes more marked at progressively lower temperatures. Inhibition of the respiratory centers which serves to prevent inhalation of water was also observed as part of this phenomenon. See Brett A. Gooden, "Drowning and the Diving Reflex in Man," *Med. J. Aust.,* 1972, 2:583–589.

There are reports of at least two recent incidents in which survival is known to have occurred despite prolonged submersion. A group of Norwegian physicians have reported the successful resuscitation and complete recovery of a five-year old boy who had been submerged in ice-cold water for a period of 40 minutes. See H. Siebke, H. Breivik, T. Rǿd and B. Lind, "Survival after 40 Minutes' Submersion Without Cerebral Sequelae", *Lancet,* June 7, 1975, 1275–1276. *Medical World News,* June 27, 1977, reports the resuscitation and recovery of an 18-year old who had been submerged in the icy waters of a Michigan lake for 38 minutes and cites the opinion of one pulmonary specialist, Morton J. Nemeroff, who believes this phenomenon to be a function of youth. Dr. Nemeroff notes that the human newborn appears to be protected during birth by the same cardiovascular reflexes which are elicited by the diving reflex and states that, in his opinion, the diving reflex becomes attenuated as part of the mammalian aging process. See also *Time,* August 22, 1977, pp. 74–75.

3. The admissibility of "brain death" criteria is also rejected emphatically by R. Eliezer Waldenberg, *Ẓiẓ Eli'ezer,* X, no. 25, chap. 4, sec. 7: "There are those who err in thinking that examination of the nose is indicative of cessation of brain activity and, on the basis of this, wish to establish that life is contingent upon the brain. . . . In truth this is an absolute error and contradicts that which our Sages, of blessed memory, have established on our behalf . . . 'And there is nothing new under the sun' (Ecclesiastes 1:9). There have already been many among those who are great in wisdom who were inclined to think that way, i.e., that life is contingent upon the brain, but greater persons came and disproved these notions as is recorded in *Teshuvot Ḥakham Zevi . . .*"

4. Rabbi Feinstein is, however, elsewhere quoted as requiring the absence of cardiac activity as a necessary condition of death. *Halachah Bulletin* no. 11, dated November, 1970, one of a series of bulletins distributed by the Rephael Society of the Association of Orthodox Jewish Scientists, is devoted to the definition of death in Jewish law and bears a legend declaring that the contents have the approval of Rabbi Feinstein. The statement reads as follows: "A patient who has no evidence of either spontaneous respiration or heart action for ten minutes or more of continuous observation is considered halakhically dead, provided resuscitation is deemed impossible." The ensuing discussion affirms that the absence of spontaneous respiration *and* the absence of any palpable pulse are the cardinal signs for ascertaining death. Parenthetically, Rabbi Feinstein's written statement requires observation for a minimum period of 15 minutes while the *Halakhah Bulletin* speaks of a ten-minute period; cf. *supra,* note 1.

5. This view is also urged in "Brain Death: A Status Report of Medical and Ethical Considerations," *Journal of the American Medical Association,* vol. 238, no. 15 (October 10, 1977), pp. 1651–55, which lists Rabbi Tendler as one of the co-authors and in another article by him, "Cessation of Brain Function: Ethical Implications in Terminal Care and Organ Transplant," *Annals of the New York Academy of Sciences,* vol. 315 (1978), pp. 394–397.

6. See also Rabbi Gerald Blidstein, *Ha-Darom,* Nisan 5733, who argues that even actual decapitation is not *ipso facto* to be equated with death. The most significant source for this position is *Sefer ha-Eshkol, Hilkhot Tum'at Kohanim,* no. 54, who categorizes a decapitated person as a *nevelah me-ḥayyim,* a "living carcass," i.e., a person who defiles while yet alive, rather than as a corpse. Cf., however, R. Jacob Reischer, *Shevut Ya'akov,* I, no. 13, who rules that decapitation is an absolute criterion of death. See also R. Ephraim Oshry, *She'elot u-Teshuvot mi-Ma'amakim,* II, no. 10.

7. Cellular decay or destruction of tissue is indeed viewed as tantamount to excision and removal by Rabbi Ḥayyim of Volozhin, *Ḥut ha-Meshullash;* no. 11, section 3; *Bet Ephra'im Even ha-Ezer,* no. 2, p. 10; *Ḥatam Sofer, Even ha-Ezer,* nos. 17 and 19; Rabbi Isaac Elhanan Spektor, *Ein Yiẓḥak, Even ha-Ezer,* no. 9,

sections 15-17; and *Shem Aryeh,* no. 6. These authorities base themselves upon *Yam shel Shelomo, Yevamot* 8:9, who develops this thesis in interpreting the position of Rambam, *Issurei Bi'ah* 16:9. Cf. also Rambam, *Hilkhot Shehitah* 7:15, and *Dagul me-Revavah Tinyana, Yoreh De'ah,* 48:5. This view is, however, disputed by Rabbi Jeruchem Judah Perilman, *Or Gadol,* no. 3, p. 32a, who dismisses Maharshal's position and the position of those who follow him as a *sevarat ha-keres,* an unsubstantiated visceral hypothesis devoid of basis in rabbinic sources. Total lysis, involving liquification of the brain tissue may, however, be tantamount to decapitation even according to *Or Gadol.*

8. See, however, *supra,* note 5, as well as a possible alternate analysis of *Oholot* 1:6 advanced in this writer's article in *Ha-Pardes.* According to that analysis, it is not the heartbeat *per se* which is a criterion of life, but the beating of the heart as causing circulation of blood throughout the body which is the indicator of life. Upon decapitation "the blood upon which the soul depends" escapes and cannot be recirculated. This would not result from even total lysis of the brain, since lysis involves no wound and causes no blood to escape.

9. See P. Braunstein *et al.,* "A Simple Bedside Evaluation for Cerebral Blood Flow in the Study of Cerebral Death," *The American Journal of Roentegenology, Radium Therapy and Nuclear Medicine,* vol. CXVIII, no. 4, August 1973, pp. 757-767, and Julius Korein *et al.,* "Radioisotopic Bolus Technique as a Test to Detect Circulatory Deficit Associated with Cerebral Death," *Circulation,* vol. 51, May, 1975, pp. 924-939.

10. Korein, p. 924.

11. In contradistinction to his presently-expressed position, in a Hebrew article which appeared in a publication of the Student Organization of Yeshiva University, Rabbi Tendler himself wrote, ". . . brain death [which] is the modern criterion for determining death has no basis whatsoever in Halakhah," *Kevi'at ha-mavet be-Halakhah, Be'er Yizhak,* 1970, p. 23 (translation mine). Rabbi Tendler further wrote, ". . . it is clear as the sun that it is impossible to establish that a person is dead on the basis of any demonstration by means of a medical instrument or physiological test if there yet remains in him a power of movement or the power of respiration or the power of pulsation. Rather, as long as one of the powers . . . remains functional the person is considered alive, for all purposes . . ." (*Ibid., p.* 22.) The identical position was reiterated by Rabbi Tendler in the context of a discussion of transplant surgery: ". . . in heart transplants the heart which was taken from the donor was still beating. Here there was certainly an act of murder. . . ." (*Ibid.,* pp. 23-24.) Cognizance is taken of *Oholot* 1:6, but with a clear awareness that death occurs only upon actual decapitation or total destruction of the brain. Rambam's ruling, *Hilkhot Shabbat* 2:18, "If he is found alive even though he has been crushed . . ." is cited by Rabbi Tendler as evidence that injury to the brain is not a criterion of death. Rabbi Tendler defines the phrase "he has been crushed" as "meaning his head has suffered a great wound such that his brain has certainly been greatly injured." (*Ibid.,* p. 23). Although the proof adduced on the basis of Rambam's choice of words is rather tenuous, the conclusion is certainly correct: Partial destruction of the brain is in no way comparable to decapitation. Curiously, in his more recent statements, Rabbi Tendler does not refer to his previously published opinion.

12. *Hatam Sofer's* criteria of death must be understood as involving the *irreversible* cessation of these vital functions. Thus a patient maintained on a heart-lung machine during the course of open heart surgery is not dead even if totally immobilized since the absence of these vital signs is reversible. See R. Moshe Sternbuch, *Ba'ayot he-Zeman be-Hashkafot ha-Torah,* I, 10.

13. *Hakham Zevi* also states, ". . . even he who maintains that (the source) of

movement is the brain agrees that life is contingent only upon the heart, for with regard to this no man has ever disagreed.'' See also Dr. Ya'akov Levi, *No'am,* XIII (5730), 9, who cites the criteria formulated by *Hatam Sofer* and concludes, ''And therefore it is clear as the sun that a moribund patient who has respiration or a heartbeat . . . is considered a living person according to Halakhah.''

14. The respirator should not be confused with a heart-lung machine. A patient maintained on a respirator suffers only from the absence of spontaneous respiration; his heart functions in a spontaneous rather than in an artificial manner.

15. Cf. *Contemporary Halakhic Problems,* pp. 380–382.

16. See *Tiferet Yisra'el, Avodah Zarah* 2:6 and *Arukh ha-Shulḥan, Yorah De'ah* 83:15 and 84:36.

20
Suicide in Jewish Law
FRED ROSNER

Introduction

Every day in the United States, about sixty people kill themselves by poisoning, hanging, drowning, shooting, stabbing, jumping from high places or other means. Although nearly 25,000 deaths from suicide are recorded annually in the United States,[1] the actual figure according to the National Institute of Mental Health is probably closer to 50,000 yearly.[2]

Worldwide, more than 500,000 suicides are registered yearly, according to the World Health Organization[3] and there are approximately eight times as many suicide attempts. The problem of suicide has reached such proportions that the United States Public Health Service created the National Center for Studies of Suicide Prevention in October 1966, headed by Dr. Edwin S. Schneidman. Presently there are 90 regional suicide prevention centers in 26 states in this country whereas in 1965 there were only 15 such centers.

The medical, psychological, psychiatric, legal and social literatures are replete with articles, monographs, symposia and other publications on suicide. Factors such as age, sex, marital status, day of week, month of year, method, religion, race, motivation, living conditions, repetitive attempts, medical and psychiatric histories of patients attempting and commiting suicide are amply covered in these writings as well as the many books published on this subject.[4] A periodical devoted exclusively to suicide is the *Bulletin of Suicidology* published by the United States Public Health Service since 1967.

Several salient features of the problem deserve mention. Sucides are three times as frequent in men than in women although there are more attempts by women than men. Twice as many white Americans commit suicide than

Reprinted from *Tradition* (Summer, 1970). Copyright © 1970 by the Rabbinical Council of America.

do black Americans and twice as many single people kill themselves than do married individuals. College students have a suicide rate 50 percent higher than non-college students of comparable age, sex and race. In industrialized countries, physicians, dentists and lawyers have a higher rate of suicide than other professionals. Although the suicide rate has remained relatively constant in the United States over the past decade or so, poisoning by drugs, especially barbiturates, has become much more popular as a method of choice.[5]

The age group with the highest suicide rate is that above 65 years. Suicide ranks third as a cause of death among teenagers.[6] It has also been estimated that the ratio of suicide attempts to actual successes in adolescents is 100 to 1.

One phase of suicide hardly discussed at all is the religious aspect. This paper attempts to organize and present in a systematic fashion the subject of suicide as found in Jewish sources. The closely related topic of martyrdom will be discussed briefly at the end.

Suicide in the Bible

During the period of the Judges in approximately the 11th or 12th century B.C.E., lived Samson of the tribe of Dan whose story is known to all. Samson's final effort in bringing down the Philistine temple upon himself as well as his enemies is vividly described in the Book of Judges (16:23-31):

> And Samson said: "Let me die with the Philistines." And he bent with all his might; and the house fell upon the lords, and upon all the people that were therein. So the dead that he slew at his death were more than they that he slew in his life.

At the end of the First Book of Samuel (31:1-7), we read of King Saul's final battle against the Philistines on Mount Gilboa in the 11th century B.C.E. Here, Saul saw his three sons Jonathan, Abinadab and Malchishua and most of his army slain. Not wishing to flee nor to be taken prisoner and exposed to the scorn of the Philistines, King Saul entreated his armor bearer to kill him. The latter refused and so the king fell upon his own sword. The Biblical passage concludes (1 Samuel 31:5)

> And when his armor bearer saw that Saul was dead, he likewise fell upon his sword and died with him.

From these events it would appear as if Saul committed suicide. However, later on when David is informed of Saul's death, we read as follows (2 Samuel 1:5-10):

And David said unto the young man that told him: "How knowest thou that Saul and Jonathan his son are dead?" And the young man that told him said: "As I happened by chance upon Mount Gilboa, behold, Saul leaned upon his spear; and lo, the chariots and the horsemen pressed hard upon him. And when he looked behind him, he saw me, and called upon me. And I answered: Here am I. And he said unto me: Stand, I pray thee, beside me, and slay me, for the agony hath taken hold of me because my life is just yet in me. So I stood beside him and slew him, because I was sure that he could not live after that he was fallen . . ."

Biblical commentators differ in their interpretation of this passage. R. David Kimḥi explains that Saul did not die immediately when he fell on his sword but was mortally wounded. In his death throes, Saul asked the Amalekite to render the final blow of mercy to hasten his death. Rashi, Ralbag and *Meẓudat David* agree with Kimḥi and consider the death of King Saul as a case of euthanasia. Others view the story of the Amalekite as a complete fabrication.

In any event, Saul did attempt suicide. Only the question of his success is debated. As to Saul's armor bearer, no one disputes that he committed suicide.

King David's faithless counsellor, Ahithophel, committed suicide by hanging himself in his native town of Giloh. One of several reasons probably prompted suicide. First, he knew that Absalom's attempt to overthrow David was doomed and that he would die a traitor's death. Second, and less likely, is the disgust of Ahithophel at Absalom's conduct in setting aside his counsel, thus wounding Ahithophel's pride and disappointing his ambition.[7] Finally, David's curse (*Makkot* 11a) may have prompted Ahithophel to hang himself.

And when Ahithophel saw that his counsel was not followed, he saddled his ass and arose, and got himself home unto his city, and set his house in order, and strangled himself; and he died and was buried in the sepulchre of his father.[8]

King Baasha of Israel reigned from 911 to 888 B.C.E. and was succeeded by his son Elah. The latter was addicted to idleness and drunkenness and passed the days drinking in his palace while his warriors were battling the Philistines at Gibbethon.[9] Zimri, a high ranking officer, took advantage of the situation, assassinated Elah and mounted the throne. His reign, however, lasted only seven days. As soon as the news of King Elah's murder reached the army on the battlefield General Omri was elected king and laid siege to the palace. When Zimri saw that he was unable to hold out against the siege, he set fire to the palace and perished in the flames. It is written in I Kings 16:18:

And it came to pass, when Zimri saw that the city was taken that he went unto the castle of the king's house, and he burnt the king's house over him with fire, and he died.

Some Biblical commentators, notably Radak and *Mezudat David,* to whom the thought of suicide was abhorrent, interpret that Omri burned the house over Zimri. Most commentators, however, interpret the Biblical passage literally.

Suicide in the Apocrypha

In the Second Book of Maccabees two acts of suicide are recorded. The first occurred when King Demetrius I of Syria (162 to 150 B.C.E.) escaped from his imprisonment in Rome and returned home as an invader.[10] Attempting to put down a rebellion of his Judean subjects, King Demetrius sent Nicanor, one of the warriors who escaped with him from Rome, to Judea, to treat the insurgents with the utmost harshness. Nicanor, in order to induce surrender from the Judeans, ordered that the most respected man in Jerusalem, Ragesh (or Razis) be seized. When the arresting soldiers were forcing open the courtyard door to Ragesh's house ". . . he fell upon his sword preferring to die nobly rather than to fall into the wretches' hands . . ." (II Maccabees 14:41–42). The ghastly tale of his lack of success in the first suicide attempt, his subsequent attempt by throwing himself down from a wall and his final success by self-disembowelment is vividly described (*ibid.* 14:43–46).

The second act of suicide is that of Ptolemy, an advocate of the Judeans at the Syrian Court, who was called a traitor before King Antiochus Eupator. Unable to maintain the dignity of his office, Ptolemy poisoned himself (II Maccabees 10:12).

Other Suicides and Near Suicides in Ancient Jewish Writings

All the suicides mentioned in the Bible and Apocrypha are psychologically understandable. Each knew what lay ahead if he remained alive, namely a prolonged, torturous martyrdom and/or disgrace to the God of Israel. All were prominent people. Except, perhaps, for King Saul, none could be accused of having experienced temporary insanity to excuse his act of self-destruction. Perhaps Ragesh and Ptolemy were influenced by the Greek philosophy of their times in which suicide was highly acceptable.

There are several individuals mentioned in the Bible, Apocrypha and other ancient Jewish writings who considered suicide and perhaps wished to attempt it, but did not.

Job, during his quest for an explanation of his wretchedness, speaks of suicide (Job 7:15):

And my soul chooseth strangling, and death rather than these my bones.

He did not attempt suicide perhaps out of either love or fear of God as he himself states (Job 13:15):

Though He slay me, yet will I trust in Him.

Possibly Job did not mean to even consider suicide but was remarking that he would prefer death to life. This question remains unresolved.

One of the most famous "near suicides" is Flavius Josephus who failed to commit suicide at Jotapata in the year 69 C.E. when all other zealots there did so in a mass suicide pact. Flavius Vespasian, successor to Nero as Emperor of Rome, had come to conquer Judea. Strong resistance was offered at the fortress of Jotapata. After a 40 day siege, the fortress fell. Many chose suicide by flinging themselves over the walls or falling on their weapons. Josephus, however, sought concealment in a huge cistern in which he found 40 of his own soldiers. They all swore to die by their own hand in a mass suicide pact. When his turn came Josephus reneged and surrendered to the Romans.[11] In Josephus' *Antiquities of the Jews,* there are numerous examples cited of suicide including the mass suicide at Masada.

Suicide in the Talmud

The Talmud is replete with stories concerning suicide and martyrdom as well as discussions relating to the laws of burial and mourning for the deceased.

Avodah Zarah 18a describes Rabbi Ḥanina ben Teradyon's death by burning at the hands of the Romans. He was wrapped in the Scroll of the Law, bundles of branches were placed around him and these were set ablaze. The Romans also brought tufts of wool which they had soaked in water, placing them over his heart to prevent a quick death. When his disciples pleaded with him to open his mouth so that the fire consume him more quickly, he replied that one is not to accelerate one's own death. The executioner asked him: "Rabbi, if I raise the flame and remove the tufts of wet wool from your heart, will I enter the world to come?" "Yes," was the reply. The executioner did as he proposed and the rabbi died speedily. The executioner then jumped into the fire and was burned to death. A voice from heaven exclaimed that Rabbi Ḥanina ben Teradyon and his executioner had been assigned to the world to come.

Another case of suicide is related in *Bava Batra* 3b. Herod was the slave of the Hasmonean house of the Maccabees and had set his eyes on a certain maiden of that house. One day he heard a voice from heaven saying that every slave that rebels now will succeed. So he killed the entire household but spared the maiden. When she saw that he wanted to marry her, she ran up to the roof and cried out: "Whoever comes and says that he is from the Hasmonean house is a slave since I alone am left of it and I am throwing myself down from this roof." Herod loved her so that he preserved her body in honey for seven years.

The suicide of a Roman officer who saved the life of Rabban Gameliel is portrayed in *Ta'anit* (fol. 29a). When Tinneius Rufus the wicked destroyed the Jewish Temple, Rabban Gamaliel was condemned to death. A high officer came to the house of study to search for him but Rabban Gamaliel hid. The officer found him and asked him secretly: "If I save you, will you bring me into the world to come?" The answer was affirmative. The officer made Rabban Gamaliel swear to it and then he (the officer) mounted the roof and threw himself down and died. The Romans annulled the decree against Rabban Gamaliel according to their tradition that the death of one of their leaders (i.e. the officer's suicide) is a punishment for an evil decree. Thereupon a voice from heaven was heard saying that this high officer was destined to enter the world to come.

Two nearly identical stories are told in *Hullin* (fol. 94a) and *Derekh Erez Rabbah* (Chapter 9, fol. 57b). Because of an incident that once occurred, it was decreed that guests may not give any of the food that is set before them to the host's son or to his servant or deputy unless they have received the host's permission to do so. The incident was that in a time of scarcity a man invited three guests to his house and only had three eggs which he set before them. When the host's (hungry) child entered and stood before them, one of the guests took his portion and gave it to him; the second guest did the same and so did the third. When the father came in and saw his son with one egg in his mouth and holding two in his hands he picked him up to his full height and flung him to the ground so that he died. When the mother saw her child dead, she went up to the roof, threw herself down and died. On seeing this, the father also went up to the roof, threw himself down and died. Rabbi Eliezer ben Jacob said: "Because of this, three souls perished."

A related incident that terminated in suicide is told in *Hullin* (fol. 94a). A man had sent his friend a barrel of wine and there was oil floating at the mouth of the barrel leading the recipient to believe that the whole barrel contained oil. He invited some guests to partake of it. When he came and found that it was only wine, he went and hanged himself out of shame because he had nothing else prepared to set before his guests. As a result, it was decreed that a man should not send to his neighbor a barrel of wine with oil floating on top of it.

Another Talmudic episode of suicide is found in the commentary of

Rashi on *Avodah Zarah* 18b. Rabbi Meir is said to have fled to Babylon. One of the reasons given is "because of the incident of (his wife) Beruryah." The incident concerns the fact that Rabbi Meir's wife once taunted him regarding the rabbinic adage that women are temperamentally light headed. He replied that one day she would testify to its truth. Subsequently she was enticed by one of her husband's disciples proving she was too weak to resist. She then committed suicide by strangulation.

A mass suicide is described in *Gittin* (fol. 57b) where 400 boys and girls are said to have been carried off for immoral purposes. They guessed what they were wanted for and said to themselves that if we drown in the sea we shall attain the life in the future world as portrayed in Psalms 68:23. The girls leaped into the sea first and the boys followed.

In *Gittin* 57b is related the story from the Second Book of Maccabees of the woman and her seven martyred sons. The sons were killed one by one by Emperor Antiochus Epiphanes for refusing to serve an idol. As the last son was being led away to be killed, his mother said to him: "My son, go and say to your father Abraham: Thou didst bind one (son to the altar, i.e., Isaac), but I have bound seven altars." Then she went up on a roof and threw herself down and was killed. A voice thereupon came forth from heaven saying, "A joyful mother of children." (Psalms 113:9).

Another incident is related in *Berakhot* (fol. 23a). A certain student once left his phylacteries on the side of the road in a hole before entering a privy. A harlot passed by and took them. She came to the house of learning and said: "See what so and so gave me for hire." When the student heard this, he went to the top of a roof and threw himself down and killed himself.

The rules and regulations governing suicide are discussed in at least two tractates of the Talmud. In *Bava Kamma* 61a is found the following: "No Halakhah may be quoted in the name of one who surrenders himself to meet death for the words of the Torah." Further in the same tractate (91b) we find: ". . . who is the Tanna that maintains that a man may not injure himself? It could hardly be said that he was the Tanna of the teaching: 'And surely your own blood of your souls will I require' (Genesis 9:5) which Rabbi Eleazar interpreted to mean that I will require your blood if shed by the hands of yourselves (i.e. suicide), for murder is perhaps different . . ." Rashi interprets this scriptural verse to mean that even though one strangles oneself so that no blood flows, still I will require it.

The major Talmudic discussion of rules governing suicide is found in chapter 2 of *Semahot*. Here we are told that we do not occupy ourselves at all with the funeral rites of someone who committed suicide wilfully. Rabbi Ishmael said: We exclaim over him "Alas for a lost (life). Alas for a lost (life)." Rabbi Akiva said to him: "Leave him unmourned; speak neither well nor ill of him." Further "we do not rend garments for him, nor bare the shoulder (as signs of mourning), or deliver a memorial address over him. We do, however, stand in a row for him (at the cemetery after the funeral to offer condolences) and recite the mourner's benediction for him because this is respectful for the living (relatives). The general rule is that we occupy ourselves with anything that is intended as a matter of honor for the living . . .''

The Talmud (*Semaḥot,* chapter 2, rule 2) defines an intentional suicide. It is not he who climbed to the top of a tree and fell down and died, nor he who ascended to the top of a roof and fell down and died as these may have been accidents. Rather, a wilful suicide is one who calls out: "Look, I am going to the top of the roof or to the top of the tree, and I will throw myself down that I may die." When people see him go up to the top of the tree or roof and fall down and die, then he is considered to have committed suicide wilfully. A person found strangled or hanging from a tree or lying dead on a sword is presumed not to have committed suicide intentionally and none of the funeral rites are withheld from him.

The Talmud (*ibid.,* rules 4 and 5) next relates two childhood suicides and considers neither an intentional suicide. One case concerns the son of Gornos of Lydda who ran away from school, and the other case is that of a child in Bene-Berak who broke a bottle on the Sabbath. In each case, the father threatened to punish the child and out of fear each child destroyed himself in a pit. Rabbi Tarfon in the former case, and Rabbi Akiva in the latter case ruled that these are not wilful suicides and therefore none of the funeral rites should be withheld.

Suicide in the Midrash

In the Midrash Ecclesiastes Rabbah (chapter 10, 7; fol. 26b) the story is told of Rabbi Akiva walking (barefoot) to Rome when met by a eunuch officer of the Emperor riding on a horse. The officer asked him whether he was the famous rabbi of the Jews and he answered yes. In order to embarrass Rabbi Akiva, the eunuch said three things: "He who rides on a horse is a king, he who rides on a donkey is a free man and he whose feet have shoes on is a human being; he who has none of these is worse than a dead person." Rabbi Akiva replied saying three things: "One's beard is one's majestic countenance, happiness of heart is one's wife and the inheritance of God is to have children; woe is the man who is lacking all three. Not only that but Scripture states, 'I have seen servants upon horses and princes walking as servants upon the earth' (Eccles. 10:7)''. When the eunuch officer heard these words, he knocked his head against a wall until he died.

Another case of intentional suicide is related in Midrash Rabbah on Genesis (65:22; fol. 130b). The case is that of Yakum of Ẓerorot, nephew of

Rabbi Yose ben Joezer of Zeredah. Yakum taunted Rabbi Joseph Meshita and, as self-punishment, subjected himself to the four modes of execution inflicted by the courts: stoning, burning, decapitation and strangulation. He took a post, planted it into the earth, raised a wall of stones around it and tied a cord to it. He made a fire in front of it and fixed a sword in the middle of the post. He hanged himself on the post, the cord was burned through and he was strangled. The sword caught him while the wall of stones fell upon him and he was burned.

Suicide in the Codes of Jewish Law

In his *Mishneh Torah* (Laws of Mourning, chapter 1, section 11), Maimonides states:

> For one who has committed suicide intentionally we do not occupy ourselves at all (with the funeral rites), and we do not mourn for him nor eulogize him. However, we do stand in a row for him and we recite the mourner's benediction and we do all that is intended as a matter of honor for the living.

Maimonides then defines an intentional suicide exactly as defined in *Semahot*. The commentators on Maimonides' code, Radbaz, *Kesef Mishneh,* and *Lehem Mishneh,* all point out that Maimonides considers mourning an honor for the dead and therefore prohibited.

Rabbi Jacob ben Asher (*Tur, Yoreh De'ah* No. 345) codifies the section of the Talmud from *Semahot* nearly verbatim. He states that we do not rend garments, bare the shoulder or eulogize the wilful suicide victim. However, we do stand in a row to offer condolences to the family at the cemetery and we utter the mourner's benediction for these are intended as a matter of honor for the living relatives. Rabbi Jacob ben Asher then continues by saying that the prohibition of rending the garments refers only to distant relatives but the immediate relatives who have to mourn the deceased should rend their garments as a sign of mourning. This is diametrically opposed to Maimonides. The *Shulhan Arukh* follows Maimonides.

The *Tur* defines a wilful suicide as it had been defined in *Semahot*. However, a child who committed suicide even wilfully is not considered to have attained his full measure of intelligence. Similarly, he continues, anyone who commits suicide in unusual circumstances, such as King Saul, is not considered a wilful suicide and he is entitled to all funeral rites. According to *Beit Yosef* and *Bayit Hadash* in their commentaries on Jacob ben Asher, the latter statement in the *Tur* is based on Nahmanides work entitled *Sefer ha-Adam.*

In the Shulhan Arukh Rabbi Joseph Caro seems to combine the Talmudic

(*Semaḥot*) and Maimonidean regulations regarding suicide. He states (*Yoreh De'ah* No. 345) that we do not occupy ourselves at all for anyone who has committed suicide wilfully. We do not mourn for him (contrary to Jacob ben Asher but in agreement with Maimonides) nor eulogize him nor rend garments for him nor bare the shoulder. However, all that is in honor of the living, such as standing in a row to offer condolences to the relatives of the deceased, is performed.

Several commentators on Caro, including *Siftei Kohen, Ba'er Hetev,* and *Pitḥei Teshuvah,* point out that Jacob ben Asher's code differs from Caro in that the former does require garment rending and mourning of close relatives of the deceased. *Siftei Kohen* also quotes Rashba, who in one of his several thousand responsa (no. 763) explains that "we do not occupy ourselves at all" as cited from the Talmud and Maimonides does not refer to burial itself. Rather, only the rites surrounding the funeral are withheld but the deceased must be buried.

Suicide in Recent Rabbinic Writings

Responsa literature on suicide is rather sparse. Rabbi Moses Schreiber (*Ḥatam Sofer—Yoreh De'ah* no. 326) was asked concerning a person found drowned in a river. Rabbi Schreiber defines in great legal detail what a wilful suicide is in Jewish law. He seeks legal technicalities such as fear, anger, emotional instability on the part of the victim which, if present, would remove the deceased from being considered an intentional suicide. He thus justifies the actions of Saul and Ahithophel. Rabbi Schreiber concludes that laws of mourning, including the recitation of the *Kaddish* prayer are observed even for an intentional suicide victim.

Rabbi Jehiel Michael Tukazinsky, in his two-volume work entitled *Gesher ha-Ḥayyim* (Jerusalem, 1960) devotes an entire chapter (no. 25) to a discussion of suicide. The person who commits wilful suicide is considered a murderer. It matters not whether he kills someone else or himself since his own soul is not his, just as someone else's soul is not his. Would we be able to bring this man to justice in this world, he would be adjudicated as any murderer. In fact, he may be so judged in Heaven above.

The thirteenth century *Sefer Ḥasidim* written by Rabbi Judah the Pious states (no. 675) that even one who neglects the preservation of his health is guilty of partially murdering himself. Rabbi Tukazinsky states that it may even be a graver sin to commit suicide than to murder someone else for several reasons. Firstly, by killing himself, a person removes all possibility of repentance. Secondly, death in most circumstances is the greatest atonement for one's sins (*Yoma* 86); however, in a suicide's death there has been committed a cardinal transgression rather than expiation. A third reason why Judaism abhors suicide is that the person who takes his own life asserts by this act that he denies the Divine mastery and ownership of his life, his body and his soul. The wilful suicide further denies his Divine creation. Our Sages compare the departure of a soul from a human body to a Torah scroll which has been consumed by fire. Thus, a person who commits suicide can be likened to one who burns a *Sefer Torah*.

He who takes his own life is also one who denies the Judaic teaching of the immortality of the soul and the eternal existence of Almighty God. Such a person will have to answer to Heavenly judgment in the world to come as our rabbis of blessed memory stated: "He who wilfully destroys himself has no share in the world to come."

Martyrdom in Judaism

The subject of suicide is intertwined with the topic of martyrdom since many suicides are committed as an act of martyrdom. The Jewish attitude toward martyrdom is based upon the following passage in Leviticus (18:5): "Ye shall therefore keep my ordinances and my judgments which, if a man do, he shall live in them: I am the Eternal." The rabbis deduce from the words "he shall live" that martyrdom is prohibited save for idolatry, adultery and murder (*Sanhedrin* 74a). All other commandments may be transgressed if life is in danger in order that "he shall live." Martyrdom includes both the ending of one's own life for the sanctification of the name of God (Levit. 22:32) or allowing oneself to be killed in times of religious persecution rather than transgress Biblical commandments. Perhaps the best known example of martyrdom in Jewish life are the ten famous scholars executed or martyred by the Roman state at different times for their insistence on teaching the Torah.

The topic of martyrdom is vast and there is a great deal of literature on it, especially from the responsa during and after the Holocaust. This subject is mentioned here only for purposes of "touching all bases" since martyrdom might be considered a special form of suicide.

Suicide and Modern Psychiatry

The preponderance of modern psychiatric thinking on the pathology of suicides is that, with rare exceptions, the act of suicide, whether or not successful, is *prima facie* evidence of mental illness. Most often the illness is depression or despondency but occasionally may manifest itself as a psychosis or schizophrenia. The rare exception can be illustrated by a person who has lived a full and good life and who feels he (or she) has nothing to look forward to. If this type of person attempts or commits suicide, it is not a sign of despondency.

Suicide may represent the act which expresses the fantasy reunion of a person with a departed loved one or a fantasy reunion with God. Such a psychiatric aberration of a person's mind cannot be classified as anything other than pathological. Suicide can accompany virtually all psychiatric illnesses or may occur during periods of life crisis and stress in persons without discernible mental illness.

Although physicians daily witness profound despair and tragedy in their patients, suicide attempts are an unusual event, and successful suicide is rarer still. The clinician should recognize the painful states of bitterness and desperation which so often raise the suicidal impulse.

At the other extreme of modern psychiatric thought is the American psychiatrist Thomas Szasz, who claims that suicide is rarely, if ever, a sign of mental illness. He further asserts that a person should have the right to commit suicide just as a person has many civil rights. Halakhah would not condone such an approach because, in Judaism, we believe that the human body is not ours to do with as we please. Man was created in the image of God and was entrusted with his body, to guard it and to watch over it. This is the philosophy behind Judaism's abhorrence of suicide. Since the vast majority of suicides are assignable to emotional stress or psychiatric illness, lenient rabbinic rulings are usually enunciated (*Gesher ha-Ḥayyim, loc. cit.*).

Summary and Conclusions

Judaism regards suicide as a criminal act and strictly forbidden by Jewish law. The cases of suicide in the Bible as well as from the Apocrypha, Talmud and Midrash took place under unusual and extenuating conditions.

In general a suicide is not accorded full burial honors. The Talmud and codes of Jewish law decree that rending one's garments, delivering memorial addresses and other rites of mourning which are an honor for the dead are not to be performed for a suicide victim. The strict definition of a suicide for which these laws apply is one who had previously announced his intentions and then killed himself immediately thereafter by the method he announced. Children are never regarded as deliberate suicides and are afforded all burial rites. Similarly, those who commit suicide under extreme physical or mental strain, or while not in full possession of their faculties, or in order to atone for past sins are not considered as wilful suicides and none of the burial and mourning rites are withheld.

These considerations may condone the numerous acts of suicide and martyrdom committed by Jews throughout the centuries, from the priests who leaped into the flames of the burning Temple to the martyred Jews in the time of the Crusades, from the Jewish suicides during the medieval persecutions to the martyred Jews in recent pogroms. Only for the sanctification of the name of the Lord would a Jew intentionally take his own life or allow it to be taken as a symbol of his extreme faith in God. Otherwise intentional suicide would be strictly forbidden because it constitutes a denial of the Divine creation of man, of the immortality of the soul and of the atonement of death.

NOTES

1. Solomon, P., "The Burden of Responsibility in Suicide and Homicide," *J.A.M.A.,* 199:321–324, 1967.

2. Nelson, B., "Suicide Prevention: NIMH Wants More Attention for 'Taboo' Subject," *Science,* 161:776–777, 1968.

3. Campaign Against Suicide, *Medical World News,* 10:7 (Jan. 3), 1969.

4. See Shneidman, E.S. and Farberow, N. L., editors, *Clues to Suicide* (New York: McGraw Hill, 1957), pp. XII and 227; Morielli, E. A., *Suicide: An Essay on Comparative Moral Statistics* (New York: D. Appleton & Co., 1903), pp. XI and 388; Bohannan, P., editor, *African Homicide and Suicide* (Princeton: Princeton Univ. Press, 1960), pp. XIX and 270 and appendix; Douglas, J. D., *The Social Meanings of Suicide* (Princeton: Princeton Univ. Press, 1967), pp. XIV and 398; Yochelson, L., editor, *Symposium on Suicide* (Washington, D. C.: George Washington Univ., 1967), pp. 150; Yap, P. M., *Suicide in Hong Kong with Special Reference to Attempted Suicide* (Hong Kong Univ. Press, 1958), pp. X and 101; Stengel, E. and Cook, N. G., *Attempted Suicide: Its Social Significance and Effects* (London: Chapman and Hall, 1958), pp. 136; Sainsbury, P., *Suicide in London: An Ecological Study* (London: Chapman and Hall, 1955), pp. 116; Hendin, H., *Suicide and Scandinavia: A Psychoanalytic Study of Culture and Character* (New York: Grune & Stratton, 1964), pp. XII and 153; Leonard, C. U., *Understanding and Preventing Suicide* (Illinois: Charles C. Thomas, 1967), pp. XII and 351; Durkheim, E., *Suicide: A Study in Sociology* (Glencoe Free Press 1951), pp. 405; Farberow, N. L. and Shneidman, E. S., *The Cry for Help* (New York: McGraw Hill, 1961), pp. XVI and 398; Murphy, G. E. and Robins, E.; "Social Factors in Suicide," *J.A.M.A.* 199:303–308, 1967; "The Burden of Responsibility," *J.A.M.A.* 199:334, 1967; "Changing Concepts of Suicide," *J.A.M.A.* 199:752, 1967; "Suicide and Suicidal Attempts in Children and Adolescents," *Lancet* 2:847–848, 1964; "Of Suicide and Folly," *Canad. Med. Ass. J.* 96:1167–1168, 1967.

5. Berger, F. M., "Drugs and Suicide in the United States," *Clin. Pharmac. and Therap.* 8:219–223, 1967.

6. Bakwin, H., "Suicide in Children and Adolescents," *J. Pediatr.* 50:749–769, 1957; Faigel, H. C., "Suicide Among Young Persons. A Review of Its Incidence and Causes, and Methods for Its Prevention," *Clin. Pediatr.* 5:187–190, 1966; Jacobziner, H., "Attempted Suicides in Adolescence," *J.A.M.A.* 191:7–11, 1965.

7. Graetz, H., *History of the Jews,* [six volumes] (Philadelphia: Jewish Publication Society), p. 143.

8. 2 Samuel 17:23.

9. Graetz, H., *History of the Jews,* p. 192.

10. *Ibid.,* pp. 482–485.

11. *Ibid.,* pp. 276–290.

12. See also *Avodah Zarah* 17b; *Ta'anit* 18b; *Ta'anit* 29a; *Berakhot* 61b; *Pesaḥim* 50a; *Bava Batra* 10b; *Sanhedrin* 11a; 14a; 74a, b; 110b. and Unterman, I. Y., *Shevet mi-Yehudah* (Jerusalem, 1955), pp. 38ff. and Jakobovits, I., *Jewish Medical Ethics* (Bloch, New York, 1959), pp. 52–54.

21

Autopsy in Jewish Law and the Israeli Autopsy Controversy

FRED ROSNER

The purpose of postmortem examination — autopsy — is to modify, elaborate, confirm or reject antemortem diagnoses, thus aiding the medical profession in understanding human illness. It is performed to correlate the clinical aspects of disease for diagnostic and therapeutic evaluations, to determine the cause of death, to evaluate incompletely known disorders or discover new disease, to serve an educational function through demonstration of tissue alterations as they relate to pathogenesis and to the therapeutically altered or natural courses of disease, and to collect data for statistical analysis of disease incidence.

In Paris in a study of 1,000 autopsies,[2] 85 percent were classified as useful and 15 percent as useless. A similar study of autopsies done in London[3] revealed that the clinical diagnosis was completely right in 53 percent of patients; the clinical diagnosis was wrong or missed in 25 percent of patients; one diagnosis was right, another wrong or missed in 15 percent of patients; and the clinical diagnosis was completely wrong in 7 percent of patients. There is little doubt that autopsies sometimes are a revelation to the physician, sometimes of the expected, at other times of unanticipated disease. Cases where autopsy disclosed unexpected findings are well documented periodically in the medical literature.[4] There is also no dispute concerning the value of autopsy as an essential component of medical education.[5] These and other overwhelming reasons for the performing of autopsies, however, still leave many questions unanswered. How many

autopsies are "needed"? How should they be done? Who should do them?[6]
It is incorrect to assume that since autopsies are good, we must have more
of them. It is also fallacious to presume that the more autopsies we perform
the better quality medicine we have. Dr. Lester King, senior editor of the
American Medical Association Journal, refutes this assumption when he
states:[7]

> It is a pernicious misconception that the mere performance of postmortem
> dissection leads to progress in medical science, or the discovery of new
> diseases, or the advancement of medical frontiers. We lose sight of the fact
> that progress depends not on the autopsy, but on the person who is
> examining the material. Those who believe that the more autopsies we
> perform, the more medical science will advance, are actually pleading not
> for more autopsies but for persons who can profitably utilize the data of
> autopsies, persons who have imagination, originality, persistence, mental
> acuity, sound education and background, the indispensable prepared mind
> without which observations are quite sterile. It is a grave disservice to
> confuse the performance of autopsies with the spark of insight which the
> autopsy may trigger. We want the insight; and autopsies alone, no matter
> how numerous, are not the equivalent. We must not confuse the
> performance of postmortem dissection with the autoptic attitude. They
> may indeed coincide, but they need not.

A recent article published in the *Journal of the American Medical
Association* (volume 233, pp. 441–443, 1975) entitled "The Postmortem
Examination: Scientific Necessity or Folly?" concludes that current
medical diagnostic techniques have decreased the value of the "routine"
autopsy and that greater stress should be placed on the postmortem
examination in selected cases rather than in a fixed percentage of deaths.
From the religious viewpoint, however, even where an autopsy is sanctioned, different answers must be provided, particularly to the question of
how an autopsy is to be done. In most religions, including Judaism, the
physical remains of a deceased person must be treated with honor and
respect. Judaism requires not only that the dead be treated with utmost
dignity and honor but that no desecration of the dead be performed except
where such an act may immediately save a life. Even in such a situation, all
organs examined and/or removed must be returned to the body prior to
burial. Burial must not be delayed. No benefit may be derived from the
dead except where a life is at stake.

Autopsy and Jewish Law

This essay will discuss the Jewish attitude towards anatomical dissection
and postmortem examinations as developed in the Biblical, Talmudic and

rabbinic literature. There is a desperate need for Orthodox Jewish physicians to obtain answers to the following perplexing questions: When, if ever, does Jewish law sanction or even demand an autopsy? When is it permissible for a Jewish physician to request permission for an autopsy from the next of kin, as required by American law? Does Jewish law require permission in the cases where autopsy is allowed? From whom must permission be sought—the bereaved family or the deceased prior to his demise? What if the deceased specifically asked that his body be dissected after his death? What constitutes desecration of the dead? Can one not use cadaver organs for transplantation to live recipients who are desperately in need of a kidney, an eye or even a heart? How do autopsies affect the double commandment of burying the dead without delay?

The earliest leading responsum on autopsy is authored by 18th century Rabbi Ezekiel Landau.[8] It is this responsum upon which all subsequent inquiries and rabbinic and legal decisions are based. Rabbi Landau was asked by the rabbinical authorities in London concerning a patient with a bladder calculus (probably urinary bladder, but possibly gallbladder) who had died following an unsuccessful operation for this condition. The question posed was whether it was permissible to make an incision into the body of the deceased at the site of the previous surgery, and to directly observe the root of the illness. The purpose was to learn what the proper therapy should be in future cases and to avoid unnecessary surgery. Rabbi Landau answered that autopsy constitutes a desecration of the dead, and is only permissible to save the life of another patient who is immediately at hand (*lefaneinu*). In the case before him, however, the life of no specific living patient was under consideration, and the autopsy was solely to learn therefrom for a future patient with a similar affliction. This possibility was too remote to permit an autopsy. Furthermore, continues Rabbi Landau, "if we would be lenient in this matter, heaven forbid, they would dissect all dead people in order to learn the arrangement of the internal organs and their functions, so as to know what therapy to give to the living."

The only other 18th century rabbinic responsum dealing with autopsy is that of Rabbi Jacob Emden[9] who was asked by a medical student whether he could participate in the dissection of dogs on the Sabbath as a part of his anatomy training. Rabbi Emden replied that numerous prohibitions relating to the Sabbath are involved. Dissection of human bodies, he continued, is prohibited because one is not permitted to derive any benefit from the deceased.

In the nineteenth century, there are five recorded rabbinic responsa dealing with autopsy by Rabbis Schreiber,[10] Ettlinger,[11] Schick,[12] Auerbach[13] and Bamberger.[14] All take an essentially negative view towards the performance of autopsy except if the lives of other existing (not future) patients might thereby be saved. Rabbi Ettlinger also allows autopsy if the deceased had willed his body for that purpose during his lifetime.

Twentieth century responsa on permitting autopsies are numerous and, rather than present an exhaustive enumeration of them, it seems more appropriate to discuss the principles upon which is based the Jewish legal attitude toward autopsy. These are described in detail by Rabbi Isaac Arieli,[15] and others.[16] The questions discussed by Rabbi Arieli include whether autopsies are permitted for the following:

> 1) the sake of studying anatomy; 2) as a general procedure to gain knowledge; 3) to determine the cause of death; 4) to save an existing seriously ill patient; 5) to save future patients who may present with a similar disease; 6) in the case of a common disease; 7) in the case of a rare disease; 8) in the case of a genetic disorder; 9) on a person who asked that this procedure be performed after his death; 10) transplantation of an organ from a dead person to a living individual; and 11) on a stillbirth.

The prohibition of desecrating or disgracing the dead is based upon the Biblical passage "And if a man has committed a sin worthy of death, and he be put to death, and thou hang him on a tree, his body shall not remain all night upon the tree but thou shalt surely bury him the same day . . ." (Deut. 21:22-23). The Talmud (Sanhedrin 47a) interprets this phrase to mean that just as hanging all night is a disgrace to the human body, so too any other action which constitutes a disgrace to the deceased is prohibited. If the Torah was concerned for the body of a convicted criminal, certainly, a fortiori, the body of a good citizen should be treated with the proper respect, and be properly interred without being subjected to shame or disgrace.

Two Talmudic passages dealing with autopsy should be mentioned, although neither deals directly with dissection of the dead for purely medical purposes. One case deals with criminal law, the other with civil law. The first case, described in Ḥullin 11b, deals with a murderer for whom the Divine Law prescribes death. The Talmud asks:

> Why do we not fear that the victim may have been afflicted with a fatal organic disease, for whose killing a person is not punishable as a murderer? Is it not because we follow the majority and most victims of murderers are not so afflicted? And should you say that we can examine the body — this is not allowed because it would thereby be mutilated. And should you say that since a man's life is at stake, we should mutilate the body, then one could answer that there is always the possibility that the murderer may have killed the victim by striking him in a place where he was suffering from a fatal wound, thus removing all traces of the wound. In such a case it is clear that no amount of postmortem examination would show that the victim was afflicted with a fatal illness.

Therefore it is proved, concludes the Talmud, that we follow the majority and do not perform an autopsy. In this case, the findings of an autopsy, even if it were permitted, would have been irrelevant to the conviction of the murderer, and insufficient to acquit him.

The second case is described in *Bava Batra* 154a where the story is told that in Bene-Berak a person once sold his father's estate and died. The members of the family, thereupon, protested that he was a minor at the time of his death and therefore not eligible to sell any of his father's estate. Hence, the property he sold should belong to the surviving members of the family. They came to Rabbi Akiva and asked whether the body might be exhumed and examined, so as to ascertain his age by performing a post mortem examination. Rabbi Akiva replied that one is not permitted to dishonor the dead; and furthermore, the signs of maturity usually undergo a change after death. Hence, the examination would not produce reliable evidence of his age. Neither Talmudic case deals with autopsy for medical purposes but both illustrate the objection to this procedure on the grounds that it would constitute a desecration of the dead, a biblically prohibited act.

The next major objection in Jewish law against autopsy is the multi-faceted problem of burial of the dead. Firstly, the Biblical phrase, "Thou shalt surely bury him . . ." (Deut. 21:23), tells us that it is a positive commandment to bury the dead (*Sanhedrin* 46b). Secondly, whoever keeps his dead unburied overnight transgresses a negative commandment. This is deduced from the earlier part of the same Biblical phrase: "His body shall not remain all night . . ." Thirdly, the body must be interred whole, for if one leaves out even a small portion, it is as if no burial at all took place (Jerusalem Talmud, *Nazir* 7:1). According to Maimonides (*Hilkhot Sanhedrin* 15:8) the infinitive "Thou shalt surely bury him . . ." indicates that the command regarding burial concerns all dead, not only those executed by the Court. A fourth facet of the burial problem is the question as to whether burial, in addition to averting disgrace (by later putrefaction of the body), also represents atonement for the sins committed during life (*Sanhedrin* 46b). If one performs an autopsy, one is in fact transgressing the prohibition of delaying burial of the dead. If one fails to return all removed organs to the body for burial, one also prevents atonement since such a burial is incomplete.

Another serious objection to autopsy in Jewish law is the prohibition of deriving any benefit from the dead as deduced in the Talmud (*Avodah Zara* 29b and *Nedarim* 48a). The question of whether observation alone constitutes a benefit, or whether parts of the deceased must be used, such as for organ transplantation in order to be considered deriving benefit from the dead, is a legal technicality, as is the question of whether the prohibition is Biblical or rabbinic in origin.

Other halakhic questions are also raised concerning autopsies. For example, can a priest ritually defile himself for the burial of a first degree relative if the deceased has had an autopsy, particularly if organs are removed? Or can mourning begin if burial is effected but parts of the body have not been buried? Thirdly, do the prohibitions regarding autopsy apply to a stillbirth? Fourthly, according to the Jewish concept of the soul being bound to the body, does not the soul suffer pain and/or disgrace if the body is dissected? Is permission for autopsy required to avoid the problem of stealing, particularly in regard to organ transplants? Who may give such consent? The deceased in his lifetime? The family? Society?

Rabbi Arieli arrives at 14 conclusions:

1. A postmortem examination is a desecration and disgrace to the dead and Biblically forbidden.
2. There is suffering to the soul which is bound to the body when the latter is desecrated.
3. The body of a Jew is holy.
4. If one leaves unburied any part of the deceased, then one transgresses the positive commandment of burying the dead, and the negative commandments of delaying the burial and defiling the land. There is no rest to the deceased until his entire body returns to the earth.
5. If the relatives are able to effect burial of the entire body then the laws of *Aninut* (time prior to the onset of mourning) apply until they have done so.
6. If any part of the body is missing, then priestly relatives may not actually defile themselves for the deceased.
7. Autopsy on a stillbirth is prohibited.
8. In addition to the reasons mentioned above, dissection for medical studies is prohibited because one derives benefit from the dead, which some but not all rabbis also state is not allowed.
9. Dissection of the dead to save another person's life is permitted, provided such a patient is available, and there is a reasonable prospect that the autopsy will directly save that life. But to save the life of some patient at a future time, autopsy is prohibited.
10. Autopsy to establish the cause of death is adjudicated like the case of a patient who may be present in the future (i.e., prohibited).
11. Autopsies are permitted in cases of hereditary diseases, just as if a patient whose life could be directly saved is at hand.
12. If the deceased in his lifetime freely consented to an autopsy, then many authorities allow it, and it is permitted.
13. Corneal grafts[16a] from the dead to the living are permitted, but the transplantation of other organs requires further investigation.
14. The family, while not empowered to permit autopsies, may prevent them. In some cases, anyone can prevent an autopsy.

Rabbi Arieli, as well as most 20th century rabbis, bases his decisions primarily on the classic responsum of Rabbi Ezekiel Landau who allows autopsies only if they would save the life of a patient immediately available (*lefaneinu*). Rabbi Jakobovits points out:

> Rabbi Arieli is prepared to extend this principle even to patients who are not locally at hand, but who — through modern means of communication — may benefit from the findings of autopsies elsewhere, provided the ailment concerned is widespread enough to warrant the assumption that some other sufferer at the same time may be cured through these findings. But in fact, adds Rabbi Arieli, while the disease may be widespread, the likelihood of a cure being discovered as a result of any particular autopsy is very remote indeed. In these circumstances, therefore, one would not be justified in setting aside the ban on disfiguring the dead for the (almost hypothetical) sake of saving life . . . Equally restrictive is Rabbi Arieli's rejection of autopsies to establish the cause of death, since he regards the link between such operations and the saving of life once again too tenuous . . . he is inclined (however) to permit autopsies on bodies or persons who gave their consent in their lifetime . . .[17]

The consensus of rabbinic opinion today seems to permit autopsy only in the spirit of the famous responsum of the *Noda bi-Yehudah,* Rabbi Ezekiel Landau, i.e., if it may directly contribute to the saving of a life of another patient at hand. In the case of hereditary diseases, the family or future offspring of the deceased are considered to represent patients at hand and thus autopsies are allowed. However, as pointed out by Rabbi Jakobovits, in applying the 18th century ruling of the *Noda bi-Yehudah,* one must take into account the following new circumstances:

1. With the speed of present-day communications, such patients are in fact at hand all over the world, and the findings of an autopsy in one place may aid a sufferer in another immediately.
2. Without autopsies, some of the worst scourges still afflicting mankind cannot be conquered.
3. Autopsies now bear a relationship to the saving of life not only in the hope they hold out for finding new cures for obscure diseases, but also in testing the effects and safety of new medications.
4. On the other hand, the very frequency of autopsies increases the danger that they will become a sheer routine, without any regard for their urgency, and without proper safeguards for the respect due to the dead.
5. With some patients in Israel refusing to be admitted to hospitals for fear of autopsies, the consideration of the saving of life now also operates in reverse.

Certain concrete proposals have already been made by Rabbi Jakobovits who stated:

> While no general sanction can be given for the indiscriminate surrender of all bodies to post mortem examinations, the area of the sanction should be broadened to include tests on new drugs and cases of reasonable suspicion that the diagnosis was mistaken; for autopsies under such conditions, too, may directly result in the saving of life . . .
>
> Any permission for an autopsy is to be given only on condition that operation is reduced to a minimum, carried out with the greatest dispatch, in the presence of a rabbi or religious supervisor if requested by the family, and performed with the utmost reverence and with the assurance that all parts of the body are returned for burial.
>
> Just as it is the duty of rabbis to urge relatives not to consent to an autopsy where the law does not justify it, they are religiously obliged to insure that permission is granted in cases where human lives may thereby be saved, in the same way as the violation of the Sabbath laws in the face of danger to life is not merely optional but mandatory.

Another step forward is the pronouncement by Rabbi Moses Feinstein that postmortem needle biopsies of various organs are permitted by Jewish law, as long as the chest or abdomen are not opened. Such needle biopsies do not constitute a desecration of the dead, because such procedures are often performed on the living in order to ascertain the proper diagnosis of disease. Similarly, continues Rabbi Feinstein, to remove a sample of blood after death, through a needle puncture, for medical examination, is certainly permissible. Finally, postmortem peritoneoscopy, where the physician looks into a body cavity with an electric instrument, is also permitted, according to Rabbi Feinstein.

The Israeli Autopsy Controversy

Nowhere has the controversy over autopsies been more intense and bitter than in the State of Israel where we have often seen Jew pitted against Jew, rabbi against physician and friend against friend. It was first raised prior to Israel's establishment when the Hadassah Hospital in Jerusalem asked whether it was permitted to perform anatomical dissections for medical student teaching. The Chief Rabbinate, in answering the inquiry, stated that no objection exists for such anatomical dissections in cases where the deceased had freely willed his body for such purposes prior to his death. Chief Rabbi Herzog's responsum on this subject was publicized in the Hebrew periodical *Kol Torah* (vol. 1, 1947). Regarding autopsy or the dissection of bodies to discover pathologic anatomy, the agreement reached between Rabbis Herzog and Frank, and Dr. Yasski, the then director of the

Hadassah Hospital, stated that the Chief Rabbinate would not oppose autopsy in the following situations:

a) if the autopsy is required by law;
b) if the cause of death cannot be established without an autopsy; and where three physicians attest to this fact;
c) to save a life, and
d) in cases of genetic or inherited disease where the family may be guided or counselled concerning future children . . .

    The deceased must be buried in accordance with Jewish Law and all organs removed for examination must be returned for burial.

On August 26, 1953, the Israel *Knesset* passed the present Anatomy and Pathology Law. One of the major provisions of this law (section 2) is that if a person agreed, in writing, that his body be used for science it is permitted to dissect that body for medical instruction and research. A second major provision of the law states that a physician may perform an autopsy to establish the cause of death, or in order to use one or more of the organs of the deceased for transplantation to a critically ill recipient (section 6). The Ministry of Health was empowered to make amendments and decrees to implement and interpret the law. The law was unclear as to who had the final word over whether an autopsy should be performed or not, the family of the deceased or the medical authorities. Some clarification emerged from the "Collected Amendments" (*Koveẓ ha-Takkanot* 10 Shevat, 5714) in which section 2 of the Anatomy and Pathology Law is explained as follows.

If a person dies without leaving written consent for autopsy, his next of kin may request that the body not be disturbed, and no autopsy should then be performed. Next of kin is specifically defined. Furthermore, if the deceased had no family, the burial society (*Hevra Kaddisha*) may also object to autopsy, in which case it is not to be done. If the body is unclaimed, then the medical school can utilize the body for teaching and research purposes. However, a panel of three physicians was still empowered to order an autopsy if the cause of death could not be established without such a procedure.

Physicians were accused of taking advantage of this ambiguity in the law, overruling the wishes of families against performing autopsies in many instances. It was alleged that blank autopsy forms were signed by two physicians even prior to the death of the patient so that only one physician would need to sign the order for an autopsy once the patient died, a practice contrary to the spirit of the law, and against the wishes of the family. Physicians were accused of desecration of the dead, because they removed internal organs and filled the body cavities with rags.

When Yiẓhak Raphael became Deputy Minister of Health late in 1961, the Israeli Parliament charged him with the formation of a committee to consider the law concerning autopsies, and to present its conclusions and recommendations to the government for action. The desires of the family of the deceased were to be considered in the committee's deliberations. In 1962 a committee was appointed by Dr. Raphael

> . . . to make a thorough study of the *de facto* and *de jure* situations, including all the relevant ordinances and operational directives and to present to the Ministry of Health conclusions to guide the Ministry's future actions in the matter. The committee is to take into consideration the needs of medical practice and research, the sensibilities of the public in the matter, the law of the land and Jewish legal (halakhic) law.

The full committee met 17 times and its sub-committees held additional meetings. It took testimony from 14 experts. All the members of the committee made a sincere effort to work in a spirit of mutual understanding, despite the differences of opinion among some of them. They found a common language, and it transpired that for the needs of real life a solution could be found in halakhic literature which provides for all contingencies. A detailed report was submitted by the committee which said in part:

> Having carefully weighed the data put before us, the testimony we have heard and the pamphlets and articles we have read, we have come to the conclusion that, despite the great gap that appears to exist between the two points of view expressed before us, there is a way of satisfying at least part of the demands of both sides.

The following recommendations were accepted unanimously:

1) The 1953 law should be amended to include halakhic principles.
   a. An autopsy should be performed only when, by thus establishing the exact cause of death, it will provide information which will make it possible to save lives, and
   b. in order to perform a transplant to treat a patient who has been specifically marked for this particular transplant.
2) An autopsy shall not be performed if the deceased had, in his lifetime, expressed opposition to it, or if, after his death, certain specified next of kin express opposition, except
   a. if there are grounds to suspect that not establishing the cause of death might constitute a danger to the public or to the family, or
   b. if there are grounds to suspect that death was caused by a medical error which, if it is not ascertained, might lead to deaths.
3) The next of kin shall be given enough time to express their opposition.

4) The section of the law concerning penalties (section 6) should be extended to apply also to false autopsy certificates.

5) A control committee should be set up consisting of a doctor, a rabbi and a Christian clergyman.

These very restrictive amendments to the 1953 Anatomy and Pathology Act also required that in a case where physicians invoke item 2 above (danger to society or a medical error), the matter should come for adjudication before a rabbi or Christian clergyman. An appeals board was also to be established by the Ministry of Health. Deputy Minister of Health Yiẓhak Raphael, writing in the Hebrew periodical *Gevilin* (vol. 25), stated that he was certain that the *Knesset* would not adopt such a restrictive law where the family has the final word. The rate of autopsy would drop to near zero, and the non-religious elements in the government would defeat any such proposal. After much deliberation and discussion with various members of the cabinet, Dr. Raphael presented to the *Knesset* on December 25, 1964, the following compromise bill:

1) The concept of objection to autopsy by the burial society or a relative to the deceased is added to the 1953 law.

2) Autopsy is permitted to establish the cause of death if this will make possible the saving of lives.

3) An organ from a deceased may be used for transplant purposes for a patient who has been specifically designated for that transplant.

4) Autopsy will not be performed if the deceased had, in his lifetime, expressed opposition to autopsy after his death.

5) Autopsy will not be performed if there is opposition to autopsy from the person whose name appears in the hospital chart, and who is to be called in case of emergency, or from certain specified relatives, or a specified burial society.

6) Items 4 and 5 above are overruled if there are grounds to suspect that not establishing the cause of death might constitute a danger to the public, or to the family, or if there is a suspicion that death was caused by a medical error which, if not ascertained, might lead to further danger to life. Such a suspicion must be certified in writing by a panel of three physicians.

7) Autopsy is not to be performed until at least 5 hours had elapsed from the time of notification of death to the responsible family member or burial society as in item 5. Sabbaths and Jewish holy days are not included in the five hour waiting period.

8) The Minister of Health will appoint a control commission to supervise the implementation of the law. Among the members of this commission should be a physician, rabbi and Christian clergyman.

9) Penalties are to be imposed upon a physician who falsely certifies

to the need for an autopsy, punishment to consist of three years imprisonment.

This new proposal was much more restrictive than the 1953 law but more moderate than the earlier proposal in that it did not require each case to be presented for rabbinic judgment. In spite of strong objections from many sides, particularly the medical profession and the non-religious elements in the government, the proposal was presented to the Israeli Parliament as the "Anatomy and Pathology Law. Revised 1965." Renewed controversy among the various factions in the government brought the debate to fever pitch. Some demanded that the earlier version of the bill, as originally proposed by the Special Wahl Commission, be brought to the floor for a vote. Yet others had intermediate or compromise suggestions, but none were adopted because the parliamentary debate took place shortly before election time, and members of the *Knesset* felt that votes might be influenced by that consideration. The whole matter was referred back to the Special Commission and to a Committee made up of members of the Coalition Parties. As a result of these new deliberations, the following modification of the earlier proposal was made:

1) To delete the concept of the burial society objecting to an autopsy, except as it was defined in the 1953 law.
2) To allow autopsy in exceptional cases, even if this means overruling the expressed wishes of the deceased before his death or the objections of the next of kin.

   The exceptional cases are where three physicians certify in writing that there exists the possibility that death was due to an unusual, unknown cause, or due to an accident, and without establishing the cause of death there may result danger to life; or where there is suspicion that a danger to society or to an individual exists which may be overcome by establishing the precise cause of death, or where a need exists to use an organ from the deceased for transplantation purposes. Corneas may be preserved in an eye bank.
3) To delete completely the paragraph dealing with a control commission to supervise implementation of the law.
4) To broaden the matter of transplantation.

This new "revision of the revision," which was now acceptable to the medical community but not to the religious elements in the Government, was presented to the fifth *Knesset* at the end of the session in 1965. In the haste of adjourning, the bill was referred back to a parliamentary committee. The sixth *Knesset* failed to act on the bill. In the meantime, autopsies continued to be performed in the major hospitals of Israel over the opposition of families of the deceased, burial societies and the Rabbinate. Polarization between the medical and religious communities reached a climax with an incident in the Kaplan Hospital in Petaḥ Tikvah. An autopsy had been performed and the family of the deceased stormed the hospital, wreaked havoc causing extensive property damage, and physically assaulted members of the medical staff of the hospital. As a result of this incident, the Ministry of Health issued a circular to all hospitals in Israel directing that patients who stipulate that their bodies not be dissected if they die, should not be admitted to the hospital.

This directive outraged both the religious and non-religious public. Demonstrations were held in Israel and throughout the world demanding that indiscriminate autopsies cease at once. Many violent incidents ensued in the various confrontations. The Chief Rabbinate of Israel published a statement on October 15, 1966 which asserted that:

> In view of the great calamity in the matter of autopsy, we express our opinion that autopsy in any form whatsoever is prohibited by the law of the Torah. And there is no way to allow it except in a matter of immediate danger to life, and then only with the approval in each instance of a brilliant rabbi who is authorized to do so.

The statement was signed by Chief Rabbis Isser Yehuda Unterman and Isaac Nissim, Rabbi Yeḥezkel Abramsky and three hundred and fifty-six rabbis from the entire State of Israel. The 14 pages of signatures end with the following pronouncement: "This judgment is a warning against the passage of any law which would negate it."

Needless to say, this extreme viewpoint of the Chief Rabbinate, generated more protest, more controversy, more violence. Accusations, counter-accusations and denials, flew between the Hadassah Medical Center in Jerusalem and *ad hoc* organizations such as the "Committee for Safeguarding Human Dignity." The Association of Orthodox Jewish Scientists, headquartered in New York, sent a letter to Prime Minister Levi Eshkol on May 5, 1967, part of which follows:

> We would like to emphasize that in spite of our appreciation of the contributions of postmortem examination to modern medicine, we are firm in our conviction that the primary rights of disposition of the remains of a deceased individual — not merely the right to object to an autopsy — must be granted to the next of kin. This practice is almost universal in scientifically advanced countries. We are certain that non-coercive means can be found to assure adequate numbers of postmortem examinations to preserve Israel's position in the medical world.
>
> We urge you to act immediately to achieve passage of legislation, vesting permission for autopsy in the hands of the family of the deceased. Until such legislation is passed, we urge you to prevail upon the medical community to declare a voluntary moratorium on autopsies, except when specific consent is obtained from the family of the deceased.

With the prevailing climate of distrust and controversy, your personal intervention is urgently needed to terminate this destructive internecine war within the Jewish community. We urge you to act now.

The controversy did not abate, however. Stories were published in the Israel lay[18] and medical[19] presses as well as in American lay[20] and medical publications.[21] Acts of incitement and provocation, slanders, derogations, disturbances and personal threats and abuse against physicians continued. On the other hand, autopsies continued to be performed at major Israeli hospitals in spite of the objections of next of kin. People were afraid to be admitted to an Israeli hospital for fear their body might be dissected if they should die.

Ten years later (i.e., in 1977), the Israeli autopsy situation was as follows:

1. There was no change in the law.
2. There seemed to have been a change in the practice in many hospitals in that far fewer autopsies were being done in opposition to the wishes of the family. In general, people were still not formally asked, but expressed opposition was much more frequently honored.
3. There seemed to be some Ministry of Health internal administrative guideline which instructed hospitals not to do autopsies against family wishes. The existence of such a guide was confirmed by the head of the ministry, but a copy thereof could not be obtained.

Thus, there was a *de facto* change in practice as a result of the realities of pressures and conflict but no change of Israeli law.

The solution can only come about when tempers subside and rational thinking is substituted for emotional panic. When physicians and rabbis will, face to face, discuss their mutual problems, then a major hurdle will have been surmounted. A new law concerning autopsy necessarily must take into account the religious and social sensitivities of the population, as well as the needs of the medical community in its dedication to provide the best possible medical care for the sick. In those circumstances where Jewish law does permit an autopsy, the procedure must be performed according to all halakhic principles including the return of all removed organs to the body for burial. Only in an atmosphere of mutual trust can the rabbinate and medical profession arrive at a compromise solution which will satisfy the requirements of both.

It is hoped that more rabbis will speak out in the near future concerning the areas of disease (i.e., genetic and infectious diseases, experimental drug therapy and others) where autopsy may be permitted and how it should be conducted. Physicians, on their part, particularly pathologists, must make arrangements to perform autopsies without undue delay. They must return all organs to the body for burial, removing only minute pieces for microscopic examination. Photographs of the gross pathology can be taken for later use rather than saving whole organs, an act prohibited by Jewish law. Only with a recognition of the problems of medicine and Jewish law by both sides — that is physician and rabbi — can progress be made towards a mutually acceptable solution. This is true not only in the United States, but also in Israel, because in the matter of autopsy, medicine and Judaism do, in fact, strive toward a common goal, the eradication of disease.

NOTES

1. The medical literature on autopsies is voluminous. The Committee on Necropsies of the American Society of Clinical Pathologists, in its bibliography on necropsies covering only a four year period, listed 158 articles. The following represents a list of the articles, textbooks and editorials on the autopsies:
Hazard, J. B., "The Autopsy," *JAMA* 193: pp. 805–806, 1965. Rosahn, P. D., "The Autopsy," (Editorial). *Amer. J. of Clin. Path.* 31: pp. 348–349, 1959. Angrist, A. A., "What Remedies for the Ailing Autopsy?: *JAMA* 193: pp. 806–808, 1965. Angrist, A. A., "A Plea for Grant Support of the Autopsy," *AMA Archives of Path.* 63: pp. 318–321, 1957. Davidsohn, I., Helwig, A., Saphir, O. and Warwick, M., Bibliography on Necropsies, 1931 to 1934. *Amer. J. Clin. Path.* 7: pp. 199–208, 1937. Saphir, O., Autopsy, Diagnosis and Technic., New York, Hoeber-Harper, 1958, 4th edit. Farber, S., *The Post Mortem Examination,* Springfield, Illinois, Charles Thomas, 1937. "Symposium on the Autopsy," *JAMA,* 193: pp. 805–814, 1965. "Medicine and the Law, Autopsy," *JAMA,* 165: 697–699, 1957. Camps, F., "Postmortem Examination from the Medicolegal Viewpoint," *Postgraduate Med.* 35: pp. 47–51, 1964. Bowden, K. M., "Medicolegal Problems Based on Experience at the Morgue," *Med. J. of Austral,* I: pp. 12–15, 1949, Davis, J. H., "Hospitals and the Autopsy: Legal and Social Elements," *Hospitals* 33: pp. 57–58, 1959. Hershey, N., "Who May Authorize an Autopsy?" *Amer. J. Nursing,* 63: pp. 103–105, 1963. Cahal, M. F. and Cady, E. L., "Invasion of Rights in Dead Bodies," *G. P.* 27: pp. 183–184, 1963. Abeshouse, B. J., "The Problem of Autopsies on Orthodox Jewish Patients," *Sinai Hosp. J.* (Balt.), 6: pp. 76–98, April, 1957. Belford, J. L., "Religious Views of Autopsies," *Long Island Med. J.,* 9: pp. 484, 1915. Gottlieb, J., "A Review of Jewish Opinions Regarding Postmortem Examinations," *Boston Med. & Surg. J.,* 196: pp. 726–728, 1929. Joslin, E. P., "Autopsies Upon Jews and Gentiles," *Boston Med. & Surg. J.,* 196: pp. 728–729, 1929. Kottler, A., "The Jewish Attitude on Autopsy," *New York State J. Med.,* 57: pp. 1649–1650, 1957. Gordon, H. L., "Autopsies According to the Jewish Religious Laws," *The Hebrew Physician (Harofe Haivri),* 1: pp. 203–201 Eng. & 130–141 (Heb.), 1937. Levinson, S. A., "The Dead Teacheth the Living," *Hospitals,* 35: pp. 81–92, August 15, 1961. Spivak, C. D., "Post Mortem Examination Among Jews," *New York Med. J.,* 99: 1185, June 13, 1914. Plotz, M., "The Jewish Attitude Toward Autopsies," *Modern Hospital,* 45: pp. 67–68, November, 1935. Saphir, O., "Religious Aspects of the Autopsy," *Hospitals,* 12: pp. 50–55, July, 1938. Ribner, H., "Jewish Law, Social Prejudice and Autopsy,"

Bull. Maryland Univ School of Med., 44: pp. 21–25, Jan., 1959. Figon, G. and Pequignot, H., *"Nouvelles Dispositions Sur Les Autopsies et Leur Intérét Pour la Recherche et la Thérapeutique,"* Sem. Hop. *Paris,* 24: pp. 193–194, 1948. Wolff, G., *"Leichen-Besichtigung Und- Untersuchung Bis Zur Carolina Als Vorstufe Gerichtlicher Sektion,"* Janus, 42: pp. 225–286, 1938. Ackerknecht, E. H., "Primitive Autopsies and the History of Anatomy," *Bull. Inst. Hist. Med.,* 13: pp. 334–339, 1943. Schmeisser, H. C. and Scianni, J. L., "Autopsy and Museum Technique: The History of the Autopsy," *J. Tech. Meth. & Bull. Intern. Ass. Med. Museums,* 15: pp. 26–33, 1936. Rabl, R., *"Die Wertung der Sektionen in Wandel der Zeiten. Eine Kulturgeschichtliche Betrachtung,"* Virch. Arch. Path. Anat., 321: pp. 142–162, 1952. Krumbhaar, E. B., "History of the Autopsy and Its Relation to the Development of Modern Medicine," *Hospitals* 12: pp. 68–74, 1938. Chavarria, A. P. and Shipley, P. G., "The Siamese Twins of Espanola. The First Known Post-Mortem Examination in the New World," *Annals Med. Hist.,* 6: pp. 297–302, 1924. Ehrhardt, H., *"Sektionsbericht und Amtsarztliches Gutachten aus dem Jahre 1722."* Mediz. Welt, 8: pp. 426–427, 1934. Sporlein, G. and Glanz, H., *"Originalberichte Uber die Obduktion von zwei Wurzburger Furstbischofen aus den Jahren 1749 und 1754,"* Virch. Arch. 330: pp. 569–573, 1957. Holzmann, A., *"Anatomische Sektionen Wurzburger Furst-bischofe aus dem 17 and 18 Jahrhundert,"* Virch. Arch. 283: pp. 513–539, 1932. Ficarra, B. J., "Eleven Famous Autopsies in History," *Annals Med. Hist.* (3rd series) 4: pp. 504–520, 1942.

2. Justin-Besançon, L., Chrétien, J. and Delavierre, P., Intérêt Clinique Des Autopsies Systématiques en Milieu Hospitalièr. *Sem. Hop.* Paris. 40: pp. 531–534, 1964. Useful was defined as confirming (55.4 percent), contradicting (6 percent) or completing (23.5 percent) the clinical diagnoses.

3. Wilson, R. R., "In Defense of the Autopsy," *JAMA.* 196: pp. 1011–1012, 1966.

4. Shaw, R. E. and Deadman, W. J., "The Clinical Value of Autopsies," *Canad. Med. Assn. J.* (new series) 42: pp. 168–171, 1940. Collis, J. S., "Permission for Autopsy — Granted," *Cleveland Clin. Quart.* 28: pp. 105–108, 1961. Marx, G. F., "Value of Autopsy," *N.Y. State J. Med.* 68: pp. 950–952, 1968. Frumin, M. J., and Fine, E., "Post Mortem or Post Hoc. The Necessity for Autopsy," *JAMA.* 208: pp. 519–520, 1969.

5. Angrist, A. A., "Effective Use of Autopsy in Medical Education," *JAMA.* 161: pp. 303–309, 1956.

6. Madden, S. C., "How Many Autopsies?" *JAMA.* 193: pp. 812–813, 1965.

7. King, L. S., "Of Autopsies," (Editorial). *JAMA.* 191: pp. 1078–1079, 1965.

8. Landau, E., Responsa *Noda bi-Yehudah, Mahadura Tanina. Yoreh De'ah,* No. 210. Paris. Lang Press, 1947.

9. Emden, J., Responsa *She'elat Yavez.* Section 1, No. 41. Altona 1739.

10. Shreiber, M., Responsa *Hatam Sofer. Yoreh De'ah,* No. 336. Grossman Press, New York 1958.

11. Ettlinger, J., Responsa *Binyan Zion,* No. 170–171, Altona 1868.

12. Shick, M., Responsa *Maharam Schick. Yoreh De'ah,* No. 347, Muncacz 1881.

13. Auerbach, B. Z., *Nahal Eshkol,* Part 2, No. 117 ff. 1868.

14. Bamberger, S., Responsa *Zekher Simhah,* No. 158.

15. Arieli, I. *Bayat Nittuhei Metim, No'am,* Jerusalem 6: pp. 82–103, 1963. Arieli, I. *Bayat Nittuhei Metim, Torah she-be-al Peh,* Jerusalem. Mosad ha-Rav Kook 1964, pp. 40–60.

16. Rubenstein, S. T., *Lishe'elat Nittuhei Metim be-Halakhah, Torah she-be-al Peh,* Jerusalem Mosad ha-Rav Kook 1964, pp. 67–74. Siberstein, V., *Nittuah*

Metim Le'ohr Korot ha-Refu'ah ve-Hitpathutah, Torah she-be-al Peh, Jerusalem Mosad ha-Rav Kook, 1964, pp. 82–86. Wilner, M.D., *Nittuah Metim le-Zorkhei Limmud ve-Shimush be-Helkei Gufot Metim le-Zorkhei Refu'ah, Ha-Torah ve-ha-Medinah,* Vol. 5–6, 1953–1954, pp. 202–212. Yisroeli, S., editor, *Beshe'elat Nittuah ha-Metim, ha-Torah ve-ha-Medinah,* Vol. 5–6, 1953–1954, pp. 213–226. Hadaya, O., *Nittuah Metim le-Zorkhei Limmud u-Refu'ah, Hatorah ve-ha-Medinah,* Vol. 5–6, 1953–1954, pp. 191–201. Hirshenson, Ch., *Nittuah ha-metim, Malki ba-Kodesh,* Part 3, pp. 6–9 and 137–152, 1923, Hoboken, New Jersey, Raphael, Y., *Li-she'elat Nittuhei Metim u-Pitronah, Or ha-Mizrah,* New York, Vol. 16, No. 1 (55), pp. 5–13, Nov. 1966. Schechter, N. S., *Be-Inyan Nittuah Metim, No'am,* Vol. 5, pp. 165–181, 1962. Wachtfogel, Y. Y., *Be-Din Pinui ha-Met me-Kivro u-Bayat Nittuhei Metim, No'am,* Vol. 5, pp. 159–164, 1962. Sharshafsky, S. *Al Nituah Metim, No'am,* Vol. 7, pp. 387–392, 1964. Feinstein, N., *Be-Inyan Nittuah Metim, No'am,* Vol. 8, pp. 9–16, 1965. Hadaya, O., *Be-Inyan 'Lo Talin' be-Met, No'am,* Vol. 8, pp. 68–74, 1965. Grossberg, H. Z., *Nittuah ha-met, No'am,* Vol. 10, pp. 204–207, 1967. Levin, Y. H., *Li-She'elat Nittuah Metim, Ha-Torah ve-ha-Medinah,* Vol. 7–8, pp. 22–227, 1955–57. Levine, S. Y., *Nittuah Metim, Ha-Pardes* (Rabbinical Monthly Journal), Jubilee Book, New York 1951, pp. 138–141. Greenwald, J. J. *Kavod ha-Met, Kol-Bo al Avelut,* New York, Vol. I, pp. 33–63, 1947. Tukazinsky, J. M., *Nittuah ha-Metim,* in *Gesher ha-Hayyim,* 2nd edit., Jerusalem, Vol. 1, 1960, pp. 70–74. Margalit, D., *Le-Ba'ayat Nettihat Gufat Niftarim, Korot* (Jerusalem), Vol. 4, No. 1–2, pp. 41–64, Dec. 1966. Globus, E. L., *She'elot u-Teshuvot al Hukei Nittuhei Metim, Ha-Refuah,* Jerusalem, Vol. 60, No. 6, pp. 196–200, March 15, 1961. Uziel, B. Z., *Responsa Mishpetei Uzi'el, Yoreh De'ah,* Part 1, No. 28–29 and Part 2, No. 110, Tel Aviv, 1935. See also A. D. Kook (*Da'at Kohen,* No. 199), M. J. Zweig (Responsa *Ohel Moshe,* Part 1, No. 4), J. Zweig (Responsa *Parat Yosef,* No. 17), D. Hoffman (Responsa *Melamed le-Ho'il, Yoreh De'ah,* No. 109), M. T. Halevy (Responsa *Divrei Malkiel,* Part 2, No. 92), E. J. Waldenberg (Responsa *Ziz Eli'ezer,* Vol. 4, No. 14), Y. M. Shapira (Responsa *Ohr ha-Meir,* Part 1, No. 74), E. H. Shapira (Responsa *Minhat Eleazar,* Part 4, No. 25), D. M. Manesh (*Havazelet ha-Sharon, Yoreh De'ah,* No. 95), A. Sofer (Responsa *K'tav Sofer, Yoreh De'ah,* No. 174), and M. Winkler (Responsa *Levushei Mordekhai, Orah Hayyim,* Part 2, No. 29), among many others.

16a. See "Heart and Other Organ Transplantation and Jewish Law," *Jewish Life,* Vol. 37, pp. 28–51, Sept.-Oct. 1969.

17. Jakobovits, I., *Ba'ayat Nittuah ha-Metim le Halakhah u-le-Ma'aseh,* in *Torah she-be-al Peh,* Jerusalem, Mosad ha-Rav Kook 1964, pp. 61–66. See also the following by Rabbi Jakobovits: "The Religious Problem of Autopsies in New York Jewish Hospitals," *Ha-Rofe ha-Ivri* 2: pp. 233–238, 1961; "The Dissection of the Dead in Jewish Law: A Comparative and Historical Study," *Tradition,* 1: pp. 77–103, Fall, 1958; "The Dissection of the Dead in Jewish Law: An Historical Study," *Ha-Rofe ha-Ivri,* 1: pp. 210–222, 1960 (Part 1) and 2: pp. 212–221, 1960 (Part 2); *Jewish Medical Ethics,* New York, Block, 1959, pp. 132–152; *Jewish Law Faces Modern Problems,* New York, Yeshiva University Press, 1965, pp. 81–87; *Journal of a Rabbi,* New York, Living Books, 1966, pp. 173–193.

18. Gillon, P., "Autopsies," *The Jerusalem Post,* Friday, March 24, 1967. Rosenthal, Y., *Nettiehat Geviyot Raq be-Hetar Rav, Ha-Arez,* December 4, 1966.

19. Resnekov, V., Editorial on Autopsies. *Quarterly Review of the Israel Medical Association.* (Tel Aviv). 23: No. 1, pp. 3–11, Jan.-April, 1967.

20. Greenberg, M. M., "The Autopsy Crisis in Israel," *The Jewish Observer,* September 1966, pp. 5–9, Chalef, M. N. and Goldberg, J., "Are Autopsies Really Prohibited?" *The Jewish Press,* Friday, Sept. 2, 1966, pp. 20–21 and Birnbaum, M., "Eye Witness to Autopsy Mill Tells of Experiences in Israel," *Ibid.,* Friday,

Oct 7, 1966. Robbins, P. "Unauthorized Autopsy on Israel Hero Performed," *The Guardian,* Vol. 3, No. 2, November, 1967, p. 1. Maeir, D. M., "An Examination of the Autopsy Problem," *Yeshiva University Alumni Review,* Vol. 7, No. 4, Summer, 1967, pp. 2 and 8.

21. Sohn, D., "Israeli Autopsy Debate," *New York State J. Med.,* 68: pp. 398–401, Feb. 1, 1968. "Autopsy Dispute Brings Israeli M.D.'s Under Fire," *Medical World News,* June 9, 1967, p. 45.

Organ Transplantation

22

What is the Halakhah for Organ Transplants?

NACHUM L. RABINOVITCH

In a recent interview, Dr. Christian Barnard is quoted as saying: "No heart condition is hopeless anymore. Anything can be treated."[1]

Whatever may be the ultimate validity of this opinion, Dr. Barnard has certainly earned a place for himself in history as the man who, contrary to the unanimous exegesis of all commentators both ancient and modern, introduced a strictly literal interpretation of the prophetic admonition: "Get yourself a new heart . . ., why should you die?" (Ezekiel 18:31). One who is given to whimsy might even adduce support from the prophet in favour of transplanted hearts rather than artificial ones. Twice Ezekiel repeats the Divine promise: "I will take the stony heart out of their flesh and give them a *heart of flesh*" (11:19 and 36:26).

The staggering dimensions of the technological revolution in medicine and the biological sciences were thrust upon the consciousness of the whole world by the exploits of the cardiac surgeons. Such is the cultural significance of the heart that the announcement of the synthesis of a self-reproducing virus raised barely a ripple of public attention in a world intently absorbed in every detail of the goings-on in Capetown's Groote Schuur Hospital.

Small wonder then that the ethical, moral and legal problems involved in these medical miracles have become the subject of spirited discussion. It is, of course, not true that the questions raised are really new. However, the novel applications and the prospect of increasing frequency of cases requiring ethical decisions of this nature lend an air of urgency to these considerations.

Reprinted from *Tradition* (Spring, 1968). Copyright © 1968 by the Rabbinical Council of America.

While practical halakhic decisions are obviously beyond the scope of this article and, furthermore, each case must be weighed on its own merits, nonetheless it seems not inappropriate to review some of the general halakhic issues which may be relevant.

It is clear that there are two types of acts involved in any transplant — those performed upon the recipient and those carried out on the donor. It seems more expedient to consider the various questions likely to be asked, under these two headings. Removing a living person's heart or other vital organ is murder. Even if it is done with the intent to implant a substitute is it not perhaps still prohibited? Dr. Barnard has admitted to being over-awed by the sight of an empty pericardial cavity. The question is especially relevant in view of the experimental nature of some of the transplant operations.

An established principle of Jewish law is that "The Torah has granted permission to the authorized physician to heal, and it is a commandment included in that to save life. He who refrains from healing is shedding blood, even if other physicians are available."[2]

The freedom of action of the physician is far wider than that granted to any other agent performing a commandment. For example, for a father who is permitted to discipline his child in order to teach him, or for an official of the court whose duty it is to administer stripes, certain actions which are ordinarily considered assault are allowed. Yet these are strictly limited, whereas a surgeon is permitted any kind of incision, or even amputation, designed to save his patient; and a physician may administer drugs which are fatal to ordinary people, if they are calculated to produce a beneficial effect on his patient.

Nonetheless, if an accused should accidentally die under the hand of a duly authorized court official, the killer is blameless and is not required to be exiled like the inadvertent murderer.[3] But if a patient dies as a result of treatment and the doctor discovers that he erred, the doctor is subject to the law of exile as an unintentional slayer.[4] Precisely because the physician, unlike others, is given complete discretion in deciding what treatment is appropriate, any error of judgment on his part renders him liable as an unwitting killer.

However, the recognition of error requires a prior definition of correct procedure. What techniques can be regarded as right and proper in an art which is constantly developing and progressing? Maimonides sets forth two categories to define admissible procedure:

1) Anything which has been proven effective in practice, even though it is not understood how it operates and why.
2) That which follows as a rational deduction from generally accepted physical theory.[5]

Naturally, the second class of treatments again depends upon the trained judgment of the seasoned practitioner. The integrity of the physician in examining and re-examining his reasoning and his conclusions is the final guarantor. Moreover the advice and opinions of his peers must always be sought.[6]

This question has often been dealt with: a patient is suffering from a condition which will certainly cause death — may one administer a treatment which will, if it fails, kill him immediately, but, if it succeeds, prolong his life? Although ordinarily it is murder to shorten the life of even a terminal patient,[7] yet where there is a possibility of improving his chances, we consider him as if he has nothing to lose.[8] In fact one authority applies this not only to a terminal case but even to one where the disease is estimated to cause death within one year.[9] Where there is only a prospect of short-term life this may be risked in favour of a possibility of extended life.

It would appear, then, that where informed judgment considers transplantation a reasonable procedure, since in such cases one is always dealing with critically ill patients, the possibility of even a partial cure is sufficient warrant to attempt a graft.

Another question that has been posed and there have even been suggestions of legislation on it, is that of priorities. Already there are waiting lists of people with renal failure who can be saved by kidney transplants, but there are no organs available. Clearly, a valid criterion is probability of success, but given two patients equally likely to respond to treatment, who should get the available organ?

Framed in this way it seems a new question. However, it is really a question of priority for survival which has many precedents. Thus when a man and a woman both need food desperately, the woman precedes the man[10] in order to preserve her dignity.[11] The same is true if they are captives and need to be ransomed.[12] On the other hand, if they are both drowning, saving the man takes precedence[13] because he is subject to more commandments.[14] In general, the Mishnah[15] rules that scholarship and meritorious deeds accord one priority, since these serve the primary needs of society.[15]

Suppose that the recipient and the likely donor have been selected. In general, the donor who is chosen is an accident victim, close to death. As soon as possible after death, the organ must be removed. In fact, in some sense, the organ must still be alive or at least be capable of living again. This poses the problem: what is the definition of death, or conversely, life?

A precise definition of death has always been important for the Halakhah for several reasons. The commandment to save life over-rides all others.[16] As long as the state of death is not confirmed, the commandment applies. An interesting Talmudic[17] precedent codified in the *Shulḥan Arukh* is that of a woman who dies in childbirth but one can still detect the movements of the foetus.[18] Even on the Sabbath, one is obligated to remove the child by section in the hope that it may yet be alive. However, some authorities raised the objection that the usual symptoms of death detectable by the gross senses may be inadequate in certain cases of stupor or coma, where there is apparent cessation of breathing and heartbeat. A hasty incision to save the child would in such an instance be murder of the mother.[19] In the absence of suitable surgical techniques to preclude this likelihood, the practice in doubtful cases was to wait. However, where death is certain, as for example, if the mother was accidentally beheaded, an immediate section is required.[20]

It would seem that the halakhic definition of death is based upon two criteria:

1) There is complete cessation of biological functions as far as can be determined by the gross senses, i.e., no breathing, no heartbeat, etc.[21]

2) The body can no longer be restored to function as an organism, although individual limbs or organs may still exhibit muscular spasms.

While the first condition is fixed and self-evident, the second is subject to constant change as medical science advances. That the first condition alone was regarded as inadequate is clear from the case already cited. Where there is even a slight possibility to restore life by natural means of resuscitation, the commandment to do so applies, even if all the observable signs of life have ceased. Thus *Tosafot*[22] maintains that Elijah was permitted to defile himself by contact with the dead child only because he knew for certain that he would revive him solely by the power of God. The implication is clear that if there was some natural means of resuscitation, he would have been obligated to risk defiling himself in order to try to save him even if the outcome were in doubt.

It is also clear from the case mentioned of the woman who was decapitated that the absence of any possibility of revival confirms the status of death even though there may still be muscular spasms. Maimonides explains that the organism is no longer considered to be alive "when the power of locomotion that is spread throughout the limbs does not originate in one center, but is independently spread throughout the body."[23] It follows that if the restoration of central control is feasible, the commandment to save life applies. Obviously then the definition of death depends upon the availability of more sophisticated techniques of resuscitation. Here again, the applicability of such methods and the consequent decision as to the onset of death is determined according to the judgment of the physicians.[24]

Crucial to the possibility of successful homografts is the drawing of the line defining death at some point before the tissues begin to deteriorate, and as we have seen, this is halakhically established.

Jewish law is very strict in its prohibition of:

1) mutilating the lifeless body[25]
2) deriving any use or benefit from a cadaver[26] and
3) delaying the interment of any part of a corpse.[27]

Do any of these prohibitions apply to transplants?

The subject of wanton mutilation and needless autopsies has recently been in the public eye in Israel and throughout the Jewish world. However, it is clear that where there is an immediate possibility of saving life, the commandment to save life makes it not only permissible, but even obligatory, to suspend all prohibitions.[28] It goes without saying that in removing an organ, meticulous care must be taken to avoid unnecessary mutilation.

Another question that has been raised is that of ritual defilement. Since the donor is dead, any organ removed from his body is a source of defilement.[29] While this is of concern only to *kohanim,* it is still a problem to consider.

In dealing with internal organs it would seem that the question of *tumah* cannot arise because anything which is absorbed within a living body does not defile.[30]

In any case, however, the status of a transplanted organ is changed. If the transplant takes, it is no longer dead: it becomes a part of the living host body. This concept has been discussed in connection with corneal transplants by Chief Rabbi Unterman and others.[31] Precedent may perhaps be found in the Talmudic case of a certain type of rodent that was thought to originate from inorganic earth. On death, this rodent defiles, while of course ordinary earth does not. However, such earth that was presumably being assimilated into the body of the rodent is considered as being part of it already and therefore is unclean.[32] Maimonides, while expressing amazement at the possibility of such generation, explains the basis of the Mishnah ruling as follows:

"The rodent in process of becoming from earth is partly flesh and partly clay but *all of it moves together.*"[33]

Thus, although to all appearances the clay in question is as yet unchanged, because it has become somehow part of the rodent's body and moves with it, its status is that of flesh. Certainly, an organ which functions within another body is no less part of it and is therefore alive when the host is living.

A new era has begun in man's never-ending struggle against death.

Millions listen daily to the bulletins on the progress of heart transplants and pray for their success. Now that it is literally possible to "get . . . a new heart," is it not time to give heed to the prophet's next sentence?

"For I have no pleasure in the death of any one, says the Lord God: so turn and live!" (Ezekiel 18:32).

NOTES

1. *Toronto Globe & Mail,* January 16, 1968.
2. *Yoreh De'ah* 336:1.
3. *Rambam, Hilkhot Roze'ah* 5:6–7.
4. *Yoreh De'ah, loc. cit.*
5. *Moreh Nevukhim* 3:37; see *Meiri, Shabbat* 67a.
6. *Tiferet Yisrael's* commentary on the Mishnah at the end of *Kiddushin* 77.
7. *Yoreh De'ah* 339:1.
8. *Shevut Ya'akov* 3:75 (cited in *Pithei Teshuvah* 339:1) on the principle in *Tosafot Avodah Zarah* 27b. s.v. *lehayai* "we set aside the certainty (of death) in favor of the possibility (of cure)"; also *Ramban* in his *Torat ha-Adam:* "We are not concerned with the life of the hour if there is a chance of prolonging life"; see also Ritva in *Avodah Zarah, loc. cit.,* s.v. *ude'aimat;* see also *Gilyon Maharsha, Yoreh De'ah* 155.
9. *Darkhei Teshuvah, Yoreh De'ah* 155:6 in the name of *Hokhmat Shelomo.*
10. *Yoreh De'ah* 251:8.
11. *Siftei Kohen, Yoreh De'ah* 251:12.
12. *Yoreh De'ah* 252:8.
13. *Ibid.,* in the gloss.
14. *Turei Zahav* 252:6.
15. End of *Horayot.*
15a. See *Horayot* 13a: "If a sage dies, there is none to replace him; if a Jewish king dies, all Jews can succeed him."
16. *Rambam, Hilkhot Yesodei ha-Torah* 5:6.
17. *Arakhin* 7a.
18. Even if it is not struggling, one desecrates the Sabbath to extricate him; *Orah Hayyim* 335:5.
19. *Ibid.* and *Magen Avraham* 335:11; "Perhaps she is only in a swoon and if her abdomen is cut open, she will die."
20. *Shevut Ya'akov* 1:13.
21. *Orah Hayyim* 329:4.
22. *Bava Mezia* 114b s.v. *omar.* See also the commentary of *Maharaz Chajes ad loc.* who questions the words of *Tosafot;* similar comments are made by other authorities. Those questions are resolved on the basis of the explanation here advanced.
23. Commentary on the Mishnah, *Oholot* 1:6.
24. *Rambam, Hilkhot Roze'ah* 2:8.
25. *Arakhin* 7a; "So that it not come to a desecration."
26. *Rambam, Hilkhot Avel* 14:21; *Yoreh De'ah* 349:2.
27. *Yoreh De'ah* 357:1; see also Ezekiel 39:15 and *Mo'ed Katan* 5b.
28. See *Noda bi-Yehudah Tinyana, Yoreh De'ah* 210: "Why do you debate this

matter so much; it is a clear rule that even for a potential danger, the Sabbath laws are set aside . . . if there is a question of danger to life as in the case of a sick patient." See also *Yoreh De'ah* 155:3; "In case of danger, one sets aside other prohibitions . . ."

29. *Rambam, Hilkhot Tumot* 3:1; *Yoreh De'ah* 369:1.

30. *Mikva'ot* 10:8; *Rambam, Hilkhot Tumat Met* 1:8.

31. *Shevet mi-Yehudah* p. 313.

32. *Ḥullin* 126b.

33. This is the textual reading as found in *Meiri:* "The rodent comes from the earth alone until it is partially flesh and partially dust and mud and all of it moves . . ." However, in the Commentary on the Mishnah found in the usual editions of the Talmud, the phrase "and all of it moves" is lacking. See the commentary of *Tiferet Yisrael (Yakhin)* 70. I have recently seen the new translation of R. Y. Kapach who translated from original Maimonidean manuscripts and who has the textual reading "and all of it moves" like *Meiri*.

This ruling can also have lenient consequences for if someone touches the earth adjacent to the flesh of this rodent and enters the Temple, he can offer a sacrifice and we are not concerned about profane items in the Temple.

23
Organ Transplantation in Jewish Law
FRED ROSNER

Introduction

Recent advances in medical knowledge and technology have made possible the transplantation of a human heart from a deceased person into another individual[1,2] stricken with severe, advanced heart disease refractory to all other medical and surgical approaches. The life and health of the recipient may thereby be prolonged considerably. These operations have raised many moral, theological, legal, social and philosophical problems which seem to cry out for answers. The present paper is an attempt to present the halakhic aspects of heart and other organ transplantation procedures as derived from classical Biblical and Talmudic sources, as well as the more recent rabbinic literature on the subject.

Theological, Moral, Ethical, Social, Legal and Philosophical Problems of Heart Transplantation

It would seem useful prior to embarking on the substance of this chapter to briefly outline some of the questions, other than those of Jewish law, revolving around cardiac transplantation in man. First, theological questions arise. For example, is one interfering with God's will by "artificially" prolonging a person's life by providing him with a new heart when God may have ordained a shorter life span for this person? Is one interfering with the patient's right to die in dignity without extraordinary heroic efforts to extend the duration of his life?

Reprinted from *Jewish Life* (Fall, 1969). Copyright © 1969 by the Union of Orthodox Jewish Congregations of America.

Moral and ethical issues also stimulate our thinking. Is the publicity surrounding heart transplants in excess of that dictated by usual medical practice and ethics? Is cardiac transplantation premature? Is it still in the experimental stages or have we reached therapeutic application? What of the physical and emotional stresses on the family of the donor at the time of their bereavement? Some of these moral issues have been discussed by Tendler[3] and Schimmel[4] and others.[5-10]

Social problems regarding heart transplantation are also self evident. Who shall pay for the enormous expense of the procedure and the pre and post operative care? The patient? Society? Are only the rich entitled to benefit from this medical advance? Who should select the recipients? Since there are many more potential recipients than donors available, who should decide "who shall live and who shall die"? The physician? A group of physicians? Society? Should not society be investing billions of dollars in medical research to attempt to find the cure for heart disease and thus obviate the need for cardiac transplantation? These questions cry out for answers.

Philosophical questions also crop up. The heart is considered to be the seat of the soul. In removing the patient's diseased heart prior to implantation of a "new" heart, has one removed his soul? The famous expression of Descartes "I think, therefore, I am" would take on new meaning. Who am I?

Finally, legal problems[7,11] are of great concern to many people. The donor heart in one instance of cardiac transplantation performed in Texas was derived from a 36 year old sailor who had been fatally beaten. The County Medical Examiner feared for the possible legal problems involved in this homicide case, problems that might affect the prosecution and autopsy procedures. Further legal stumbling blocks include the fact that only 36 states currently have laws allowing the donation of an entire body and 5 additional states allow an individual to will his eyes. Donation of a heart specifically is not dealt with in the legal statutes of any state. A Uniform Anatomical Gift Act reforming the current legal structure relating to the donation and use of organs and tissues for transplantation and other medical purposes has been formulated[11a] and endorsed by the American Bar Association. In Italy, a new law governing kidney transplants was recently adopted.[11]

The answers to some of the above questions seem to be forthcoming. Medical and ethical guidelines for heart transplantation have been established by numerous hospitals, states, medical societies and also the prestigious American Medical Association[12] and National Academy of Sciences.[13] Recommendations in these guidelines include the requirements that the surgical team shall have had extensive laboratory experience in cardiac transplantation, that death of the donor shall be certified by an independent team of physicians and that the information and knowledge gained should be rapidly disseminated to the medical world. All aspects of cardiac transplantation were considered at a meeting held on September 29 and 30, 1968 at Bethesda, Maryland under the sponsorship of the American College of Cardiology. Present at the meeting were surgeons, internists, biomedical scientists concerned with transplantation and immunology, government representatives, private philanthropists and lawyers concerned with cardiac and other organ transplantation. The proceedings of that conference have been published[13a] and cover the following subjects: scientific background of cardiac transplantation, clinical and experimental status of cardiac transplantation, procurement of organs and their storage, tissue matching, and the "nature of the regional and national effort required for realization of the full potential of this new approach to heart disease."

Halakhic Questions in Heart Transplants

The problems in Halakhah concerning transplantation of the human heart may be conveniently subdivided into those which pertain to the recipient, those that concern the donor and those which primarily affect the physician.

Recipient: Is the recipient allowed to subject himself to the danger of the operative procedure? We know that it is not proper for someone to wound himself.[14] Does this apply to the surgical cut of an operation in general, and of a heart transplant operation in particular? Furthermore, does the recipient transgress the commandment of *Take heed to thyself and keep thy soul diligently* (Deut. 4:9) or *Take ye therefore good heed unto yourselves* (Deut. 4:15) which both the Talmud[15] and Maimonides[16] interpret to mean the removal of all danger to one's physical well being?

Another halakhic problem concerning the recipient revolves around the need for burial of his "old" heart. This problem is not unique to heart transplants but applies to any organ removed from the body of a live human being. Thus, a gallbladder, stomach, lung or other diseased internal organ may require burial by Jewish law (there is some dispute on this point) and so might the excised "old" heart.

A third halakhic question regarding the recipient is the status of his new heart after he dies. Does the new heart revert back to the original owner?

Another problem concerns the recipient who happens to be a priest *(kohen)*. Does the question of avoidance of ritual defilement[17] apply to the heart of the dead donor which is now to be implanted into a priest?

Finally, what halakhic priorities are there in choosing a recipient? We know, for example, that a woman takes precedence over a man when both desperately need food[18] because it would be less dignified and more shameful for a woman to go begging than a man.[19] A woman is ransomed before a man if both are captives,[20] but a man takes precedence over a woman if both are drowning[21] because he is subject to more commandments.[22] Additional priorities are enumerated in the Talmud[23] and mentioned by Rabinovitch.[24] Do any of these priorities apply to heart transplant recipients? Should medical criteria be used exclusively in the selection of recipients?

Physician: After the recipient's old heart has been removed and prior to the implantation of the new heart, the patient is without a heart. Is he considered halachically dead during this interim? If so, is the surgeon guilty of the Biblical prohibition of *Thou shalt not kill* (Exod. 20:13 and Deut. 5:17) as enunciated in the decalogue?

Does heart transplantation constitute human experimentation or is it a therapeutic procedure? The former would only be sanctioned under specific regulations and conditions,[25] whereas the latter would fall under the purview of the physician's permissibility to heal: *And heal he shall heal* (Exod. 21:19). From this verse we deduce the physician's license to practice medicine.[26]

Donor: The major considerations from the Jewish legal viewpoint in cardiac transplantation are the halakhic questions that concern the donor. These are five in number. First, there is a prohibition of deriving any benefit whatsoever from the dead.[27] Second, there is a prohibition of desecrating or mutilating the dead body.[28] A third problem regarding the donor is the prohibition of delaying the burial of the dead[29] and the positive commandment of burying the dead.[30] Another halakhic consideration is that of ritual defilement *(Tumah)* for priests in the same room with either the donor or only with the donor's heart.[31] Does this heart transmit ritual defilement? The final and perhaps most crucial question concerns the establishment of the death of the donor. Since the chances of successfully resuscitating a transplanted heart diminish with time following death of the donor, it is imperative to define the criteria for death in order for physicians not to be accused of "heart snatching" from donors prior to their demise. This would constitute an act of murder on the part of the physician who is bound to prolong life but not to prolong the act of dying.[32] The halakhic definition of death has recently been reviewed.[33] This classic definition of death in the Talmud[34] and codes[35] would be set aside if prospects for resuscitation of the patient, even remote, are deemed feasible.[36]

The Halakhah in Eye Transplants

Most of the rabbinic responsa literature concerning organ transplantation deals with eye (cornea) transplants. The basic halakhic principles governing eye transplants, however, are applicable to nearly all other organ transplants and will thus be considered here. Kidney and heart transplants involve several additional unique questions and these will be discussed separately below.

The classic responsum on eye transplants is that of the late Chief Rabbi of Israel, Isser Yehuda Unterman.[37] Rabbi Unterman states that the prohibitions of deriving benefit from the dead, desecrating the dead and delaying the burial of the dead are all set aside because of the consideration of saving a life *(Pikku'ah Nefesh)*. These prohibitions would remain if there is no threat to life involved for which the transplant is being done. For example, there is no *Pikku'ah Nefesh* involved in a bone or nose transplant. The question then arises: is an eye transplant in the category of *Pikku'ah Nefesh?* Attempting to answer this question, Rabbi Unterman cites the Talmud (*Avodah Zarah* 28b) where it states: "If one's eye gets out of order, it is permissible to paint it on the Sabbath because the eyesight is connected with the perception of the heart." Thus, eye damage does seem to constitute *Pikku'ah Nefesh* since one may desecrate the Sabbath to save an eye. Rabbi Unterman argues, however, that this case deals with preventing blindness whereas in eye transplantation one attempts to restore vision, a totally different matter.

On the other hand, Rabbi Unterman does agree that blindness is considered a life-threatening situation since the person so afflicted may fall down a flight of stairs or into a ditch and be killed. Thus, since blindness constitutes a true *Pikku'ah Nefesh,* the problems of desecrating and benefiting from and delaying the burial of the dead are put aside.

What of a person blind in one eye? The concept of *Pikku'ah Nefesh* does not apply and thus on what grounds would corneal transplants be permitted? To answer this question, Rabbi Unterman provides us with an enlightening and original pronouncement. Once the eye is implanted into the recipient, it is not considered dead but a living organ. Thus, the prohibitions of deriving benefit from the dead and delaying the burial of the dead are not applicable since no dead organ is involved. Furthermore, the problem of ritual defilement *(Tum'ah)* is non-existent since *Tum'ah* relates only to a dead organ or a dead body. Confirmation of this last point can be found in the Talmud (*Niddah* 70b) where it states "The men of Alexandria asked R. Joshua . . . was the (dead) son of the Shunammite woman (revived by Elijah the Prophet) unclean? He replied: "A corpse is unclean, but a living person is not." Thus, when the boy came back to life, the problem of *Tum'ah* was eliminated.

One problem remains, however, in Rabbi Unterman's dissertation and that is the prohibition of desecrating the dead to obtain an eye for a person with unilateral blindness. One still has to make an incision into the donor and one doesn't have the concept of *Pikku'aḥ Nefesh* to set the question of desecration aside. A brilliant answer is offered by Rabbi Unterman who states that since the eyes of a deceased person are always closcd, removing one or both would not constitute a desecration. Only a visible incision into the body or the removal of externally visible or internal organs represents a true desecration and this would be permitted for a real *Pikku'aḥ Nefesh* such as blindness in both eyes or advanced renal disease requiring a kidney transplant. An exhaustive review of the rabbinic literature on eye transplants is beyond the scope of this paper and does not seem to be desirable or necessary since it would probably add little if anything to the halakhic principles enunciated in Rabbi Unterman's book.[37] However, the following additional rabbinic responsa dealing primarily with eye transplants have been selected because each makes a new point.

Rabbi Jekuthiel Judah Greenwald[38] states that the prohibition of deriving benefit from the dead applies only to flesh *(basar)* or organs but not to skin *(or)*. The cornea of the eye, according to Rabbi Greenwald, is considered as skin and not as flesh. This is based on a passage in the Talmud (*Niddah* 55a) and the commentary of *Tosafot (s.v. shema ya'aseh shetikhin)* thereon. Rabbi Unterman and many others, however, reject this difference between skin and flesh.

Another point brought out by Rabbi Greenwald is that the engrafted or transplanted cornea becomes nullified on the recipient. An analogous situation is described in the Talmud (*Sotah* 43b) where it states: "If he grafted a young shoot on an old stem, the young shoot is annulled by the old stem and the law of *Orlah*[39] does not apply to it." Similarly, when a cornea is transplanted, it does not retain its original status but becomes annulled on the recipient.

The conclusion to be drawn from Rabbi Greenwald's arguments is that one cannot remove the whole eye from a deceased donor for transplantation; only the cornea may be used since a whole eye represents flesh whereas the cornea alone is considered skin. Furthermore, one cannot overcome the problems of desecrating and delaying the burial of the dead without invoking the concept of *Pikku'aḥ Nefesh*. Thus, Rabbi Greenwald, as most authorities, would only permit eye grafts for a person blind in both eyes.

Rabbi Isaac Glickman[40] reiterates and agrees with all of Rabbi Unterman's theses described above. Rabbi Glickman adds, however, that one may only perform a transplant if the donor gave permission prior to his death. Otherwise the donor is hindered from achieving atonement *(kapparah)* for his sins through his death since one of his organs remains alive. If he gave permission, then he has voiced his acquiescence to delaying his atonement until his organ is later buried following the eventual death of the recipient. In the meantime, he has performed a charitable act *(gemilat ḥesed).* Most other rabbinic responsa agree with the need for permission from the donor or his family. There is one dissenting viewpoint.[41]

Rabbi Meyer Steinberg[42] raises the problem of eye banks. Is the permissibility for corneal transplantation only applicable to an immediate transfer of the cornea from donor to recipient or may one place an eye in an eye bank for later use? Since the permissibility of organ transplantation rests primarily on the overriding consideration of *Pikku'aḥ Nefesh,* it would seem that the recipient would have to be at hand (*lefaneinu,* literally: before us). Rabbi Steinberg answers that since the number of blind people is so large, it is as if there is always a recipient at hand. The Chief Rabbi of the British Commonwealth, Dr. Immanuel Jakobovits, also permits[43] "organs or blood to be donated for deposit in banks provided there is a reasonable certainty that they will be eventually used in life-saving operations (including the restoration or preservation of eye-sight)." Even Rabbi Unterman had already stated at the end of his remarks on eye transplants[37] that blood donations to blood banks are permissible for the same aforementioned reason.

Rabbi Moses Feinstein, in a lengthy responsum[44] devoted exclusively to the prohibition of deriving benefit from the dead, raises the problem of a Gentile donor for an eye transplant. Rabbi Feinstein's conclusion is that it is permissible.

Rabbi Jacob Weinberg[45] takes exception to nearly all of Rabbi Unterman's arguments[37] but concludes that since rabbinic authorities that preceded him permitted eye transplants, he would also be in accord with this ruling, providing, however, that the recipient is blind in both eyes.

Most other rabbinic responsa on our subject agree with Rabbi Unterman's ruling.[37] One outstanding exception is Rabbi Shmuel Huebner[46] who admits that most rabbis permit eye transplants but he himself does not consider a blind or deaf person to be in the category of a dangerously ill person (*ḥoleh sheyesh bo sakkana*). Therefore, the concept of *Pikku'aḥ Nefesh* cannot be invoked and thus, states Rabbi Huebner, the prohibitions of desecrating, deriving benefit from, and delaying the burial of the dead cannot be set aside.

The Halakhah in Kidney Transplants

All the halakhic principles discussed above relating to eye transplants are equally applicable to kidney transplants. In fact, many of the responsa deal with both eye and kidney transplants. A kidney transplant is only undertaken when both kidneys of the recipient are so diseased that life cannot continue without the removal of the body's waste products that accumulate in the blood. Elimination of such wastes can be accomplished by the intermittent use of an artificial kidney or its equivalent, or by the definitive implantation of a healthy human kidney to replace the non-functioning patient's own kidneys. All rabbinic authorities would agree that such a case constitutes *Pikku'aḥ Nefesh* and, therefore, the prohibitions revolving around the dead donor would all be set aside for this overriding consideration of saving a life.

In addition to cadaver kidneys, physicians also employ kidneys from live donors for transplantation. Here, new halakhic questions arise. Is the donor allowed to subject himself to the danger, however small, of the operative procedure to remove one of his kidneys in order to save the life of another? Does the donor transgress the commandment of "Take heed to thyself and keep thy soul diligently" (Deut. 4:9) or "Take ye therefore good heed unto yourselves" (Deut. 4:15)? We have already mentioned that the Talmud[15] and Maimonides[16] interpret these verses to refer to the removal of all danger to one's physical well being. We have also already stated that it is not permitted to intentionally wound oneself.[14] We also know that one may not set aside one person's life for that of another.[47] The question then remains: may one endanger one's own life by donating a kidney in order to save another's life?

The answer is found in commentaries on Maimonides[48] and on Caro[49] and later codes[50] in nearly identical language:

> The Jerusalem Talmud concludes that one is obligated to place oneself even into a possibly dangerous situation (to save another's life). It seems logical that the reason is that the one's (death without intervention, i.e., the kidney recipient) is a certainty whereas his (the donor's) is only a possibility.

Some authorities claim that since many of the codes including Maimonides, *Alfasi, Tur,* and *Asheri,* omit this passage from the Jerusalem Talmud, the final ruling is not in accord therewith. However, based upon this passage, Rabbi Jakobovits[43] has stated that a donor may endanger his own life or health to supply a "spare" organ to a recipient whose life would thereby be saved only if the probability of saving the recipient's life is substantially greater than the risk to the donor's life or health. This principle is applicable to all organ transplantation where live donors are used as a source of the organ in question.

Rabbi Eliezer Yehuda Waldenberg[51] discusses at length the question of whether a healthy person must or may donate one of his organs for transplantation into a desperately ill individual in order to save the latter from certain death. Rabbi Waldenberg concludes that kidney transplants from a live donor are only permissible if a group of trustworthy physicians testify that there is no danger to life to the donor and if the donor is not coerced into consenting to the procedure. If one were to understand Rabbi

Waldenberg literally, then it would be impossible ever to use a live donor as a source for an organ, for there is always a very small risk involved. Fortunately, anesthetic and surgical deaths in this type of operation are exceedingly rare, but they do occur. Perhaps Rabbi Waldenberg means that one is not obligated to endanger one's life to save another, but one may do so on a voluntary basis.

The majority viewpoint [43,48,50] seems to be that a small risk may be undertaken by the donor if the chances for success in the recipient are substantial. Even a major risk may be undertaken if otherwise the death of the recipient is certain.

The Halakhah in Heart Transplants

In the case of transplantation of a human heart from a dead donor, the prohibitions dealing with desecrating the dead, delaying the burial of the dead and ritual defilement are all set aside by the overriding consideration of *Pikku'ah Nefesh,* saving a life. The major halakhic problem remaining is the establishment of the death of the donor. Prior to death, the donor is in the category of a *goses* (hopelessly ill patient) and one is prohibited from touching him or moving him or doing anything that might hasten his death.[52]

There are many types of death: intellectual death when a person's intellect ceases to function; social death when a person can no longer function in society; spiritual death when the soul leaves the body; and physiological or medical death. We are concerned with the halakhic definition of death. (The Jewish legal definition of death based upon Talmudic and rabbinic sources has already been reviewed and summarized earlier in this book.) Cessation of respiration and absence of a heartbeat for a given time period represents the classical halakhic interpretation of death. Today, an additional halakhic criteria is the impossibility of resuscitation.[36]

On the assumption that the donor is absolutely and positively dead, many rabbinic authorities permit heart transplants. Rabbi Jakobovits states:

> An organ may never be removed for transplantation from a donor until death has been definitely established. The prohibition of *nivul ha-met* (desecration of the dead) would then be suspended by the overriding consideration of *pikku'ah nefesh.* Hence, in principle, I can see no objection in Jewish law to the heart operations recently carried out, provided the donors were definitely deceased at the time the organ was removed from them.[43]

Rabbi Isaac Arieli is also quoted[53] as having said that heart transplants are permissible if the donor is definitely dead, but only with the family's consent. A similar pronouncement was made by Rabbi David Lifshutz[54] of the Rabbi Isaac Elchanan Theological Seminary of Yeshiva University.

A published responsum dealing specifically with heart transplants is that of Rabbi Unterman[55] who begins by stating that consent from the family of the donor must be obtained. Otherwise, the doctors and the recipient would transgress the prohibition of "Thou shalt not steal" (Exod. 20:13 and Deut. 5:17). The Chief Rabbi then reviews the halakhic definition of death. He states that under ordinary circumstances, death occurs when respiration ceases. However, sudden unexplained death in young otherwise healthy individuals should be followed by resuscitative measures. A *goses* need not be resuscitated when respiration ceases. Rabbi Unterman then briefly mentions the problem of organ banks by stating that freezing organs for later use is allowed provided there is a good chance they will be used to save a life. Then, the situation would be comparable to having the recipient at hand (*lefaneinu*).

A novel pronouncement by the Chief Rabbi is that heart transplants may not be halakhically sanctioned until such time that the chances for survival from the surgery are greater than those for failure. That is, we invoke the requirement that the probability of success of the surgery shall be greater than the risk to the recipient. This ruling seems to be contrary to the pronouncements of earlier rabbis[56] who allow a sick person to submit to very dangerous surgery or a very dangerous medication if there is a small chance for cure even if the risk of the operation or the treatment is much greater than the chance for cure.

Rabbi Unterman explains that the recipient of a new heart is in a different situation from all other desperately ill (but not necessarily dying) people. After his diseased heart is removed and before the new heart is implanted, the recipient has lost *ḥezkat ḥayyim* (hold on life, or presumption of still being alive). Once he loses his *ḥezkat ḥayyim,* the heart transplant recipient is no longer permitted to risk his life if the chances for success are not greater than the chances of failure. A person dying of cancer, on the other hand, never loses his *ḥezkat ḥayyim* and, therefore, may subject himself to any risk, however great, if there is a small chance for cure.

The definition of *ḥezkat ḥayyim* is exemplified in the Talmud (*Gittin* 28a) where it states that if a messenger brings a divorce from a distant place and the husband was an old man or sick at the time the messenger left, he should still deliver it to the wife on the presumption that the husband is still alive. Thus, unless we have positive information to the contrary, a person retains his *ḥezkat ḥayyim* until he is pronounced dead. There are numerous other examples of *ḥezkat ḥayyim* in the Talmud.[55]

That the heart is the seat of life and that its removal causes one to lose one's *ḥezkat ḥayyim* is exemplified by the well known case of a chicken that was slaughtered in accordance with Jewish law and was found to have no heart. Two sages gave diametrically opposing rulings regarding this chicken. Rabbi Zevi ben Jacob Ashkenazi, known as the *Hakham Zevi,* decreed that the chicken is kosher because without a heart, there is no life and, since the chicken walked and ate in a normal manner, the heart must have been present. After the chicken was opened, a cat must have snatched the heart away and eaten it. The *Hakham Zevi* also cites the *Zohar* in which it is written that without a heart, life cannot exist for even a moment. Furthermore, says the *Hakham Zevi,* Rabbi Joseph Caro, in the *Kesef Mishneh* (commentary on *Mishneh Torah*), points out that Maimonides omits absence of the heart from his list of animals with defects which cannot be slaughtered for food (*terefot*) because such an animal would not be viable. Finally, says the *Hakham Zevi,* even if witnesses were to come and say that they saw the chicken at all times and nothing was removed from it, they are not believed since that is impossible and against nature. The opposing viewpoint is that of Rabbi Jonathan Eyebeschuetz, author of *Kereti u-Feleti.* This rabbi ruled that the chicken is not kosher and the witnesses are believed. He also claims that physicians in Prague assured him that another piece of flesh that did not look like a heart might in fact have functioned as a heart. Thus, without a normal heart, the chicken is a *terefah* (non-kosher).

In either event, we see from both sages involved in this case that the heart is essential to life, and life is impossible without it. Therefore, concludes Rabbi Unterman,[55] in the case of a human heart transplant recipient, removing the patient's old heart removes from him his *hezkat hayyim,* and thus the removal of the recipient's heart can be sanctioned only if the risk of death resulting from the surgery is estimated to be smaller than the prospect of lasting success. On the other hand, one must desecrate the Sabbath to rescue someone from under a collapsed building[57] even if the person may be already dead because he retains his *hezkat hayyim* until proven otherwise. Similarly, a patient dying of an incurable illness may subject himself to a potentially lethal medication or operation[56] on the small chance that cure might be achieved, because this patient never lost his *hezkat hayyim.*

This original concept of Rabbi Unterman regarding the loss of the *hezkat hayyim* by the heart transplant recipient after his diseased heart is removed raises numerous questions. What is the status of this "lifeless" patient until the new heart is implanted? Is he legally dead? Is his wife considered a widow? Can she remarry? Are his children considered orphans and how do the inheritance laws apply here, if at all? After he receives his new heart, he is certainly alive again. Does he have to remarry his wife? All these questions have already been answered negatively by Rabbi Azriel Rosenfeld.[58] Rabbi Rosenfeld discusses the case of a person who has just died of an incurable disease and whose body is stored at a very low temperature for eventual thawing out and revival when the cure for the disease will be found. If the answer to all the above questions is no, as Rabbi Rosenfeld proves for a refrigerated person who "is certainly dead — by any ordinary definition — once he has been frozen,"[58] then certainly a heart transplant patient who has only lost his *ḥezkat ḥayyim* temporarily should be considered not to have lost his status as husband and father. He might be considered lifeless during this interim period between heart exchanges but certainly not legally dead.

Dissenting from Rabbi Unterman's permissiveness towards heart transplants under the conditions described above is Rabbi Isaac Jacob Weiss of Manchester, England. Rabbi Weiss, answering an extensive inquiry from Rabbi Jakobovits, strongly condemns cardiac transplants.[59] Rabbi Jakobovits wrote to Rabbi Weiss that a transplant operation may require artificial extension of the donor's life by the use of a respirator until the recipient can be prepared to receive the new heart. As a result, the following halakhic question arises: Is it lawful to artificially prolong the life of the donor solely to preserve his heart long enough to effect the transplant and, having done so, is it lawful to then shut off the respirator thus, in effect, manipulating the life and death of the donor at will? This question, which Rabbi Jakobovits believes is highly relevant to the whole problem,[60] was answered negatively by Rabbi Weiss.

Another responsum dealing with heart transplantation is that of Rabbi Chaim Dov Gulewski of Brooklyn, New York.[61] Rabbi Gulewski discusses the question of whether a person can renounce his desire to live in order to give his heart to another and, if this is permissible, whether the potential recipient is allowed to accept this heart and whether the surgeon is guilty of murder if he performs the transplantation. Rabbi Gulewski further offers legal definitions for a person who is considered a *terefah* (suffering from a serious organic disease and who cannot live more than twelve months) and a dying individual *(goses)*. The law differs whether this person is dying by Divine decree (*goses bi-yedei shamayim*) such as from incurable cancer or old age, or by human intervention (*goses bi-yedei adam*) such as a car accident or homicide victim. At the end of his article, Rabbi Gulewski offers a rebuttal to Rabbi Unterman's responsum.[55]

Another published responsum on heart transplants is that of Rabbi Aryeh Leib Grossnass of the London *Bet Din* (Court of the Chief Rabbi). Rabbi Grossnass writes[62] that a person is still alive by Jewish law if his breathing is maintained either spontaneously or artificially even if all cerebral function has ceased. Such an individual is classified as a *terefah* upon whom one may not operate save to heal him but not to use his heart even with his permission to save another. Once a person reaches the status of a *nevelah* as defined in the Talmud (*Ḥullin* 21a), then one may remove his heart and transplant it into another. Rabbi Grossnass also discusses the status of the recipient after his diseased heart was removed and before his "new heart" is implanted. Although legally dead, if the operation is successful, then the matter becomes clear that the patient was never really dead at all. A long discussion follows in Rabbi Grossnass' responsum dealing with the question as to whether one is required or allowed to donate an organ such as a kidney to save another if there is a risk involved to the donor.

Rabbi Moses Feinstein added his voice[63] to those condemning heart transplantation. Rabbi Feinstein considers this procedure to involve a double murder. However, a personal interview with Rabbi Feinstein by this writer as well as careful reading of Rabbi Feinstein's lengthy responsum[64] on this subject discloses the following clarification of his position. If the donor is absolutely and positively dead by all medical and Jewish legal criteria, then no murder of the donor would be involved and the removal of his heart or other organ to save another human life would be permitted. He reiterates this view at the end of his responsum defining death.[65]

Concerning the recipient, when medical science will have progressed to the point where cardiac transplantation becomes an accepted therapeutic procedure with reasonably good chances for success, then murder of the recipient would no longer be a consideration. Additional animal experimentation, continues Rabbi Feinstein, is essential to overcome major obstacles such as organ rejection, tissue compatibility typing and immunosuppressive therapy before heart transplantation in man can be condoned. In the present state of medical knowledge, however, where chances for success are minuscule and the recipient's life is probably shortened rather than lengthened by this procedure, heart transplantation must still be considered murder of the recipient.

Another recent responsum on cardiac transplantation is by Rabbi Yehuda Gershuni of Yeshiva University.[66]

The major concern of most, if not all, the rabbis attempting to give legal rulings in heart transplant cases is the establishment of the death of the donor. This is the identical problem that the medical and legal professions are now wrestling with. The majority of rabbinic opinion expressed to date in regard to heart transplants is of a permissive nature *provided* the donor was definitely deceased at the time his heart was removed. Even Rabbis Feinstein and Weiss who voice the most stringent opposition might also agree under these conditions.

Final Note

On December 3, 1967, Dr. Christian Barnard performed the world's first cardiac transplant at Groote Schuur Hospital in Capetown, South Africa. Exactly one year and two days later, on December 5, 1968, Professor Morris Levi at the Belinson Hospital in Petaḥ Tikvah performed Israel's first heart transplant and the world's one hundredth. Because the donor's name was not revealed, a furor of speculation and religious dispute emerged with reverberations throughout the world press.[67] The major concern seemed to have been the possible lack of permission from the donor's family to use his heart for transplantation thus raising the issue of "organ stealing." The operation itself was sanctioned by Chief Rabbi Unterman under the conditions described in his responsum.[55] Sephardic Chief Rabbi Nissim said that transplants are acceptable "in the case of danger to life and as long as clinical death is insured."

Heart transplantation is probably here to stay, although it must still be considered an experimental procedure. As of November 1976, according to the International Registry of Organ Transplantation, there had been 316 heart transplants worldwide. Of that total, 107 had been performed at Stanford University Medical Center in Stanford, California. One year survival had increased progressively by calendar year from 22 percent in 1968 to 62 percent in 1974. Among the 71 patients who received transplants at Stanford since January 1, 1972, 57 percent have survived at least one year and 43 percent for five years.

Many medical problems such as availability of donors, tissue typing, and rejection control remain to be solved. However, just as answers to the legal, moral and religious issues seem to be forthcoming, so too, it is hoped, strict medical evaluation and careful consideration of the prerequisites before a transplantation is performed, will improve the likelihood of successes.

As a motto to our survey of Jewish legal attitudes toward heart and other organ transplantation, we might cite the prophecy of Ezekiel as promised by Almighty God: "And a new heart will I give you and a new spirit will I put within you, and I will take away the stone heart out of your flesh and I will give you a heart of flesh" (Ezekiel 11:19 and 36:26). Although this scriptural reference is obviously meant in a purely figurative and spiritual sense, it seems to vividly depict the present epoch of cardiac transplantation.

Addendum

Since the original publication of this essay, several additional rabbinic responsa on heart transplantation have appeared by leading authorities in Israel including the former chief Rabbi, Rabbi Unterman, and the armed forces Chief Rabbi, Rabbi Goren, later to become the country's Chief Rabbi himself.[68] Finally, an exposition on brain transplants and the Jewish legal questions involved has also been published.[69]

NOTES

(Titles of Articles in Hebrew periodicals are given in English.)

1. Barnard, C. N., "A Human Cardiac Transplant: An Interim Report of a Successful Operation Performed at Groote Schuur Hospital, Capetown," *S. Afr. Med. J.,* 41:1271–1274, (Dec. 30) 1967.

2. Cooley, D. A., Bloodwell, R. D., Hallman, G. L. and Nora, J. J., "Transplantation of the Human Heart. A Report of Four Cases," *J.A.M.A.,* 205(7):479–486, (Aug. 12) 1968.

3. Tendler, M. D., "Medical Ethics and Torah Morality, *Tradition,* 9(4):5–13, (Spring) 1968.

4. Schimmel, E. D., "Medical Ethics and Torah Morality. A Rejoinder," *Tradition,* 9(4):14–19, (Spring) 1968.

5. Hamburger, J. and Crosnier, J., *Moral and Ethical Problem in Transplantation.* In *Human Transplantation.* Edit. by F. T. Rapaport and J. Dausset, New York, Grune and Stratton, 1968, pp. 37–44.

6. Elkinton, J. R., "Moral Problems in the Use of Borrowed Organs, Artificial and Transplanted." Editorial. *Annals of Int. Med.,* 60(2):309–313, (Feb.) 1964 and 61(2):355, (Aug.) 1964.

7. Appel, J. A., "Ethical and Legal Questions Posed by Recent Advances in Medicine," *J.A.M.A.,* 205(7):513–516, (Aug. 12) 1968.

8. Reemtsma, K., *Ethical Problems with Artificial and Transplanted Organs: An Approach by Experimental Ethics. In Ethical Issues in Medicine. The Role of the Physician in Today's Society.* Edit. by E. F. Torrey, Boston, Little, Brown and Co., 1968, pp. 263–294.

9. Wolstenholme, G. E. W. and O'Connor, M., *Ethics in Medical Progress: With Special Reference to Transplantation.* Ciba Foundation Symposium. Boston, Little, Brown and Co., 1966, x and 257 pp.

10. Ladimer, I. and Newman, R. W. Editors: *Clinical Investigation in Medicine: Legal, Ethical and Moral Aspects, an Anthology and Bibliography.* Boston University Law-Medicine Research Institute. 1963, XXIII and 517 pp.

11. "Organ Transplantation and Our Laws: A Warning and a Need," Medical News Section, *J.A.M.A.,* 203(2):31–32, 38, (Jan. 8) 1968.

11a. Sadler, A. M., Sadler, B. L. and Stason, E. B., "The Uniform Anatomical Gift Act. A Model for Reform," *J.A.M.A.,* 206(11):2501–2506, (Dec. 9) 1968.

12. Judicial Council, "Ethical Guidelines for Organ Transplantation," *J.A.M.A.,* 205(6):341–342, (Aug.5) 1968.

13. "Cardiac Transplantation in Man." Statement Prepared by the Board on Medicine of the National Academy of Sciences. *J.A.M.A.,* 204(9):805–806, (May 27) 1968 and editorial comment thereon in the same issue, pp. 820–821.

13a. Moore, F., Burch, G. E., Harken, D. E., Murray, J. E. and Lillihei, C. W. "Cardiac and Other Transplantation In the Setting of Transplant Science as a National Effort,: *J.A.M.A.,* 206(11): 2489–2500, (Dec. 9) 1968.

14. *Bava Kamma* 91b; Maimonides' *Mishneh Torah: Hilkhot Shevu'ot* 5:17 and *Hilkhot Hovel u-Mazik* 5:1.

15. *Berakhot* 32b.

16. *Mishneh Torah: Hilkhot Roze'ah u-Shemirat ha-Nefesh* 11:4.

17. *Shulhan Arukh, Yoreh De'ah* 369:1 and 374:2.

18. *Ibid.* 251:8 and Mishnah *Horayot* 3:7.

19. *Shakh* on Caro 251:8.

20. *Shulhan Arukh, Yoreh De'ah* 252:8 and Mishnah *Horayot* 3:7.

21. *Ibid.*

22. *Taz* on Caro 252:8.

23. Mishnah *Horayot* 3:7 and the Talmud *Horayot* 13a, 13b and 14a.

24. Rabinovitch, N. L., "What is the Halakhah for Organ Transplants?", *Tradition,* 9(4):20–27, (Spring) 1968 (reprinted above in this volume).

25. Jakobovits, I., "Medical Experimentation on Humans in Jewish Law," *Proc. Ass'n. Orthodox Jewish Scientists.* New York, 1:1–7, 1966 (reprinted below in this volume).

26. *Bava Kamma* 85a; *Shulḥan Arukh, Yoreh De'ah* 336:1.

27. *Avodah Zarah* 29b; *Shulḥan Arukh, Yoreh De'ah* 349:1–2; *Mishneh Torah, Hilkhot Avel* 14:21.

28. *Arakhin* 7a; *Hullin* 11b; and *Bava Batra* 154b.

29. *Sanhedrin* 46b; *Shulḥan Arukh, Yoreh De'ah* 357:1; based on "His body shall not remain all night upon the tree" (Deut. 21:23).

30. Jerusalem Talmud *Nazir* 7:1; Babylonian Talmud *Sanhedrin* 46b; *Mishneh Torah: Hilkhot Avel* 12:1; based on "but thou shalt certainly bury him on that day" (Deut. 21:23).

31. *Mishneh Torah: Hilkhot Tumat Met* 3:1; *Shulḥan Arukh, Yoreh De'ah* 369:1.

32. Rosner, F., "Jewish Attitude Toward Euthanasia," *New York State J. Med.,* 67(18):2499–2506, (Sept. 15) 1967 (reprinted above in this volume).

33. Rosner, F., "The Definition of Death in Jewish Law," *Tradition,* 10(4):33–39, (Fall) 1969.

34. Mishnah *Yoma* 8:6–7; Babylonian Talmud *Yoma* 85a; Jerusalem Talmud *Yoma* 8:5.

35. *Mishneh Torah: Hilkhot Shabbat* 2:19; *Shulḥan Arukh, Oraḥ Ḥayyim* 329:4.

36. Jakobovits, I., Personal Communication. Aug. 1, 1968.

37. Unterman, I. Y., *Shevet mi-Yehudah.* 1955, Jerusalem, pp. 313–322.

38. Greenwald, J. J., *Kol Bo al Avelut.* Vol. 1, New York, 1947, pp. 45–48.

39. Prohibition of using fruit during the first three years after planting a tree (Levit. 19:23).

40. Glickman, I., "Regarding the Law of Grafting Organs from the Dead onto the Sick," *No'am,* Vol. 4, pp. 206–217, Jerusalem 5721 (1961).

41. Pirer, B. Z., "In the Matter of Grafting an Organ from the Dead to a Living Person," *No'am,* Vol. 4, pp. 200–205, Jerusalem 5721 (1961).

42. Steinberg, M., "In the Matter of Grafting an Eye from the Dead to a Blind Person," *No'am,* Vol. 3, pp. 87–96, Jerusalem 5720 (1960).

43. Jakobovits, I., Personal Communication. Jan. 8, 1968.

44. Feinstein, M., "In the Matter of Attaching an Organ or Flesh or Bone from a Dead to a Live Person, Whether This is Prohibited Because of the Law Prohibiting the Derival of Benefit from the Dead, if the Dead Person is a Jew or if He is a Gentile." *Responsa Iggerot Moshe, Yoreh De'ah* no. 229, New York, 1959, pp. 459–469.

45. Weinberg, J., *Responsa Seridei Esh, Yoreh De'ah* no. 120, vol. 2, Jerusalem, 1962, pp. 276–277.

46. Huebner, S., "The Utilization of Eyes from a Dead Person to Restore the Vision of the Blind," *Ha-Darom.* vol. 13, New York, Nisan 5721 (1961), pp. 54–64.

47. Mishnah *Oholot* 7:6; *Mishneh Torah, Hilkhoth Roze'aḥ u-Shemirat ha-Nefesh* 1:9; *Shulḥan Arukh, Yoreh De'ah* 425:2.

48. *Kesef Mishnah* on *Mishneh Torah, Hilkhot Roze'aḥ u-Shemirat ha-Nefesh* 1:14.

49. *Me'irat Einayim* on *Shulhan Arukh, Hoshen Mishpat* 426:1.

50. *Arukh ha-Shulhan, Hoshen Mishpat* 426:4.

51. Waldenberg, E. Y., "Whether there is an Obligation or any sort of Commandment for a Healthy Person to Donate one of his Organs for Transplantation into the Body of a Dangerously Ill Person and to thereby Save the Latter from Death." *Responsa Ziz Eli'ezer,* vol. 9, no. 45, Jerusalem, 1967, pp. 179–185. See also vol. 10, no. 25, 1970, pp. 120 ff. for a lengthy discussion of organ transplants.

52. Mishnah *Semahot* 1:2; Babylonian Talmud *Shabbat* 151b; *Mishneh Torah, Hilkhot Avel* 4:5; *Shulhan Arukh, Yoreh De'ah 339.*

53. Arieli, I.: cited by Abraham Ben Melech in *Panim el-Panim* no. 458, March 1, 1968, p. 16.

54. Lifshutz, D., Personal Communication. Feb. 16, 1968.

55. Unterman, I. Y., "Points of Halakhah in the Question of Heart Transplantation" (From an address to the Congress of Oral Law), Jerusalem, Elul, 5728 (August, 1968).

56. Rabbi Jacob Reischer, *Shevut Ya'akov,* part 3, no. 75 and Rabbi Hayyim Ozer Grodzinski, *Ahi'ezer, Yoreh De'ah,* chapter 16.

57. Mishnah *Yoma* 8:6–7; Babylonian Talmud *Yoma* 85a; *Mishneh Torah, Hilkhot Shabbat* 2:19; *Shulhan Arukh, Orah Hayyim* 329:4.

58. Rosenfeld, A., "Refrigeration, Resuscitation and the Resurrection," *Tradition,* vol. 9, No. 3, pp. 82–94, (Fall) 1967.

59. Weiss, I. J., "Whether It is Permissible to Transplant the Heart of a Sick Person about to Die into Another Ill Person as Therapy," *Ha-Ma'or,* no. 178, Elul, 5728 (Aug.-Sept.) 1968, pp. 3–9.

60. Jakobovits, I., Personal Communication. December 18, 1968.

61. Gulewski, C. D., "Regarding the Law of the Pursuer Who Commits No Act, The Problems of Heart Transplantation and the Laws of a *Goses* and a *Terefah,*" *Ha-Ma'or* no. 179. Tishri-Heshvan, 5729 (Oct.-Nov.) 1968, pp. 3–16.

62. Grossnass, A. L., *Lev Aryeh,* vol. 2.

63. Feinstein, M., "Final Legal Judgment in the Matter of Heart Transplantation," *Ha-Pardes,* 43(6):4, March-April, 1969.

64. Feinstein, M., "Concerning Heart Transplantation for a Patient," *Iggerot Moshe, Yoreh De'ah,* part 2, New York 1973, no. 174, pp. 286–294.

65. Feinstein, M. "Concerning the Signs of Death," *ibid.,* no. 146, pp. 247–252.

66. Gershuni, Y., "Heart Transplantation in the Light of Jewish Law," *Or ha-Mizrah,* 18(3):133–137, April, 1969.

67. "Heart Transplant Spurs Dispute in Religious Circles in Israel," *New York Times,* December 9, 1968.

68. Levi, J., "In the Matter of Transplanting Organs from the Dead," *No'am,* vol. 12, pp. 289–313, Jerusalem, 5729 (1969); Unterman, I. Y., "The Problem of Heart Transplantation from the Viewpoint of Halakhah," *No'am,* vol. 13, pp. 1–9, Jerusalem, 5730 (1970); Kasher, M. M., "The Problem of Heart Transplantation," *No'am,* vol. 13, pp. 10–20, Jerusalem, 5730 (1970); Goren, S., "Heart Transplantation in the Light of Halakhah," *Mahanayim,* no. 122, pp. 7–15, Marheshvan, 5730 (1969).

69. Rosenfeld, A., "The Heart, the Head and the Halakhah," *New York State Journal of Medicine,* vol. 70:2615–2619, (Oct. 15) 1970.

Human Experimentation

24
Medical Experimentation on Humans in Jewish Law

IMMANUEL JAKOBOVITS

The widespread allegations of unethical practices in medical experimentations on humans have recently been substantiated and carefully documented in a report published in the *New England Journal of Medicine*.[1] The article, which was extensively quoted in the daily press, cited twenty-two examples, out of fifty originally submitted, of "unethical or ethically questionable studies" involving hundreds of patients. In the view of the author, "it is evident that in many of the examples presented, the investigators have risked the health or the life of their subjects." In many cases no "informed consent" was obtained either at all or under conditions which would render such consent meaningful. Some of the experiments were performed for purely academic purposes or "for frivolous ends," occasionally on healthy subjects or organs "with nothing to gain and all to lose." All the examples are taken from "leading medical schools, university hospitals, private hospitals, governmental military departments and institutes, Veterans Administration hospitals, and industry." Most people involved in these studies were "captive groups" — charity ward patients, civil prisoners, mental retardees, members of the military services, the investigators' own laboratory personnel, and the like.

Reprinted from *Proceedings of the Association of Orthodox Jewish Scientists* (1966). Copyright © 1966 by the Association of Orthodox Jewish Scientists.

Such practices obviously raise grave ethical and moral problems. At issue here is not only the impropriety of physicians or researchers administering possibly hazardous treatments without the proper consent of the subject. Equally questionable is the right of the subject to submit to such experiments even with his consent. On the other hand, a certain amount of experimentation is patently indispensable for the advance of medicine and in the treatment of innumerable patients. How far, and under what circumstances, can such experimentation be ethically justified?

The author, therefore, scarcely comes to grips with the gravamen of the problem when he suggests that "greater safeguard for the patient than consent is the presence of an informed, able, conscientious, compassionate, responsible investigator, for it is recognized that patients can, when imperfectly informed, be induced to agree, unwisely, to many things," or when he recommends "the practice of having at least two physicians (the one caring for the patient and the investigator) involved in experimental situations," or even when he proposes the presentation of difficult ethical problems "to a group of the investigator's peers for discussion and counsel."

These suggestions are valuable as far as they go. They certainly would help to prevent some current abuses, such as the excessive zeal of young ambitious physicians seeking promotion by proving themselves as investigators, or the inordinate rewards, functioning as bribes, held out to participating prisoners, not to mention more common pressures, inducements and misrepresentations which destroy the whole concept of free consent. But these suggestions are inadequate on two major counts. Firstly, they limit the problem to securing the subject's free and informed consent, whereas in fact the subject may have neither the right nor the competence to grant any consent, even if freely given. Second, they assume that the physician or the investigator or their peers can pass such critical ethical judgments, whereas in fact the assessment of ethical and moral values is completely outside the purview of medical science, being properly within the domain of the moral, not medical, expert. No amount of medical erudition or expertise can by itself provide the ethical criteria necessary for verdicts that may involve life-and-death decisions or the sacrifice of one life or limb for the sake of another. Competent medical opinion is essential to supply the factual data on which such decisions are based; but the decisions themselves, since they involve value judgments, require moral specialists or the guidance of independent moral rules. Ability, conscientiousness, compassion and responsibility are no substitute for competent and reliable knowledge of what is right or wrong, ethical or unethical, particularly when human life is at stake—possibly both the life of the subject and the lives that might be saved through the experiment.

At least this certainly is the Jewish view. It emphatically maintains that moral questions of such gravity cannot be resolved simply by reference to the fickle whims of the individual conscience or of public opinion, but only by having recourse to the absolute standards of the moral law which, in the case of Judaism, has its authentic source in the Divine revelation of the Holy Writ and its duly qualified interpreters.

What cannot be stated with the same certainty and precision is the definition of the Jewish attitude to the problem at hand. Since this is a rather new question, there are as yet too few relevant rabbinic rulings published for a firm opinion to be crystallized and authoritatively accepted. All that can here be attempted is to scan the sources of Jewish law for views and judgments bearing on our issue. But it must be stressed that the resultant conclusions are entirely tentative, and any verdict in a practical case would be subject to endorsement or revision by a competent rabbinical authority duly considering all the facts and circumstances involved.

To this writer there appear to be ten basic Jewish principles affecting the issue and ultimately determining the solution. We will list them *seriatim,* adding to each item the relevant sources and considerations.

1. *Human life is sacrosanct, and of supreme and infinite worth.*

Life is of itself the *summum bonum* of human existence. The Divine law was ordained only "that man shall live by it."[2] Hence any precept, whether religious or ethical, is automatically suspended if it conflicts with the interests of human life,[3] the exceptions being only idolatry, murder and immorality (adultery and incest)—the three cardinal crimes against God, one's neighbor and oneself—as expressly stipulated in the Bible itself.[4] The value of human life is infinite and beyond measure, so that any part of life—even if only an hour or a second—is of precisely the same worth as seventy years of it, just as any fraction of infinity, being indivisible, remains infinite. Accordingly, to kill a decrepit patient approaching death constitutes exactly the same crime of murder as to kill a young, healthy person who may still have many decades to live.[5] For the same reason, one life is worth as much as a thousand or a million lives[6]—infinity is not increased by multiplying it. This explains the unconditional Jewish opposition to deliberate euthanasia as well as to the surrender of one hostage in order to save the others if the whole group is otherwise threatened with death.[7]

2. *Any chance to save life, however remote, must be pursued at all costs.*

This follows logically from the preceding premises. Laws are in suspense not only when their violation is certain to lead to the preservation of life, but even when such an outcome is beset by a number of doubts and improbabilities.[8] By the same token, in desperate cases even experimental and doubtful treatments or medications should be given, so long as they hold out any prospect of success. (But see also no. 9 below.)

3. *The obligation to save a person from any hazard to his life or health devolves on anyone able to do so.*

Every person is duty bound not only to protect his own life and health,[9] but also those of his neighbor.[10] Anyone refusing to come to the rescue of a person in danger of losing life, limb or property is guilty of transgressing the Biblical law "Thou shalt not stand upon the blood of thy neighbor."[11] It is questionable, however, how far one must, or may, be prepared to risk one's own life or health in an effort to save one's fellow; the duty, and possibly the right, to do so may be limited to risking a less likely loss for a more likely gain.[12] In any event, when there is no risk involved, the obligation to save one's neighbor from any danger is unconditional. Hence the refusal of a doctor to extend medical aid when required is deemed tantamount to bloodshed, unless a more competent doctor is readily available.[13]

4. *Every life is equally valuable and inviolable, including that of criminals, prisoners and defectives.*

In the title to life and its value, being infinite, there can be no distinction whatever between one person and another, whether innocent or guilty (except possibly persons under final sentence of death[14]), whether healthy or crippled, demented and terminally afflicted. Thus, even a person's inviolability after death and his rights to dignity are decreed in the Bible specifically in relation to capital criminals, created like everyone else "in the image of God."[15] Insane persons can sue for injuries received, even though they cannot be sued for inflicting them because of their legal incompetence.[16] The saving of physically or mentally defective persons sets aside all laws in the same way as the saving of normal people.[17]

5. *One must not sacrifice one life to save another, or even any number of others.*

This follows from the preceding principle (see also no. 1 above). The Talmud deduces the rule that one must not murder to save one's life (except in self-defense) from the "logical argument" of "how do you know that your blood is redder than your neighbor's?", i.e., that your life is worth more than his.[18] This argument is also applied in reverse: "How do you know that his blood is redder than yours?" to explain why one must not surrender one's own life to save someone else's.[19] For reasons given above (no. 1), there also cannot be any difference between saving one or more lives.

6. *No one has the right to volunteer his life.*

In Jewish law the right to expose oneself to voluntary martyrdom is strict-ly limited to cases involving either resistance to the three cardinal crimes (see no. 1 above) or "the sanctification of God's Name," i.e. to die for one's re-ligious faith. To lay down one's life in any but these rigidly defined cases is regarded as a mortal offense, [20] certainly when there are no religious consid-erations involved. [21] The jurisdiction over life is not man's (except where such a right is expressly conferred by the Creator), and killing oneself by suicide, or allowing oneself to be killed by unauthorized martyrdom, is as much a crime as killing someone else. [22]

7. *No one has the right to injure his own or anyone else's body, except for therapeutic purposes.*

Judaism regards the human body as Divine property, [23] surrendered merely to man's custody and protection. It is an offense, therefore, to make any incisions [24] or to inflict any injuries on the body, whether one's own or another person's. [25] One may not as much as strike a person, even with his permission, since the body is not owned by him. [26] Such injuries, including even amputations, [27] can be sanctioned only for the overriding good of the body as a whole, i.e. the superior value of life and health.

8. *No one has the right to refuse medical treatment deemed necessary by competent opinion.*

In view of the ban on the voluntary surrender of life (no. 6 above), the patient's consent is not required in Jewish law for any urgent operation. [28] His lay opinion that the operation is unnecessary, or his declared desire to risk death rather than undergo the operation, can have no bearing on the medical expert's duty to perform the operation if he considers it essential. His obligation to save life and health is ineluctable (see no. 3 above) and is altogether independent from the patient's wishes or opposition. The con-scientious physician may even have to expose himself to the risk of malprac-tice claims against him in the performance of this superior duty.

9. *Measures involving some immediate risks of life may be taken in attempts to prevent certain death later.*

Jewish law specifically permits the administration of doubtful or experi-mental cures if safer methods are unknown or not available. In fact, the authorities encourage giving a terminal patient a possibly effective drug even at the grave risk of hastening his death should it prove fatal, if the alternative to this risk is the patient's certain death from his affliction later. In that case, the chances of the drug either bringing about his recovery or else accelerating his death need not even be fifty-fifty; and any prospect that it may prove helpful is sufficient to warrant its use, provided the majority of the specialists consulted are in favor of its employment.[29] The same considerations would of course apply to doubtful surgical operations in a desperate gamble to save a patient.

10. *There is no restriction on animal experiments for medical purposes.*

The strict Jewish law against inflicting cruelty on animals[30] is inoperative in respect of anything done to promote human health.[31] This sanction clearly includes essential animal vivisection too,[32] provided always that every care is taken to eliminate any avoidable pain and that such experiments serve practical medical ends, and not purely academic investigations into animal psychology or other purposes without any bearing on human welfare.[33]

From these principles we may now tentatively reach the following conclusions in regard to medical experimentation:

1. Possibly hazardous experiments may be performed on humans only if they may be potentially helpful to the subject himself, however remote the chances of success are.

2. It is obligatory to apply to terminal patients even untried or uncertain cures in an attempt to ward off certain death later, if no safe treatment is available.

3. In all cases it is as wrong to volunteer for such experiments as it is unethical to submit persons to them, whether with or without their consent, and whether they are normal people, criminals, prisoners, cripples, idiots or patients on their deathbed.

4. If the experiment involves no hazard to life or health, the obligation to volunteer for it devolves on anyone who may thereby help to promote the health interests of others.

5. Under such circumstances it may not be unethical to carry out these harmless experiments even without the subject's consent, provided the anticipated benefit is real and substantial enough to invoke the precept of "Thou shalt not stand upon the blood of thy neighbor."

6. In the treatment of patients generally, whether the cures are tested or only experimental, the opinion of competent medical experts alone counts, not the wishes of the patient; and physicians are ethically required to take whatever therapeutic measures they consider essential for the patient's life and health, irrespective of the chance that they may subsequently be liable to legal claims for unauthorized, "assault and battery."

7. Wherever possible, exhaustive tests of new medications or surgical procedures must be performed on animals. These should, however, be guarded against experiencing any avoidable pain at all times.

NOTES

1. Henry K. Beecher, "Ethics and Clinical Research," in *New England Journal of Medicine,* vol. 274, no. 24 (June 16, 1966), pp. 1354–1360.

2. Lev. 18:5.

3. *Yoma* 85b.

4. *Pesaḥim* 25a and b; *Yoreh De'ah,* 195:3; 157:1; based on Deut. 6:5 and 22:26.

5. Maimonides, *Hil. Roẓe'aḥ,* 2:6.

6. Cf. "Whoever saves a single life is as he saved an entire world" (*Sanhedrin* 4:5).

7. *Yoreh De'ah* 157:1, gloss, end. For further details, see my *Jewish Medical Ethics,* 1962, p. 45 ff.

8. *Oraḥ Hayyim,* 329:2–5.

9. *Yoreh De'ah,* 116; *Ḥoshen Mishpat,* 427:9–10.

10. *Ḥoshen Mishpat* 426:1: 427:1–10.

11. Lev. 19:16 and *Rashi a.l.*

12. *Bet Yosef, Ḥoshen Mishpat,* 426; for details, see *Jewish Medical Ethics,* p. 96f.

13. *Yoreh De'ah,* 336:1.

14. See *Oraḥ Hayyim, Mishnah Berurah, Bi'ur Halakhah,* 329:4.

15. Deut. 21:23 and *Naḥmanides a.l.;* see also *Ḥullin* 11b.

16. *Bava Kamma* 8:4.

17. See note 14 above.

18. *Yoma* 82b; but see also *Kesef Mishneh, Hil. Yesodei ha-Torah,* 5:5.

19. *Haggahot Maimuniyyot, Hil. Yesodei ha-Torah* 5:7; see *Jewish Medical Ethics,* p. 98.

20. Maimonides, *Hil. Yesodei ha-Torah,* 5:4.

21. See *Jewish Medical Ethics,* p. 53.

22. Based on Gen. 9:5 and commentaries.

23. Maimonides, *Hil. Roẓe'aḥ,* 1:4.

24. Lev. 21:5 and commentaries.

25. *Ḥoshen Mishpat,* 420:1 ff, 31.

26. *Tanya, Shulḥan Arukh, Ḥoshen Mishpat, Hil. Nizkei ha-Guf,* 4.

27. Maimonides, *Hil. Mamrim,* 2:4.

28. Jacob Emden, *Mor u-Keẓi'ah,* on *Oraḥ Hayyim,* 228; see my *Journal of a Rabbi,* 1966, pp. 158 f.

29. Jacob Reischer, *Shevut Ya'akov,* part 3, no. 75; Solomon Eger, *Gilyon Maharsha* on *Yoreh De'ah,* 1155:5; see *Jewish Medical Ethics,* p. 263, note 69.

30. *Ḥoshen Mishpat,* 272:9, gloss; based on Ex. 23:5.

31. *Even ha-Ezer,* 5:14, gloss.

32. *Sh'evut Ya'akov,* part 3, no. 71; J. M. Breisch, *Ḥelkat Ya'akov,* nos. 30 and 31. See also *Journal of a Rabbi,* p. 170.

33. See responsa cited in preceding note, and my "The Medical Treatment of Animals in Jewish Law," in *Journal of Jewish Studies,* London, 1956, vol. v, pp. 207 ff.

25

Experimentation on Human Subjects

J. DAVID BLEICH

Is a person obligated, or even permitted, to place his life in danger in order to preserve the life of his fellow man? A number of authorities[1] record a view attributed to the Palestinian Talmud which *requires* a person to jeopardize (but not sacrifice) his life in order to save his fellow.[2] R. Joseph Caro amplifies this position by stating that it is predicated upon the reasoning that "certainty" takes precedence over "possibility" *(Bet Yosef, Ḥoshen Mishpat* 426). The effect of this rationale is to limit the obligation posited by the Palestinian Talmud to situations in which it is reasonably justified to assume that the procedure will *certainly* save the life of the beneficiary.

However, the requirement to risk one's life in order to save the life of another is not cited in any of the codes of Jewish law. This has led a number of rabbinic authorities to advance arguments designed to demonstrate that the Babylonian Talmud differs with the Palestinian Talmud and posits no such requirement.[3] Accordingly, most authorities do not regard the jeopardization of one's own life to be obligatory. While at least one scholar of the sixteenth century, R. David ibn Zimra, considers one who does so to be a "pious fool",[4] no authority forbids the assumption of such a risk. The matter is best summed up in the words of Rabbi Jehiel Michael Epstein, author of an early twentieth century compendium, *Arukh ha-Shulḥan* who, paraphrasing an earlier source, writes, "However, everything depends upon the circumstances; it is necessary to weigh the matter on a scale and not to safeguard oneself more than necessary."[5]

It would appear that the question of hazardous experiments which have no anticipated therapeutic benefit to the subject can be analyzed in much the same manner. There is no obligation to volunteer for such hazards; yet, although an individual subjecting himself to such risks may, perhaps, be a "pious fool", the person doing so commits no transgression. Rabbi Jakobovits' statement that, "Possibly hazardous experiments may be performed on humans only if they may be potentially helpful to the subject himself. . ." is not compatible with the sources which have been cited.[6] As has been shown, a person may subject himself to hazards for the immediate benefit of another. Of course, from the point of view of Jewish teaching, it is unconscionable to subject a person to such hazards without fully apprising him of all possible risks and obtaining his informed consent. Moreover, as is evident from the discussions of various authorities concerning the donation, by living donors, of organs to organ banks, the risk assumed by the subject is warranted only if it is anticipated that information derived from the experimentation will be of value in the treatment of a *holeh lefaneinu,* a patient already affected by a disease or physiological disorder. This concept was first articulated by R. Ezekiel Landau of Prague in the 18th century in his celebrated responsum on autopsies (*Noda bi-Yehudah, Yoreh De'ah,* II, no. 210). This concept was expanded by a renowned 20th century scholar, R. Abraham I. Karelitz *(Hazon Ish)* to include potential victims of a plague or epidemic[7] and applied by Rabbi I. Y. Unterman to battlefield situations in permitting the erection and supplying of field hospitals on the Sabbath even prior to the firing of the first shot.[8] The reasoning is that epidemics invariably claim victims and war situations forebode casualties.

Organ transplants involving a living donor are certainly not obligatory insofar as the donor is concerned. There are strong grounds for arguing that, even according to the view attributed to the Palestinian Talmud, there is no obligation to sacrifice an organ. To subject oneself to danger from which one may emerge unscathed is one thing; to sacrifice a limb or an organ which will not under any circumstances be regenerated is quite another. A person may avail himself of property belonging to another in order to save his own life but with the anticipation of making restitution at some future time. Insofar as organs are concerned, this is patently impossible. R. David ibn Zimra adds that it is inconceivable that the Torah "whose paths are paths of pleasantness" (Proverbs 3:17) would demand such a great sacrifice of any person as a matter of *obligation.*

By the same token, there is no provision of Jewish law which forbids the donor to assume the risks attendant upon donation of an organ in order to save a life. Indeed, according to many authorities, his act may be highly laudable.

NOTES

1. See *Kesef Mishneh, Hilkhot Roze'ah* 1:14.
2. *Terumot* 8:4; cf., however, *Ziz Eli'ezer,* IX, no. 45, sec. 5.

3. See *Teshuvot Radbaz,* III, no. 1052; *Peri Megadim, Mishbeẓot Zahav, Oraḥ Ḥayyim* 328:7; *Pitḥei Teshuvah, Ḥoshen Mishpat* 426:2; *Or Same'ah, Hilkhot Roẓe'aḥ* 7:8; and *Shulḥan Arukh ha-Rav.* VI, *Hilkhot Nizkei Guf va-Nefesh* 7.

4. *Teshuvot Radbaz, loc. cit.*

5. *Arukh ha-Shulḥan, Ḥoshen Mishpat* 426:4. Cf. also *Ha'amek She'elah, She'ilta* 147:4; *Teshuvot Amudei Or,* no. 96, sec. 3; and *Ẓiẓ Eli'ezer,* IX, no. 45 and X, no. 25, chap. 7.

6. Cf., however, R. Eliezer Waldenberg, *Ẓiẓ Eli'ezer,* IX, no. 45, sec. 13. Rabbi Waldenberg's concluding remarks are not substantiated by the sources which he cites.

7. *Ḥazon Ish, Ohalot* 22:32.

8. See Rabbi I.Y. Unterman, *Torah she-be-al Peh,* XI (5729), 14 and *No'am,* XIII (5730), 4.

26
Judaism and Human Experimentation

FRED ROSNER

We have heard much of the concept known as the "sanctity of life." My understanding of this concept is that

> the value of human life in infinite and beyond measure, so that any part of life — even if only an hour or a second — is of precisely the same worth as seventy years of it, just as any fraction of infinity being indivisible, remains infinite. Accordingly, to kill a decrepit patient approaching death constitutes exactly the same crime of murder as to kill a young, healthy person who may still have many decades to live. For the same reason, one life is worth as much as a thousand or a million lives— infinity is not increased by multiplying it.[1]

In light of this, how do we approach the problem of human experimentation? Recent technical developments and new medications have made human experimentation a virtual necessity for medical progress.[2] Yet the ethical, moral, philosophical, sociological and religious implications have not kept pace with these medical advances. The worst possible situation that one could foresee is "the onerous threat of a dehumanized medical science that implacably considers humans — infants, pregnant women, the retarded, the dying, the well and the sick, as laboratory animals."[3] Rational justifications and explanations for such a position are intolerable to most human beings including a God-fearing scientist such as I.

Reprinted from the *New York State Journal of Medicine* (vol. 75, April 1975). Copyright © 1975 by the Medical Society of the State of New York.

American law offers very little help in the dilemma of proper human experimentation other than its principal concern for the protection of the individual patient. Very little legislation exists to guide the investigator. The United States Public Health Service has promulgated regulations on human experimentation[4] as has the Food and Drug Administration concerning the use of humans in the testing of new drugs.[5] The Nuremberg Code[6] and the Declaration of Helsinki[7] provide recommendations and guidelines for doctors and other health workers in clinical research.

Perhaps more important than the legal regulations of clinical investigation on human subjects in testing new drugs, new surgical procedures and basic biologic concepts, are the moral, ethical and religious issues. Respect for the sanctity of human life is the basic moral and religious presupposition in regulating physicians in their scientific studies of human patients, just as in their day to day practice of medicine.[8] Ethical physicians from the time of antiquity, from the Talmudic physician-sages (Mar Samuel and others) to the ancient Greek physicians (Hippocrates, Galen and others), have always held to this moral precept. The ethical and moral responsibilities of the physician as a divine agent in the alleviation of human suffering have been enunciated in the deeply pious and moving prayers of Asaph,[9] Judah Halevi,[10] Jacob Zahalon[11] and Abraham Zacutus[12] as well as the physician's prayer attributed to Moses Maimonides.[13]

The sanctity of life is a concept which appears throughout Judaic-Christian traditions and bespeaks life to be God's creation over which we have no ultimate authority. Hence, suicide,[14-15] mercy killing[16] or other human violations of this principle are prohibited. An even more basic question is the moral and religious license of a physician to practice medicine. Since God said: "For I am the Lord that healeth Thee" (Exodus 16:26), is a mortal permitted to become a physician and practice medicine? Does such an act constitute interference with the deliberate designs of Providence? Does a physician play God when he practices medicine? It is clear primarily from a phrase in Exodus 21:19, "And heal he shall heal," that the Bible gives specific sanction to the physician to heal[17] and, when called upon in a situation of danger, makes it obligatory upon him to provide his medical skills to cure disease. It is just as clear that the patient must not rely on miracles but is duty bound to seek out a physician to heal him.

If the physician's predominant or exclusive concern is the healing of his patient, then the standards of good medical practice will dictate the course of treatment. If there is a sure cure available in a given situation, the physician will certainly employ it first, in preference to a treatment of doubtful efficacy. The problem which concerns us here, however, is the situation in which the physician proposes to use a treatment which is not yet fully established scientifically. Such medical experimentation might expose the patient to a significant degree of risk or inconvenience, for if these elements are lacking there is little or no moral problem involved. The experiment might merely consist in giving the treatment to a particular patient or series of patients in a controlled fashion, and of observing and recording what follows. This is human experimentation. Somebody must be the first to try such a new treatment and some patient must be the first to be exposed to it.

Before such a controlled clinical trial of a new treatment is undertaken, many basic questions must be considered and solved, among which are the following[18]: Is the proposed treatment relatively safe or is it likely to do harm to the patient? Can a new treatment ethically be withheld from any patient in the doctor's care? Which patients may or should be admitted to a controlled clinical trial and randomly allocated to different treatments? Is it necessary to obtain the patient's consent before including him in the treatment trial? Is it ethical to use a placebo treatment? Is it proper for the doctor not to know whether his patient is receiving the experimental treatment or a placebo?

In spite of the voluminous literature on ethical problems in medicine, [19] there are no easy answers. There are at least eight books dealing specifically with human experimentation[20-27] as well as many individual papers. After reviewing all this literature, at least one writer was impressed with the difficulty of solving definitively many of the specific issues involved in the basic question of what is right in the use of human subjects for experimental purposes. The only unanimity of opinion seems to be in the desirability of obtaining informed consent freely given. But there is no unanimity at all about the definition of informed consent. Several studies indicate that the act of consenting is not necessarily a token of informed understanding.[28]

One eminent authority and prolific writer in the field of medical ethics states that the bland assumption that consent is ours for the asking is a myth.[29] He further asserts that if the investigator says he obtained consent, all is not necessarily well. Far more dependable evidence of right or wrong can be found in an examination of the investigation or treatment trial undertaken. A study on human beings does not become moral or ethical merely because it turned up useful data.

Catholic and Jewish teachings differ somewhat on the matter of consent for human experimentation. In Catholicism, of primary importance is the informed consent of the patient. As a rule, this consent shall be explicit, especially if the subject is to be exposed to any appreciable risk or inconvenience for the benefit of others.[30] Presumed consent remains a speculative possibility in some cases. The position of Judaism, on the other hand, as enunciated by Britain's Chief Rabbi Jakobovits is as follows:

> In the treatment of patients generally, whether the cures are tested or only experimental, the opinion of competent medical experts alone counts, not the wishes of the patient; and physicians are ethically required to take whatever therapeutic measures they consider essential for the patient's life and health, irrespective of the chance that they may subsequently be liable to legal claims for unauthorized 'assault and battery'.

This position is based on the Judaic-Christian doctrine that the patient is not absolute master of himself, his body or his soul. He, therefore, cannot freely dispose of himself as he sees fit. To deny himself a potentially helpful treatment for an otherwise hopelessly fatal illness would be classified in the category of suicide, a cardinal prohibition both in Judaism and in Catholicism. Perhaps such a viewpoint is meant in the following statement from the Declaration of Helsinki:

> In the treatment of the sick person, the doctor must be free to use a new therapeutic measure, if in his judgment it offers hope of saving life, re-establishing health, or alleviating suffering. If at all possible, consistent with patient psychology, the doctor should obtain the patient's freely-given consent after the patient has been given a full explanation.

There is thus no supreme goal called informed consent.[31] It is a guideline that must be kept in mind by the physician in trying to help the patient reach the goal of his total well being. The patient's greatest safeguard in experimentation, as in therapy, is the presence of a skillful, informed, intelligent, honest, responsible, compassionate and hopefully God-fearing physician.

The Declaration of Helsinki has been accepted by the major clinical investigative and medical organizations in the United States[32] and an enlarged version thereof was adopted by the House of Delegates of the American Medical Association in 1966. In England the British Medical Association published a set of rules in 1963,[33] and the Medical Research Council of Great Britain provided a detailed discussion of responsibility in investigations on human subjects in its annual report in 1964.[34] This was followed by a statement of the Royal College of Physicians of London which promulgated certain general principles of policy on the supervision of clinical investigations.[35] The major impact of the regulations of the United States Public Health Service, first promulgated by the Surgeon-General in 1966 and revised in 1969, as well as the requirements of the Food and Drug Administration concerning the use of human beings in the testing of new drugs, have already been mentioned.

What about research on minors, the mentally ill or retarded and other legally incompetent persons? How does one obtain consent from them? The legal issue is very easily solved in that in American law, consent is required from parents, guardians or next of kin.[36-37] English law forbids experimentation on children, even if both parents consent, unless done specifically in the interests of each individual child,[38] a viewpoint which has been strongly criticized.[39] The moral issue is infinitely more complex. The famous Willowbrook experiments on New York's Staten Island were headlined in *Medical World News* (Oct. 15, 1971, pp. 20ff.) in a feature article entitled "Was Dr. Krugman justified in giving the children hepatitis?'' The outcry was exemplified by New York State Senator Harrison J. Goldin *(Wall Street Journal,* March 24, 1971): ''The tests were irresponsible and reprehensible. I consider it an outrage that mentally retarded children should be used for medical research.''

Furthermore, groups whose availability can be controlled are more likely to be chosen for medical research than others. Examples are prisoners, medical students, hospitalized patients and institutionalized patients. New regulations to cover these specific situations have been proposed by the former director of the National Institutes of Health.[40] From the religious standpoint, every life is equally valuable and inviolable including that of children, medical students, criminals, prisoners and defectives. As Rabbi Jakobovits points out

> In the title to life and in its value, being infinite, there can be no distinction whatever between one person and another, whether innocent or guilty, whether healthy or crippled, demented or terminally afflicted. Thus, even a person's inviolability after death and his rights to dignity are decreed in the Bible specifically in relation to capital criminals, created like everyone else in the image of God.

I would now like to turn to a discussion of experimentation on the unborn and the unconceived. I will not speak of abortion or contraception or artificial insemination or sterilization since these procedures are not, strictly speaking, experimental in nature.

Let us then examine the ethical and religious implications of genetic screening and amniocentesis, of genetic manipulation and engineering, of *in-vitro* fertilization of a human egg by human sperm, of the implantation of an *in-vitro* conceptus into a woman's womb, of the implantation of a naturally fertilized egg from the womb of a pregnant woman into the womb of another so-called ''host mother'' who serves as an incubator, and of experimentation on fetuses. These new areas of consideration have been made possible by the extraordinary advances in biomedical research and technology in the past fifty years.[41] Of such great importance are the ethical, social and legal problems associated with these advances that not only governmental agencies but also private organizations are beginning to inquire into the ethical propriety of performing procedures such as genetic engineering and *in-vitro* fertilization and growth of human embryos.[42]

Public disquiet over the use of fetuses from abortion clinics in Britain resulted in the formation of an Advisory Group on the Use of Fetuses and Fetal Material for Research in May 1970.[43] In its report[44] the group recommends that research on fetuses should continue, subject to safeguards and control. The major provisions of their suggested code of ethics are that no procedure should be undertaken on a viable fetus (20 weeks gestation or weighing 400 to 500 grams) which is inconsistent with the sustenance of its life; that parents should be able to declare their wishes about the disposal of a dead or non-viable fetus; that there should be no monetary exchange for fetuses or fetal material, and that research on pre-viable fetuses should be subject to additional safeguards and limited to fetuses weighing less than 300 grams.

We need to remind ourselves at this point that Catholic teaching preaches that life begins at conception and that any direct attack on the unborn fetus is considered murder, even if it is carried out with the best of intentions. In Jewish law, although technically life begins at birth, the destruction of the unborn fetus is considered "moral murder" and is prohibited for a variety of reasons, except to save the mother's life or prevent a serious deterioration of her physical or mental health.[45]

Turning next to genetic screening, we are faced with the problem of possibly undertaking large scale screening programs to detect diseases or the carrier state of diseases for which there is no cure. Should advanced cancer not be diagnosed because it cannot be cured? Should individuals have the knowledge they are carriers of the gene for sickle cell anemia or hemophilia or Tay-Sachs disease? Are their procreational and reproductive activities to be decided for them or by them on the basis of such genetic information?

The Institute of Society Ethics and the Life Sciences has recently pointed out[46] that the advent of widespread genetic screening raises new and often unanticipated ethical, psychological and sociomedical problems. The Institute proposes a set of principles to

> include the need for well-planned program objectives, involvement of the communities immediately affected by the screening, provision of equal access, adequate testing procedures, absence of compulsion, a well-defined procedure for obtaining informed consent, safeguards for protecting subjects, open access of communities and individuals to program policies, provision of counseling services, an understanding of the relation of screening to realizable or potential therapies, and well-formulated procedures for protecting the rights of individual and family privacy.

Religious implications of such genetic screening programs are exemplified by Tay-Sachs disease, an illness afflicting mostly Jews. The carrier rate among Jews of Central and East European ancestry is believed to be about one person in thirty. Should two carriers marry, one quarter of their children will suffer from the disease and die therefrom in the first few years of life. In Jewish law, the obligation with regard to procreation is not suspended simply because of the statistical probability that some children of the union may die of a lethal disease.[47] Although genetic counselling is desirable, the choice *not* to have children is unacceptable in Judaism.

Equally important in Jewish law is the matter of amniocentesis whereby fetal monitoring is carried out with the intent of terminating the pregnancy if the fetus is identified as having full-blown Tay-Sachs disease. Recourse to abortion in such a circumstance is not permissible unless a threat to the mother's life exists. Furthermore, since no therapeutic advantage is obtained by amniocentesis carried out solely for the purpose of diagnosing a severe genetic defect such as Tay-Sachs disease, it poses an unnecessary risk to both mother and fetus and would hence be prohibited. Although still considered an experimental procedure by some people,[48] amniocentesis performed to diagnose a condition such as blood group incompatibility, for which medical therapy is available, not only may but in Jewish law, must be performed by the physician, even repeatedly, as part of good medical practice.

Concerning experimentation on human embryos *in-vitro* and the "test-tube" fertilization of a human ovum, two major articles in leading medical journals present opposing views. Fletcher[49] claims that neither abortion nor genetic control should be condemned. His feeling that human needs are more important that fetal rights was criticized by numerous correspondents writing in the columns of the same journal.[50] Another writer[51] also disagrees and states that one cannot ethically choose for a child the unknown hazards that he must face, and simultaneously choose to give him life in which to face them. He finds it immoral to discard or terminate the lives of the zygotes, the developing cluster of cells, the blastocysts, the embryos and the fetuses which will need to be killed in the course of developing the implantation procedure. Many others also condemn *in-vitro* fertilization as unethical experimentation on future possible human beings.[51-53]

Some had called for a moratorium on experiments that would attempt to implant an *in-vitro* conceptus into a woman's womb.[54] Such implantation was first accomplished in 1978 (see J. David Bleich, "Test-Tube Babies," above in this volume). The Jewish views on host-mothers[55] as well as genetic manipulations for cloning purposes[56] have recently been enunciated.

In all these areas of medical advance, we should remind ourselves that human procreation is an act which engages two people physically and spiritually and not merely rationally, as in a laboratory procedure. With artificial insemination we have already de-humanized the act involved in conceiving a human being by making it a merely rational act.[57] Human beings should not be reproduced or manufactured, but "called into being" and given the breath of life by Divine intervention.

But what is human? Is an unborn fetus human so as to prohibit its destruction? In both Catholicism and Judaism the answer is a resounding yes. Is the fertilized ovum human? If it is not human it is potentially human; that is, if left alone it will develop into a human being. Some authorities even consider the egg and the sperm *prior* to fertilization to be potential human subjects. Hence, all experimental work in the area of genetic engineering must be considered as human experimentation and treated as such from religious, moral and legal standpoints.

The law defines what is permissible, but what is permissible is not always ethical. Legal permissibility is not synonymous with moral license. In the Judeo-Christian tradition the morality of human experimentation is based on the principle that man is responsible to God for his spiritual and physical life, since man was created by God in His image. The money value of a man was once calculated from his composition of iron, calcium, phosphorus and other elements. He turned out to be worth less than a dollar.[58] His money value as an economic social entity is much higher, but still infinitely inadequate for characterizing his value as a human being.

Medical and surgical human experimentation in Jewish law has been the subject of several recent writings. Rabbi Moses Feinstein was asked about a patient where the medical assessment was that without a dangerous surgical operation, the patient would die, but the operation itself, if unsuccessful, might hasten the patient's death. Rabbi Feinstein responded that one is permitted to submit to dangerous surgery even though it may hasten death, because of the potential, however small, of the operation being successful and effecting a cure.[59]

Israel's Chief Rabbi Shlomo Goren, writes about the following situation:[60]

> There presents to us a patient who is extremely ill and whose prospects, under ordinary circumstances, are such that he will not live more than a very short time, perhaps only a few days or weeks. There is, however, a therapy or method available to treat the illness wherein, if successful, the patient would be healed and could live for a prolonged period of time. If the therapy would not succeed, the patient would die immediately. How should the physician conduct himself in such a case? Should he risk the definite short period of life remaining for the patient by administering the drastic remedy with the hope that perhaps the patient may be rescued from danger and live a prolonged period? In other words, should the physician abandon the *definite* short life span of the patient in favor of the *possible* significant prolongation of his life? Or do we invoke the principle that a possibility does not set aside a certainty[61] and we are prohibited from relinquishing the certainty of the brief period of survival of the patient in favor of the doubt that we might succeed in completely curing him and giving him long life?

Citing sources from the Bible, Talmud and rabbinic responsa, Rabbi Goren concludes without doubt that Halakhah requires that one give precedence to the possibility of saving the patient's life by using the experimental therapy. It must be understood, adds Rabbi Goren, that this ruling applies only if the case concerns a physical ailment where the patient will certainly die without the medication or the surgical intervention and the choice is between the certainty of the "life of the hour" versus the doubtful possibility of long life.

In the Hebrew periodical *No'am* (vol. 13, pp. 77 to 82; Jerusalem 1970), Jacob Levy discusses the questions of whether or not a healthy Jew is allowed to participate in human experimentation by taking medications not previously used in man, whether or not a Jewish physician is permitted to conduct such experiments, and whether or not one can administer new drugs to or perform new operations on seriously ill patients hoping these new approaches might be beneficial. Levy answers the last of the three questions in the affirmative using the same reasoning as Rabbi Goren. However, to experiment on healthy people without need of medical intervention purely for the sake of gaining knowledge for future patients may not be permissible in Jewish law if a significant risk exists to the volunteer.

Two much earlier rabbinic sources also clearly enunciate the Jewish legal view concerning human experimentation. Rabbi Hayyim Ozer Grodzinski was asked about the permissibility of performing a dangerous surgical procedure on a seriously ill patient. He answered that if all the attending physicians, without exception, recommend such an operation, it should be performed, even if the chances for success are smaller than those for failure.[62] A similar pronouncement is made by Rabbi Jacob Reischer in regard to dangerous medical therapy for a seriously ill patient. Rabbi Reischer permits such therapy since it may cure the patient although it may hasten the patient's death.[63] He also requires a group of physicians to concur in the decision.

Numerous additional rabbinic references on this subject are cited in a recent book on medicine and Jewish law.[64] If all illness and affliction would no longer exist, it would obviate the need for human experimentation. Let us hope and pray that God will fulfill his promise to the children of Israel as found in Exodus (chapt. 23:25): "And I will take sickness away from the midst of thee."

NOTES

1. Jakobovits, I. "Medical Experimentation on Humans in Jewish Law," *Proceedings AOJS,* New York 1966, pp. 1–7 (reprinted above in this volume).

2. King, L. S. "Medical Ethics," *J.A.M.A. 212:* 1042–1044, 1970.

3. Ratnoff, O. D. & Ratnoff. M. F. "Ethical Responsibilities in Clinical Investigation." *Persp. Biol. Med. 11:* 82–90, 1967.

4. United States Department of Health, Education and Welfare. Public Health Service, Division of Research Grants, *"Protection of the Individual as a Research Subject."* Washington, D.C. Government Printing Office 1969 (Publication No. 0–348–095).

5. 32 Federal Register 3994 (March 11, 1967).

6. *Trials of War Criminals Before the Nuremberg Military Tribunals Under Control Council Law No. 10* (vol. 11), Washington, D.C., U.S. Government Printing Office 1949 pp 181 ff.

7. World Medical Association. Declaration of Helsinki. Recommendations Guiding Doctors in Clinical Research. *World Med. J. 11:*281, 1964.

8. Visscher, M. B. "Medical Research & Ethics," *J.A.M.A. 199:* 631–636, 1967.

9. Rosner, F. & Muntner, S. "The Oath of Asaph," *Ann. Int. Med. 63:* 317–320, 1965.

10. Friedenwald, H. *The Jews & Medicine.* Baltimore, Johns Hopkins Press 1944, vol. 1 p. 27.

11. Savitz, H. "Jacob Zahalon and his book *The Treasure of Life,"* *New Engl. J. Med. 213:* 167–176, 1935.

12. Ref. 10 pp. 295–321.

13. Rosner, F. "The Physician's Prayer Attributed to Moses Maimonides." *Bull. Hist. Med. 41:*440–454, 1967.

14. See my essay "Suicide in Jewish Law" above in this volume.

15. Pius XII. "Address to the First International Congress on the Histopathology of the Nervous System," Sept. 13, 1952. *Catholic Mind 51:* 305–313, 1953.

16. See my essay "Jewish Attitude Toward Euthansia" above in this volume.

17. See my essay "Physician & Patient in Jewish Law" above in this volume.

18. Hill, A. B. "Medical Ethics and Controlled Trials," *Brit. Med. J. 1:* 1043–1049, 196.

19. Elkinton, J. R. "The Literature of Ethical Problems in Medicine," *Ann. Int. Med. 73:* 495, 498; 662–666; 863–870, 1970.

20. Beecher, H. K. *Research & the Individual: Human Studies,* Boston, Little Brown & Co., 1970, 358 pp.

21. Ladimer, I. & Newman, R. W. (editors) *Clinical Investigation in Medicine: Legal, Ethical & Moral Aspects. An Anthology & Bibliography,* Boston, Law-Medicine Research Institute, Boston Univ. 1963, 517 pp.

22. Freund, P. A. (editor) *Ethical Aspects of Experimentation with Human Subjects,* Daedalus, Spring 1969, 597 pp.

23. *Deuxième Congrès International De Morale Medicale, Paris, Ordre National Des Mèdecins 1966,* 2 vol. 777 pp.

24. Fattorusso, V. (editor) *Biomedical Science and the Dilemma of Human Experimentation,* Paris, Council for International Organizations of Medical Sciences, Unesco House, 1967, 123 pp.

25. Weber, H. R. (editor) *Experiments with Man: Report of an Ecumenical Consultation,* World Council of Churches Studies no. 6, Geneva World Council of Churches; New York. Friendship Press 1969, 100 pp.

26. Ladimer, I. (editor) "New Dimensions in Legal & Ethical Concepts for Human Research." *Ann. N.Y. Acad. Sci. 169:* 293–593, 1970.

27. Pappworth, M. H. *Human Guinea Pigs: Experimentation on Man,* London, Routledge & Kegan Paul Ltd., 1967; Boston, Beacon Press 1968, 228 pp.

28. Martin, D. C., Arnold, J. D., Zimmerman, T. F. & Rickart, R. H. "Human Subjects in Clinical Research. A Report of Three Studies," *New Eng. J. Med. 279:* 1426–1431, 1968.

29. Beecher, H. K. "Consent in Clinical Experimentation: Myth & Reality" (editorial), *J.A.M.A. 195:* 34–35, 1966.

30. Lynch, J. J. "Symposium on the Study of Drugs in Man. Part 3. Human Experimentation in Medicine, Moral Aspects," *Clin. Pharmac. & Therap. 1:* 396–400, 1960.

31. Bean, W. B. "Some Moral & Ethical Problems in Human Experimentation" (editorial), *Current Medical Digest 34:* 1487–1490, 1967.

32. "Human Experimentation: Declaration of Helsinki." *Ann. Int. Med.* *65:*367–368, 1966.

33. British Medical Association: Experimental Research on Human Beings, *Brit. Med. J. 2* (suppl). 57, 1963.

34. Medical Research Council: Responsibility in Investigations on Human Subjects, *Brit. Med. J. 2:* 178–179, 1964.

35. Royal College of Physicians: Supervision of Clinical Investigations, *Lancet 2:* 357–358, 1967.

36. Curran, W. J. "New Public Health Service Regulations on Human Experimentation," *New Engl. J. Med. 281:* 781–782, 1969.

37. Curran, W. J. & Beecher, H. K. "Experimentation in Children. A Reexamination of Legal Ethical Principles," *J.A.M.A. 210:* 77–83, 1969.

38. Pappworth, M. H. "The Willowbrook Experiments," *Lancet 1:* 1181, 1971.

39. Beecher, H. K, "Experiments on Children," *Lancet 1:* 1181, 1971.

40. Marston, R. Q. "Research on Minors, Prisoners and the Mentally Ill," *New Engl. J. Med. 288:* 158–159, 1973.

41. Duval, M. K. "Duplications of Advanced Biomedical Research & Technology," *J.A.M.A. 220:* 247–249, 1972.

42. "Bioscience-Bioethics" (editorial), J.A.M.A. *220:* 272–273, 1972.

43. "Research on Fetuses," (editorial), Lancet *1:* 1222–1223, 1972.

44. *The Use of Fetuses and Fetal Material for Research. Report of the Advisory Group,* London, H.M. Stationery Office 1972, 18 pp.

45. See the essays on abortion in this book.

46. Lappé, M., Gustafson, J. M. & Roblin, R. "Ethical and Social Issues in Screening for Genetic Disease," *New Engl. J. Med. 286:* 1129–1132, 1972.

47. Bleich, J. D. "Tay-Sachs Disease," *Tradition 13:* 145–148 (Summer) 1972.

48. Nadler, H. L. "Prenatal Detection of Genetic Defects," *J. Ped. 74:* 132–143, 1969.

49. Flatcher, J. "Ethical Aspects of Genetic Controls. Designed Genetic Changes in Man," *New Engl. J. Med. 285:* 776– 783, 1971.

50. Guttentag, O. E., Lappé, M., Fitzgerald, J. A., Schweitzer, P. E. and Arena, F.P. "Genetic Control," *New Eng. J. Med. 286:* 48–50, 1972.

51. Kass, L. R. "Babies by Means of *In-Vitro* Fertilization: Unethical Experiments on the Newborn?" *New Engl. J. Med. 285:* 1174–1179, 1971.

52. Ramsey, P. "Shall We 'Reproduce'? I. The Medical Ethics of *In-Vitro* Fertilization," *J.A.M.A. 220:* 1346–1350, 1972.

53. Ramsey, P. Shall We 'Reproduce'? II. Rejoinders and Future Forecast," *J.A.M.A. 220:* 1480–1485, 1972.

54. "Genetic Engineering in Man: Ethical Considerations" (editorial), *J.A.M.A. 220:* 721, 1972.

55. Bleich, J. D. "Host-Mothers," *Tradition 13:* 127–129 (Fall) 1972.

56. Rosenfeld, A. "Judaism and Gene Design," *Tradition 13:* 71–80 (Fall) 1972, reprinted below in this volume.

57. "Genetic Engineering: Reprise" (editorial), *J.A.M.A. 220:* 1356–1357, 1972.

58. Stern, K. "Genes & People," *Perspect. Biol. Med. 10:* 500–523, 1967.

59. Feinstein, M. *Iggerot Moshe, Yoreh De'ah,* II, no. 58, New York 1973.

60. Goren, S. In *Shanah be-Shanah.* Published by *Hechal Shlomo,* Jerusalem 5736 (1976), pp. 149–155.

61. *Pesaḥim* 9a and *Yevamot* 19b.

62. Grodzinski, H. O. *Aḥi'ezer, Yoreh De'ah,* no. 16:6, Jerusalem 1946.

63. Reischer, J. *Shevut Ya'akov,* section 3, no. 75, Lemberg 1860.

64. Steinberg, A. (editor), *Assia,* Jerusalem 1976, p. 273.

Genetic Engineering

27
Judaism and Gene Design
AZRIEL ROSENFELD

Introduction

Genetics — the study of the mechanisms of heredity — is a well-established branch of biological science. As these mechanisms become better understood, it may become possible to tamper with them and so to alter heredity. For example, hemophilia — inability of the blood to clot properly — is a hereditary condition; a woman who is a carrier of this condition is likely to have sons who are "bleeders" and daughters who are "carriers." If one could identify the specific genes that transmit hemophilia, it might be possible to remove an ovum from such a woman, operate on it to repair these genes (or perhaps replace them with genes from a normal woman), and return the ovum to her body. A child that she conceived by fertilization of this ovum would then be neither a bleeder nor a carrier.

Modification of genes to correct hereditary defects such as hemophilia would seem to be a desirable goal. However, once such techniques of "genetic engineering" are developed, they will be used for many other purposes and will have enormous social implications. Prospective parents would demand improvements in their potential offspring — they would want their children to be tall, strong, handsome, intelligent. Perhaps demands of this sort are reasonable, but where would we draw the line? It might not be objectionable if a couple wanted a six-foot son, but what if they wanted a seven-foot son who could become a basketball player, or an eight-foot son who could become a circus freak? What if they wanted their son to be a piano virtuoso, and demanded that he be given six fingers on each hand, or two pairs of arms?

Reprinted from *Tradition* (Fall, 1972). Copyright © 1972 by the Rabbinical Council of America.

The present article will consider genetic engineering from a halakhic standpoint. Is gene surgery permissible? If so, what sorts of modifications would be allowed? Is it permitted to transplant genes from one person to another? If so, do we regard the resulting child as related to the donor?

Gene Surgery

In gene surgery an ovum is removed, some of its genes are modified by microsurgical techniques, and the ovum is then replaced in the body. No donor is involved here. One could also consider the possibility of performing gene surgery on a sperm cell. However, this would require artificial insemination of the mother-to-be with the modified sperm; if it were instead somehow replaced in the man's body, there would be odds of millions to one against the particular sperm being involved in fertilization. Those who forbid artificial insemination even with the husband as donor would thus certainly not allow gene surgery on sperms. On the other hand, there seems little reason to object to the removal and replacement procedures that would be required when doing gene surgery on an ovum. Assuming, for the sake of argument, that these procedures could be carried out without rendering the woman ritually unclean, so that after replacement of the ovum (in the Fallopian tube?), normal fertilization would be permissible.

As regards the surgical process itself, we assume that it has been perfected to the point where it is (almost) always successful. Otherwise, it might be regarded as "destruction of the seed," which, according to many authorities, applies to a woman's seed as well as to a man's.[1]

Another, and perhaps stronger argument for permitting all gene surgery is that the ovum (or sperm) is not a person, since conception has not yet taken place. Thus in performing gene surgery, we are not tampering with an existing human being, but only with a potential one; we are only "cutting meat," not doing surgery on a person. One might argue that we are destroying a potential person if we bring about the conception of a sufficiently altered creature, but in fact this is not so — even if there are drastic departures from the normal human form, the child is still halakhically human.[2]

Whether or not one accepts the arguments just given, the following principle seems indisputable: Any surgery that is permitted on a person must certainly be permitted on an ovum or sperm before conception. If a surgical cure for hemophilia were possible, it would surely be permissible; thus it would certainly be permissible to cure hemophilia by gene surgery. Cosmetic plastic surgery is permitted by many authorities in order to relieve psychological distress; they should thus also permit achieving cosmetic effects through gene surgery — assuming, of course, that the surgical procedures are safe and reliable.

Our sages recognize, and perhaps even encourage, the use of prenatal (or better, pre-conceptional) influences to improve one's offspring:

> R. Yoḥanan used to go and sit at the gates of the place of immersion, saying: "When the daughters of Israel come out from their required immersion, they look at me and may have sons who are as handsome as I, and as accomplished in Torah as I."[3]

This concept might well be extended to allow the use of gene-surgical techniques to produce physically and mentally superior children.

On the other hand, turning a person into a monster by surgical means would very likely be forbidden, unless it were necessary to save his life; and creating monsters through gene surgery might thus also be forbidden.[4]

Gene Transplants

We now consider the case where the gene surgery involves transplanting genes from another person into the ovum or sperm. Would this be forbidden, perhaps as constituting some sort of perverted sex act between the gene donor and the recipient? Would it be forbidden, in particular, if they were close relatives? Would a child conceived from that ovum or sperm be regarded as related to the gene donor?

Regarding the question of permissibility, an important point should be made: The transplanted genes need not come from a reproductive cell (sperm or ovum) of the donor; they can come from any cell of his or her body. On the recipient's side too, it should be noted that the sex organs are not immediately involved, since the transplanting is done outside the body. In view of this, it seems very unlikely that the transplantation process could, by any stretch of the imagination, be regarded as a sex act.

The problem of the child's relationship to the donor, on the other hand, seems at first glance to be more complicated. Our sages recognize the concept of a heredity mechanism in which different parts of the body are formed out of different parts of the reproductive material:

> R. Ḥanina b. Papa taught: "What is the meaning of the scriptural 'You have winnowed my going and my lying' (Psalms 139:3)? It teaches that man is not formed from the entire drop, but only from its clearest part" (*Niddah* 31a).
>
> R. Yoḥanan said: "The Holy One, blessed be He, forms man from a mere drop of white matter; 'You have winnowed' — like a man who winnows and puts the straw by itself, the stubble by itself, until he has purified the grain."
>
> R. Simeon b. Lakish said: "Nor does He waste the drop; rather, He winnows out part of the drop for the brain, part of the drop for the bones, and part of the drop for the sinews.

True, the parts of the "drop" are not normally regarded as having separate origins. Here, however, where we know that parts of the "drop" have come from a donor, is it possible that we might regard the child as having been generated in part by the donor?

Before discussing these problems further, let us consider an analog of gene transplantation on a much grosser scale. Suppose that ovaries are transplanted from one woman to another, or testicles from one man to another.[6] Would this be forbidden from the recipient's standpoint? (If done from a living donor, it would surely be forbidden from the donor's standpoint, since it constitutes "castration";[7] but this problem should not arise if the organs are removed from the donor posthumously.) Would we regard a child conceived after such a transplant as being related to the donor? If we could answer these questions in the negative, we could then certainly give negative answers to our analogous questions about gene transplants. It is impossible that transplanting submicroscopic parts of a single sperm or ovum could be more objectionable, or could have more effect on the status of a child, than transplanting entire testicles or ovaries.

Sex Organ Transplants

Remarkably, the problem of sex organ transplants was actually raised in the halakhic literature during the early 20th century. (It is possible that this discussion was stimulated by the then current interest in "monkey gland" transplants for men.) A series of responsa on the subject was published in the halakhic periodical *Vayelaket Yosef,* edited by R. Joseph Schwartz of Bonyhad, Hungary, vol. 10, nos. 3, 4, 6, and 9 (5668). (The help of the Harvard University Library in providing photostats of these responsa is gratefully acknowledged.)

The following quotations are taken from these responsa:

> [From R. Jacob Gordon of Southport (?), England]: I present here a problem about which I am in doubt as to the Halakhah. The doctors here have developed a method of putting a woman's generative organs in a barren woman, so that she should be able to have children. Are we permitted to take the generative organs from a mother and put them in a daughter? And if you say that it is permitted, what is the law regarding the first born, which depends on being first to emerge from the womb, and here the womb is another woman's? And in general, who is the mother in this case, the first woman or the second?
>
> [Answer by R. Eliezer Deutsch, head of the rabbinical court of Bonyhad]: It seems obvious to me that a prohibited sex act (*ervah*) is certainly not involved here. Indeed, even with an entire body, when dead, the laws of prohibited sex acts do not apply (*Yevamot* 25b) . . . And although it

seems at first glance that [in that case], while there is no punishment, there is still a prohibition; nevertheless, one can say that this is only for a dead person, where the body is complete, and it is reasonable to rule [that sex acts are forbidden] . . . But for a single organ, such a ruling is not appropriate, and there should not even be any prohibition.

And one can convince oneself that sex act prohibitions surely apply only to a living body, not to the sex organs. For if we say that these prohibitions refer to the sex organs, then if they took generative organs from a woman who is not forbidden [to someone], and put them in a woman who is forbidden [to him], and he had sexual relations with her, he would be exempt from punishment. But if so, how could there ever be a death penalty for sexual offense? . . . If we follow the sex organs, then in any case of prohibited sex, it is possible that they have put [in the woman] generative organs from a woman who is not prohibited, and the witnesses [to the sex act] could not know this. *The Torah surely prohibited [only] the woman herself, and it makes no difference where the generative organs are from. For once the generative organs have been joined to her body, they are like her body itself.* And the same for a woman who is permitted to him —there too we follow only the vitality [*hiyut*] and body of the woman, and we do not care about the generative organs, for once they have been joined to her body, they are like her body.

Aside from this, sex act prohibitions do not apply to an organ, which has no life of its own, and is like a mere piece of meat; there is not even a rabbinical prohibition . . . The story of the Arab who bought a haunch in the market, made a hole in it and performed a sex act with it (*Avodah Zarah* 22a) . . . is cited only to show that they are so bound up in sexual lust that he performed a sex act with a mere haunch . . . But it is obvious that sexual prohibitions do not apply to a piece of meat. If so, in our case there is no possibility of a sexual prohibition; this is obvious, in my humble opinion . . . And similarly regarding generative organs from a woman who is sexually prohibited [that are put] into another woman, it is obvious that there is no sexual prohibition here for it is like mere meat; there is no need to enlarge on this . . .[8]

To tell the truth, however, it is difficult for me to believe that a naturally barren woman could be helped by generative organs from another woman. It is explicit in tractate *Yevamot* (64b), on the verse "And Sarah was barren." — She did not even have a place for a child. But if we say that generative organs from another woman can help, then the Holy One, blessed be He, did not have to perform a miracle for her!

Surely the doctors are lying; if not out of respect for the questioner, I would not have replied at all. I have written on the basis of limited thought, in the time available, and only as regards the [theoretical] halakhah, not for practical application.

[Answer by R. Benjamin Aryeh ha-Kohen Weiss, chief of the rabbinical court of Tchernowitz and vicinity[9]]: Regarding the method that the doctors have developed to cut generative organs from a living woman and to attach them to the body of a barren woman, so that she should be able to have children, the halakhic question has been asked: Who is the child's mother, the first [woman] or the second? And there are many legal matters that depend on this.

I am far from believing this report; nevertheless, suppose that the story can be verified. It is certainly forbidden to do this in the first place, even if there is no danger involved, because the first woman is being "castrated" . . . But if they transgressed and did it, in my humble opinion *the child is the second woman's in all respects.* And the source from which this halakhah can be derived, in my opinion, is the explicit Talmudic law (*Sotah* 43b) regarding a [branch of a] young tree that has been grafted onto an old tree, in connection with *orlah* [the prohibition of the fruit of a tree during the first three years].

Rabbi Deutsch's responsum begins by stating that the act of sex organ transplantation is not a sex act. His reasoning seems to apply not only to the case at hand, where the donor and recipient are women, but also to the case where they are men — and perhaps even to the case of a sex change operation, where a man's organs are transplanted to a woman or vice versa.[10] And surely his arguments hold where only genes are being transplanted.

Rabbi Deutsch further rules that once the donor's sex organs are in the recipient's body, they become part of that body. In particular, the recipient is not forbidden to marry the donor's relatives. This would presumably be true even for sex change operations; although the recipient's sex changes, his/her family relationships do not change. However, Rabbi Deutsch's principle that "we follow only the vitality and body" can lead to complications in the more extreme hypothetical case of a brain transplant. There is much evidence to support the conclusion that when A's brain is put in B's body, the halakhic identity follows the brain — the person is A, not B. But according to Rabbi Deutsch's reasoning, the person should be forbidden to marry B's relatives, not A's.[11]

In Rabbi Deutsch's responsum there is no ruling on whether a child born to the recipient of a sex organ transplant is related to the donor. Rabbi Weiss, however, rules explicitly that the child has no relationship to the donor.

This ruling too would surely apply in a gene transplant case.

Heredity and Halakhah

As we have seen, genetic mechanisms and their manipulation can be treated from a halakhic standpoint. In doing so, however, let us not forget that besides the physical machinery of heredity, there is also a spiritual machinery:

Our sages have taught: There are three partners in a man — the Holy One, blessed be He; his father; and his mother. His father sows the white matter, from which comes bones, sinews, nails, the brain in his head and the white of the eye. His mother sows the red matter, from which come skin, flesh, blood, hair, and the black of the eye. The Holy One, blessed be He, puts into him breath, spirit, facial appearance, sight, hearing, speech, mobility, knowledge, wisdom and understanding.[12]

Moreover, this spiritual heredity is at least as important as the physical:

> One who raises an orphan in his house is regarded by Scripture as if he had given birth to him . . . One who teaches his friend's son Torah is regarded by Scripture as if he had given birth to him.[13]
>
> A father endows (*zokheh*) a son with beauty, strength, wealth, wisdom, and longevity.[14] But the sages say: Until he comes of age, his father endows him; thereafter, he endows himself.[15]

The father's influence on his son is not a mere matter of physical heredity or fiscal inheritance — it is also a matter of spiritual merit (*zekhut*). As we move into an era of genetic engineering, when fathers may be able to choose and control the qualities of their children, let us hope that we do not forget our ultimate dependence on the merit of our forefathers and on our Father in Heaven.

NOTES

1. See commentaries on *Niddah* 13a, particularly Ramban and Rashba.

2. On this point see *Teshuvah me-Ahavah,* no. 53 quoted in my article "Religion and the Robot," *Tradition,* Fall 1966, pp. 15–26.

3. *Berakhot* 20a; *B.M.* 84a. The Roman notables used to hold beautiful figures while engaging in sexual relations (*Gittin* 58a. See also *Midrash Numbers Rabbah* 9:34, where the fact that an Ethiopian couple produced a white child is ascribed to their house having white figures in it. On analogous procedures involving animals see Genesis 30:37 ff. and *Avodah Zarah* 24a).

4. See, incidentally, Responsa *Tashbez* pt. IV, no. 49: "The doctors have said that when the material [in the womb] becomes abundant, it is a sign of twins or of an extra finger; and if the material is bad, the form of a frog may be added there — may Ha-Shem save us!"

5. *Leviticus Rabbah* 14.

6. See *Hullin* 69a: R. Jeremiah asked, "Does organ generate organ, or is it the seed mixed?" He later said, "Obviously the seed is mixed; otherwise the blind would have blind children and the lame would have lame children."

7. *Shulhan Arukh, Even ha-Ezer* 5:11.

8. In a passage not quoted here, Rabbi Deutsch also discusses the status of the child as regards the law of the firstborn. The Talmud is in doubt (*Hullin* 70a) whether it is contact with the womb or containment within the womb that sanctifies the firstborn. In our case, the child touches only the donor's transplanted womb but

is also contained in the recipient's body; thus the child is only a doubtful (*safek*) firstborn.

9. This responsum appears also as no. 29 in Rabbi Weiss' collected responsa *Even Yekarah,* published in 1911.

10. On the possibility that the Halakhah would recognize the effectiveness of a functional sex change operation see my article "The Heart, the Head, and the Halakhah," *New York State Journal of Medicine* 70, October 15, 1970, pp. 2615–2619. See also *Yerushalmi Berakhot* 9:3; *Genesis Rabbah* 72; and especially *Tanḥuma Va-Yeẓe* 8: "It is not difficult for the Holy One, blessed be He, to make females into males and males into females."

11. See my article cited in note 10.

12. *Niddah* 31a; see also *Yerushalmi Kilayim* 8:3.

13. *Sanhedrin* 19b.

14. *Eduyyot* 2:9.

15. *Tosefta Eduyyot* 1:14.

28
Genetic Engineering and Judaism
FRED ROSNER

And God blessed Noah and his sons, and said to them: Be fruitful, and multiply, and replenish the earth (Genesis 9:1).

Introduction & Background

The nucleus of every cell in the human body contains twenty-three pairs of chromosomes. One chromosome of each pair is derived from the maternal egg and the other from the paternal sperm. Each chromosome is composed of thousands of genes which are the functional units of heredity. The science of genetics is the study of heredity or the transmission of genes for particular traits or characteristics (e.g. hair color, height, intelligence etc.) from parent to offspring.

The basic genetic material of all chromosomes is deoxyribonucleic acid or DNA for short. DNA consists of two interwining strands which form the famous double helix structure of genes. Each strand is composed of a long sequence of nucleotides. Each nucleotide is made up of a pentose sugar and phosphate linked by combinations of four bases: cytosine, thymine, adenine and guanine. The pentose sugar and phosphate are constant but the sequence of base pairs varies. It is this sequence which provides the messages or code (the so-called "genetic code") for translation of the inherited information into the production of various proteins in the cell. When a cell divides, the DNA must be replicated so that every daughter cell receives a precise copy of the DNA of the parent cell of that individual. Meanwhile, an enzyme in the nucleus of the cell transcribes the coded message in the DNA into a messenger molecule which goes into the cytoplasm of the cell to be translated into protein production. Proteins are the effector molecules of the cell; examples include enzymes, hormones, antibodies, hemoglobin, cell membranes, etc.[1]

A single change in the normal sequence of approximately 1500 nucleotides in a strand of DNA can result in a major difference in the clinical characteristics of an individual. A change in a gene is called a mutation.

Many mutations are spontaneous occurrences. Others can be induced by chemicals or radiation or other external influences. A single gene mutation may result in an absence or malfunctioning of a vital protein or enzyme leading to the toxic accumulation of metabolic products which this enzyme ordinarily detoxifies. Tay-Sachs disease exemplifies this occurrence. A mutation which produces a malfunctioning clotting protein results in the disease called hemophilia. A mutation in the gene for hemoglobin, the oxygen carrying protein of red blood cells, can lead to sickle cell anemia.

Primitive attempts by man to change the genetic makeup of certain lower forms of life involved the removal of the nuclei from frog cells and their transplantation into fertilized frog eggs whose nuclei had been previously removed. Viable tadpoles have developed, all of whom had the precise features of the original frog from whom the nuclei were obtained. This process is called nuclear cloning because a whole clone of genetically identical creatures is produced.

The technical problems surrounding nuclear cloning by nuclear transplantation in man have not yet been surmounted.

On a more basic level, the genetic material within the nucleus, DNA, can be enzymatically cut into smaller sequences of genes, and these small segments can be spliced or recombined. This recombinant DNA technology has now made it possible to transfer genes to totally unrelated hosts. A vector (usually a virus) is needed to transfer this DNA material into the animal, plant or bacterial cell of choice. Hereditary material from virtually any plant or animal cell can now be propagated in bacteria, and bacterial genes can be inserted into animal cells. Various terms have been used to describe these revolutionary methods including "gene splicing", "gene grafting", "gene cloning", "gene transplantation", "genetic manipulation" and "genetic meddling". The two most widely accepted terms are "recombinant DNA research" and the broader phrase "genetic engineering". Medical science now has the capacity to rearrange the genetic heritage of thousands of years.[2]

The purely scientific interest in cloning and recombinant DNA research is exemplified by the flood of papers on this subject which have appeared in the recent literature. An entire issue (April 8, 1977) of the prestigious journal *Science,* official publication of the American Association for the Advancement of Science, was devoted to this new area of technology. The present paper explores some of the moral, ethical and Jewish legal implications of genetic engineering and recombinant DNA research.

Moral & Ethical Considerations

Concern about the possible deleterious effects on society of genetic engineering research and application is being voiced by many scientific bodies and governmental agencies. One example is the "Conference on Ethical and Scientific Issues Posed by Human Uses of Molecular Genetics" sponsored by The New York Academy of Sciences and the Institute of Society, Ethics and the Life Sciences.[3]

The potential advantages of recombinant DNA research are several. Some genes can now be copied and thus their precise structure can be more easily studied. Bacteria can be directed by the gene transplanted into it to assemble a protein valuable to man. Insulin, antibiotics, antiviral agents and numerous other drugs, chemicals and vaccines might be synthesized in large quantities by the technology of genetic engineering. Patients with absent or defective genes suffering from such genetic disorders as Tay-Sachs disease, hemophilia, sickle cell anemia and their like, might be given a replacement gene. Clones of nitrogen-producing bacteria might be useful for agriculture. Bacteria that concentrate trace elements such as uranium or platinum could be cloned to increase the supply of such elements. Other commercial applications of recombinant DNA research such as the manufacture of methane gas and the production of pollution-eating bacteria also exist. Specially engineered bacteria are thus envisioned as factories for the production of numerous important substances for medicine and industry.

On the other hand, huge potential hazards of recombinant DNA research exist. Genes for pathogenic products might be transplanted into bacteria deliberately or inadvertently. Unexpected alterations may occur. One must contemplate the possibility of accidental release into the environment of organisms carrying extraneous genetic material and/or the infection of plant or animal life with these bacteria. Recombinant DNA may be taken up by human cells in such a way as to produce cancer or other diseases. One writer in a popular magazine[4] cautions that "pollution-gobbling bugs might go on uncontrolled binges, eating every chemical in sight; nitrogen-fixing bacteria could possibly devastate soil ecology. Possibly worst of all is the fact that, once created, the new bugs cannot be destroyed".

Cloning in man raises other moral and ethical issues. According to a prominent ethicist[5] cloning is one of eight methods of human reproduction. He lists them as follows: (a) The coital-gestational way; (b) Artificial insemination of a wife with her husband's sperm, without any assistance or input from a third party; (c) Artificial insemination of a woman with a donor's sperm; (d) Egg transfer from a wife, inseminated by her husband and then transferred to another woman's womb for substitute gestation; (e) Egg transfer from a donor to a wife or unmarried woman's womb, before or after insemination — sometimes called prenatal adoption; (f) Egg transfer from a female donor, then inseminated by a male donor, and finally transferred to the recipient's womb; (g) Artificial gestation or nurture of a fetus in a glass womb or similar artifact — which is just a refinement of the incubator and isolette already in use for premature infant — plus an artificial placenta; this is often spoken of as ectogenesis; (h) Nuclear transplant or cloning, whereby an egg (one's own or another's) is enucleated or denucleated; the original nucleus with its genetic code is removed and replaced with the nucleus of either a donated unfertilized egg or the nucleus from a body cell (either a man's or a woman's), which is then implanted and brought to term in one's own or another's womb — and all this without conception. Only a male or a female seed is used, not both. It is birth from only one parent, artificial virgin birth.

As a result of cloning, some horrifying thoughts come to mind; thoughts put into words by Vance Packard in his best seller, *The People Shapers:*

> Professional athletic organizations might well be attracted to the idea of making direct multiple copies of their basketball stars. What professional ball team wouldn't want to produce a dozen copies of Pele or O. J. Simpson? Some marriageable girls might feel honored to offer their wombs for the nurture of these prospective superstars. In any case, surrogate mothers could be hired.
>
> Similarly, military leaders with billions of dollars available for research might well be interested in mass-producing humans high in endurance, strength, or proneness to obedience. Dictators might justifiably see universal cloning as a way to achieve a more efficient, predictable, regulatable populace. Other arguments:
>
> If you had a hundred clones or a thousand clones in a community there would be one clear medical advantage. Their organs could be freely transplanted among fellow clones without the still very bothersome problem of graft rejection.
>
> If a husband and wife were in deep distress because a greatly beloved child was dying, they could arrange to create another child that would be genetically identical.
>
> A woman who wanted a baby but had not come across a satisfactory mate could have by virgin birth a baby of her own flesh. The baby, though younger, would be the mother's identical twin.
>
> People interested in personal immortality could assure themselves of at least a start. They could arrange, through cell banking, to have persons of their exact genotype live on. Not for eternity, perhaps, but for at least a couple of hundred years.
>
> If and when cloning (in man) does become a reality . . . .
>
> How long would it be before we would see movie-production empires ordering up hundreds of facsimiles of sex goddesses of the Raquel Welch type?

There would be problems right from the start. Who would decide what individuals were to be mass-produced by cloning? Would it be left to the free enterprise market mechanism? Or would the state take over? If so, there would probably be black-marketing. Or would a nervous world set up the International Commission for Genetic Control to license clonists?

. . . A new set of human ethics would seem to be required.

The ramifications of cloning, both in man and in animals, are endless. Men would feel castrated. Women would feel as if they were reduced to incubators. A child who is an identical twin of a parent might be psychologically unbalanced. Cloning and recombinant DNA research have been compared to a Dr. Frankenstein producing biological monsters[6] and characterized as a Faustian bargain.[7] The eugenic aspects of cloning are beyond the scope of this essay but must also be considered. Critics[8-9] as well as proponents[10] of such research all agree that regulation of some type is necessary since this technology of genetic engineering is so potent that even a slight deviation from the intended path may cause grievous consequences to society and to the individuals concerned.

Legislative Control

With the launching of recombinant DNA technology in 1973, scientists at a meeting on nucleic acids called the Gordon conference, held in New England in the summer of that year, expressed their concerns in an open letter. The letter was published in *Science* in July, 1974 and requested the National Academy of Sciences to recommend specific actions or guidelines in the light of potential hazards.

The scientists also asked their colleagues to voluntarily defer action on certain experiments because of the possible hazards. Individual investigators responded by voluntarily halting such research pending further discussion and the development of adequate guidelines, but this moratorium was not observed everywhere.

A meeting was held subsequently at the Asilomar Conference Grounds, Pacific Grove, California, in 1975 where 150 international scientists discussed the future of recombinant DNA research. A provisional statement was issued that proposed a tentative classification of experiments by risk and specified appropriate safeguards for low-, moderate-, and high-risk experiments. Research continued although adherence to the recommendations was voluntary.

In July, 1976 the National Institutes of Health (NIH) issued a comprehensive set of guidelines governing recombinant DNA research.[11] Compliance is mandatory for NIH laboratories and all projects supported by NIH grants and contracts. The regulations attempt to reduce the risks associated with such investigation by means of stringent safeguards that prohibit certain types of experimentation and impose standards for physical and biological containment of possibly dangerous organisms. The guidelines, however, do not apply to research performed in the private sector which is not funded by NIH.

On a state and local level, New York State held public hearings in the fall of 1976 on recombinant DNA research. Bills have been introduced in the legislatures of New York and California to regulate the research. In many cities throughout the United States, discussions and local hearings have taken place. At the University of Michigan, the Regents voted to allow such research. Princeton University's Subcommittee on Biohazardous Research unanimously recommended that certain types of moderate risk genetic research be permitted there. In Cambridge, Massachusetts, Mayor Alfred Vellucci and the city council imposed a moratorium on the building of a recombinant DNA laboratory at Harvard University. The moratorium was overturned in January 1977 by a special citizens' commission. A number of environmental groups are also actively involved in the issue. The American College of Physicians has endorsed the concept of recombinant DNA research but urges that it be subject to stringent national standards to insure the public's welfare and a safe environment and emphasized the need for public accountability and participation in the review and regulation of such investigation.

In the United Kingdom, a working party, chaired by Sir Robert Williams, made recommendations on a code of practice and on a procedure whereby experiments on genetic manipulation could be carried out with appropriate safeguards.[12] In the Senate of the United States, Senator Dale Bumpers, on February 4, 1977, introduced a bill that would require the government to issue licenses to those doing gene-splicing research. A similar bill was introduced in the House of Representatives by Congressman Richard Ottinger. These bills would extend the physical and biological containment requirements of the NIH Recombinant DNA Research Guidelines to all facilities regardless of funding source; provide for an annual review of the regulations to determine their adequacy; establish local Biohazard Committees to monitor the activities of facilities conducting such research and assure adherance to the regulations; create a National Recombinant DNA Advisory Committee; and authorize the formation of a Commission for the Study of Recombinant DNA Activities. State and local laws limiting recombinant DNA research would be pre-empted, although localities could apply for exemptions upon evidence that tighter regulations were needed.

The Jewish View

How does Halakhah view genetic manipulation or engineering, recombinant DNA technology and research or gene splicing, nuclear transplants (cloning), egg transfer from a wife inseminated by her husband and then transferred to another woman's womb which serves as an incubator (host mothers), artificial gestation in a glass womb, artificial fertilization and the like? These are new areas of concern made possible by the enormous recent advances in medical technology.

The subject of eugenics is only indirectly involved in the above questions and will not be further discussed here. Artificial insemination in Jewish law has been discussed in detail elsewhere[13-14] but is summarized below to illustrate the basic principles in Jewish law which are applicable.

Artificial insemination using the semen of a donor other than the husband is considered by most rabbinic opinion to be an abomination and strictly prohibited for a variety of reasons, including the possibility of incest, lack of genealogy and the problems of inheritance. Some authorities regard such insemination as adultery, requiring the husband to divorce his wife and her forfeiture of the *ketubbah,* and even the physician and the donor are culpable when involved in this act akin to adultery. Most rabbinic opinion, however, states that without a sexual act involved, the woman is not guilty of adultery and is not prohibited to cohabit with her husband.

Regarding the status of the child, rabbinic opinion is divided. Most consider the offspring to be legitimate as was Ben Sira, the product of conception *sine concubito;* a small minority of rabbis consider the child illegitimate, and at least two authorities take a middle view and label the child a *safek mamzer.* Considerable rabbinic opinion regards the child (legitimate or illegitimate) to be the son of the donor in all respects (i.e., inheritance, support, custody, incest, Levirate marriage, and the like). Some regard the child to be the donor's son only in some respects but not others. Some rabbis state that although the child is considered the donor's son in all respects, the donor has not fulfilled the commandment of procreation. A minority of rabbinic authority asserts that the child is not considered the donor's son at all.

There is near unanimity of opinion that the use of semen from the husband (A.I.H.) is permissible if no other method is possible for the wife to become pregnant. However, certain qualifications exist. There must have been a reasonable period of waiting since marriage (2, 5 or 10 years or until medical proof of the absolute necessity for A.I.H.), and, according to many authorities, the insemination may not be performed during the wife's period of ritual impurity.

It is permitted by most rabbis to obtain sperm from the husband both for analysis and for insemination, but difference of opinion exists as to the method to be used in the procurement of it. Masturbation should be avoided if at all possible and *coitus interruptus,* retrieval of sperm from the vagina, or the use of a condom seem to be the preferred methods.

The case of host motherhood in Jewish law has been considered in some detail in at least two publications.[15-16] Rabbi Azriel Rosenfeld[15] discusses the permissibility of transplantation of a fetus from one mother to another and the legal parenthood of the child. There is a serious question in Jewish law whether or not the biological mother is allowed to give up her child for transplantation into another "womb" and whether or not the host mother is allowed to accept it. Rabbi Rosenfeld declares that if a married woman has become a host mother, Jewish law would probably require her to abstain from sexual relations with her husband for ninety days, in order to insure that the child is not his, that is to say, that she did not miscarry the implanted fetus and become pregnant by her husband; but he would certainly not have to divorce her.

In order to apply the laws pertaining to the first-born, it is important to know whether the biological or host mother is regarded as having given birth to the infant. Based on several Jewish sources, Rabbi Rosenfeld concludes that if fetal transplantation is performed after forty days post conception, the child is considered to be the legal offspring of its biological parents since the child became "completed" while still in the biological mother's body and she is regarded as having given birth to it.

Jewish law may view differently the situation of a fetal transplant prior to forty days after conception. Rabbi J. David Bleich[16] addresses this question by drawing on sources which discuss Jewish legal aspects of ovarian transplants. A case is described in which the ovary of a fertile woman was transplanted into the body of a previously barren woman to enable her to become pregnant and bear children. Adultery is not involved here on the part of the recipient woman even if the donor of the ovary was a married woman. A transplanted organ is deemed to become an integral part of the body of the recipient. For this reason, the recipient of an ovarian transplant must also be considered the legal mother of any child subsequently conceived and born.

Another view cited by Rabbi Bleich is that the ovary alone is an inert organ and incapable of reproduction were it not for the physiological contributions of the recipient. Furthermore, in the case of fetal transplantation, the host mother nurtures the embryo and sustains gestation and, perhaps, should be considered the legal mother of the offspring. According to other authorities, the donor-mother alone may be viewed as the mother in the eyes of Jewish law since the prohibition against feticide is applicable from the moment of conception. These authorities deem the fetus to be a human being with identity and parentage from the earliest stages of gestation. Rabbi Bleich also raises the possibility of two maternal relationships existing simultaneously, the child thus having two mothers, the donor or biological mother and the host mother. The question remains unresolved.

The above considerations of ovarian transplants (testicular transplants are not discussed in Jewish sources but similar principles would probably apply), fetal transplants and host mothers relate to a medical situation where the conception and birth of a child is not possible in any other manner. To abort a mother's naturally fertilized egg and to re-implant it in a host mother for reasons of "convenience for women who seek the gift of a child without the encumbrance and disfigurement of pregnancy" is, according to Britain's Chief Rabbi Immanuel Jakobovits,[17] "offensive to moral susceptibilities." Furthermore, says Rabbi Jakobovits, "to use another person as an 'incubator' and then take from her the child she carried and delivered for a fee is a revolting degradation of maternity and an affront to human dignity."

The literature on cloning, recombinant DNA research and technology and genetic engineering as viewed in Jewish law is very sparse indeed. Genetic screening and amniocentesis is a related subject but beyond the scope of this paper. The interested reader is referred elsewhere for further discussion of general[18] and Jewish aspects.[19] (Various halakhic problems relating to gene surgery, gene modification and gene transplantation are discussed in Rabbi Azriel Rosenfeld's article entitled "Judaism and Gene Design" above.[20]) The medical problems of removing the ovum, modifying some of its genes by microsurgical techniques and replacing the viable ovum in the mother have not yet been surmounted. However, assuming such surgery can be successfully performed, Rabbi Rosenfeld contends that gene surgery might be permissible in Jewish law because genes are submicroscopic particles and no process invisible to the naked eye could be halakhically forbidden. Laws of forbidden foods do not apply to microorganisms. The priest only declares ritually unclean that which his eyes can see.

Another argument of Rabbi Rosenfeld for the permissibility of gene surgery is the fact that the ovum (or sperm) is not a person since conception has not yet taken place. Thus, gene manipulation would not be considered as tampering with an existing human being but only with a potential one. Some authorities, however, would argue that the destruction of even a potential human being (either the unborn fetus or the unfertilized human seed) is prohibited in Jewish law.[21]

Rabbi Rosenfeld considers the following principle indisputable: any surgery performed on a person must certainly be permitted on an ovum (or sperm) before conception. For example, if a surgical cure for hemophilia or Tay-Sachs disease were possible, it would surely be permissible; hence, it would certainly be permissible to cure hemophilia or Tay-Sachs disease by gene surgery.

Rabbi Rosenfeld then proceeds to discuss gene transplants involving the transplantation of genes from one person into the ovum or sperm of another. The following halakhic questions arise. Are gene transplants considered to be a type of perverted sex act between the gene donor and the recipient? Would such transplants be forbidden, in particular, if donor and recipient were close relatives? Would a child conceived from such a manipulated ovum or sperm be regarded as related to the gene donor? Rabbi Rosenfeld draws parallels from the rabbinic responsa dealing with ovarian transplants and concludes that no sex act is involved in a gene transplant, the recipient is not forbidden to marry the donor's relatives and the child conceived and born following a gene transplant is not related to the gene donor. In most organ transplants (kidney, cornea, heart, ovary, ''gene'') the organ becomes an integral part of the recipient. The only exception, according to Rabbi Rosenfeld,[22] may be the brain since there is evidence to support the position that the halakhic identity of a person follows the brain.

Conclusion

The explosion of medical knowledge and technology in the past decade have made organ transplants, genetic engineering, cloning, artificial fertilization and host mothers and their like a reality of the present and not a dream for the future. Tampering with the very essence of life and encroaching upon the Creator's domain are considerations worthy of extensive discussion from the Jewish standpoint. Are we creating artificial human beings bordering on golems? The Talmud (*Sanhedrin* 65b) describes an artificial man *(golem)* created by Rabba. Is such a golem human? What is man being reduced to? The Talmud (*Niddah* 31a) tells us that:

> There are three partners in man, the Holy One, blessed be He, his father and his mother. His father supplies the semen of the white substance out of which are formed the child's bones, sinews, nails, the brain in his head and the white in his eye. His mother supplies the semen of the red substance out of which is formed his skin, hair, blood and the black of his eye. And the Holy One, blessed be He, gives him the spirit and the breath, beauty of features, eyesight, the power of hearing and the ability to speak and to walk, understanding and discernment.

The spiritual and theological aspects of genetic engineering and DNA recombinant research also require exploration. Rabbis must examine these issues from the Jewish standpoint and offer halakhic guidance to the medical and lay communities. In the meanwhile, Rabbi Jakobovits[23] expresses sentiments which we should all take to heart:

Without prior safeguards, there is no justification for the experiments already undertaken in this sacred sphere, and a strict moratorium should be declared on further tests until the complex moral issues involved have been thoroughly examined, and some firm ethical guidelines are established to prevent abuses and excuses incompatible with the sanctity with the sanctity of life and its generation.

It is indefensible to initiate controlled experiments with incalculable effects on the balance of nature and the preservation of man's incomparable spirituality without the most careful evaluation of the likely consequences beforehand . . .

"Spare-part" surgery and "genetic engineering" may open a wonderful chapter in the history of healing. But without prior agreement on restraints and the strictest limitations, such mechanisation of human life may also herald irretrievable disaster resulting from man's encroachment upon nature's preserves, from assessing human beings by their potential value as tool-parts, sperm-donors or living incubators, and from replacing the matchless dignity of the human personality by test-tubes, syringes and the soulless artificiality of computerized numbers.

Man, as the delicately balanced fusion of body, mind and soul, can never be the mere product of laboratory conditions and scientific ingenuity. To fulfill his destiny as a creative creature in the image of his Creator, he must be generated and reared out of the intimate love joining husband and wife together, out of identifiable parents who care for the development of their offspring, and out of a home which provides affectionate warmth and compassion.

NOTES

1. Omenn, G. S. "Genetic Engineering: Present & Future," in *To Live and To Die: When, Why and How.* R. H. Williams (edit.) New York. Springer-Verlag, 1974, pp. 48–63.

2. Goldstein, R. "Public Health Policy & Recombinant DNA," *New England Journal of Medicine 296:* 1226–1228, 1977.

3. Lappé, M., & Morison, R. S. (edit.) "Ethical & Scientific Issues Posed by Human Uses of Molecular Genetics," *Annals of the New York Academy of Sciences 265:* 1–208, 1976.

4. Gwynne, P. "Caution: Gene Transplants," *Newsweek* March 21, 1977, p. 57.

5. Fletcher, J. *The Ethics of Genetic Control.* New York. Doubleday-Anchor, 1974, pp. 40–41.

6. Chargoff, E. "On the Dangers of Genetic Meddling," *Science 192:* 938–940, 1976.

7. Siekevitz, P. "Recombinant DNA Research: A Faustian Bargain?" *Science 194:* 256–257, 1976.

8. Wade, N. "Recombinant DNA: A Critic Questions the Right to Free Inquiry," *Science 194:* 303–306, 1976.

9. Wald, G. "The Case Against Genetic Engineering," *The Sciences 16:* 6–11, 1976.

10. Cohen, S. N. "Recombinant DNA: Fact & Fiction," *Science 195:* 654–657, 1977.

11. *Federal Register.* vol. 41, no. 313, July 7, 1976 part 2, pp. 27902–27943.

12. Williams, R. *Report of the Working Party on the Practice of Genetic Manipulation.* CMND 6600. H. M. Stationery Office, 50 p. 1976.

13. Rosner, F. "Artificial Insemination in Jewish Law," *Judaism 19:* 452–464, 1970 (reprinted above in this volume).

14. Jakobovits, I. "Artificial Insemination," in *Jewish Medical Ethics,* New York, Bloch, 1975, pp. 244–250.

15. Rosenfeld, A. "Generation, Gestation & Judaism," *Tradition 12:* 78–87 (Spring) 1971.

16. Bleich, J. D. "Host Mothers," in *Contemporary Halakhic Problems,* New York, Ktav & Yeshiva Univ. Press, 1977, pp. 106–108.

17. Jakobovits, I. "Test Tube Babies" and "Host Mothers," in *Jewish Medical Ethics,* pp. 264–266.

18. Committee for the Study of Inborn Errors of Metabolism. *Genetic Screening: Programs, Principles & Research,* Wash. D. C., National Academy of Sciences, 1975, XV and 388 pp.

19. Rosner, F. "Tay-Sachs Disease: To Screen or not to Screen," *Journal of Religion & Health 15:* 271–281, 1976 (reprinted above in this volume).

20. Rosenfeld, A. "Judaism & Gene Design," *Tradition 13:* 71–80 (Fall) 1972.

21. See Rosner, F. "The Jewish Attitude Toward Abortion," *Tradition 10:* 48–71 (Winter) 1968, & Bleich, J. D. "Abortion in Halakhic Literature," *ibid.* pp. 72–120 (reprinted above in this volume).

22. Rosenfeld, A. "The Heart, the Head and the Halakhah," *New York State Journal of Medicine 70:* 2615–2618, 1970.

23. See note 17 above.

Biographical Notes

Biographical Notes

J. David Bleich is a Rosh Yeshiva at Yeshiva University and Visiting Professor of Law at the Benjamin Cardozo School of Law. He is the author of *Providence in the Philosophy of Gersonides, Contemporary Halakhic Problems,* and *With Perfect Faith: The Foundations of Jewish Belief* (forthcoming).

Menachem M. Brayer is Professor of Education and of Biblical Literature, and Consulting Psychologist, at Yeshiva University. He has written extensively in the field of Jewish studies.

Immanuel Jakobovits, Chief Rabbi of the British Commonwealth, is the author of *Jewish Medical Ethics, Journal of a Rabbi,* and *The Timely and the Timeless.*

Norman Lamm, President of Yeshiva University, is the author of *Faith and Doubt* and *The Good Society* among other works.

Nachum L. Rabinovitch is Principal of Jews' College, London. He has written widely in the field of Jewish studies.

Azriel Rosenfeld is Professor of Computer Science at the University of Maryland and the author of many scholarly studies on medicine and Halakhah.

Fred Rosner is Director of Medicine at the Queens Hospital Center and Professor of Medicine at the State University of New York. Among his many books are *Modern Medicine and Jewish Law* and an English translation of Julius Preuss' *Biblical and Talmudic Medicine.*

David S. Shapiro is rabbi of a community in Milwaukee, Wisconsin. He is the author of *Studies in Jewish Thought.*

Aaron Soloveichik is Dean and Rosh Yeshiva of Brisk Rabbinical College in Chicago, Illinois.

Moshe HaLevi Spero, a child psychotherapist in Ann Arbor, Michigan, is associate editor of the *Journal of Psychology and Judaism.*

Moses D. Tendler is Professor of Talmud and chairman of the department of Biology at Yeshiva University. He has written widely in the fields of Jewish studies and medicine.